TRANSFORMING MASCULINITIES
IN AFRICAN CHRISTIANITY

Transforming Masculinities in African Christianity
Gender Controversies in Times of AIDS

ADRIAAN S. VAN KLINKEN
University of Leeds, UK

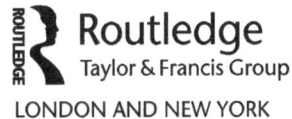
Routledge
Taylor & Francis Group
LONDON AND NEW YORK

First published 2013 by Ashgate Publishing

Published 2016 by Routledge
2 Park Square, Milton Park, Abingdon, Oxfordshire OX14 4RN
711 Third Avenue, New York, NY 10017, USA

First issued in paperback 2016

Routledge is an imprint of the Taylor & Francis Group, an informa business

Copyright © Adriaan S. van Klinken 2013

Adriaan S. van Klinken has asserted his right under the Copyright, Designs and Patents Act, 1988, to be identified as the author of this work.

All rights reserved. No part of this book may be reprinted or reproduced or utilised in any form or by any electronic, mechanical, or other means, now known or hereafter invented, including photocopying and recording, or in any information storage or retrieval system, without permission in writing from the publishers.

Notice:

Product or corporate names may be trademarks or registered trademarks, and are used only for identification and explanation without intent to infringe.

British Library Cataloguing in Publication Data
Klinken, A. S. van.
 Transforming masculinities in African Christianity : gender
 controversies in times of AIDS.
 1. Masculinity--Religious aspects--Christianity.
 2. Masculinity--Africa.
 I. Title
 261.1'0811'096-dc23

The Library of Congress has cataloged the printed edition as follows:
Van Klinken, A. S.
 Transforming masculinities in African Christianity : gender controversies in times of AIDS / by A.S. van Klinken.
   p. cm.
  Includes bibliographical (p.   ) references and index.
  ISBN 978-1-4094-5114-3 (hardback) 1. Men (Christian theology)
 2. Sex role--Religious aspects--Christianity. 3. Theology, Doctrinal-
 -Africa. 4. AIDS (Disease)--Africa. I. Title.
  BT703.5.V35 2013
  276'.0830811--dc23
                                                                    2012029565

ISBN 13: 978-1-138-25319-3 (pbk)
ISBN 13: 978-1-4094-5114-3 (hbk)

Contents

Acknowledgements		*vii*
List of Abbreviations		*ix*
1	Intersecting Masculinities, Religion and AIDS: An Introduction	1
2	Transforming Masculinities towards Gender Justice: African Theologians	25
3	Shaping Responsible Family Men: Masculinities in a Catholic Parish	61
4	Promoting 'Biblical Manhood': Masculinities in a Pentecostal Church	103
5	Comparing the Trajectories and Theologies to Transform Masculinities	149
6	Understanding Transformations of Masculinity: Patriarchy, Male Agency and Gender Justice	179
Bibliography		*201*
Index		*221*

Acknowledgements

This book has its origins in the research project 'Intersecting Religion, Masculinities and HIV/AIDS: Case Studies in African Christianity'. I carried out this project in the period 2007–2010 as a PhD research fellow in the Department of Religious Studies and Theology at Utrecht University, with funding from the Dutch faith-based organisations for development cooperation ICCO, Kerk in Actie and Prisma. The dissertation that resulted from this project formed the basis for what is now *Transforming Masculinities in African Christianity*, but has undergone substantial revision. Working on the project I have benefited enormously from the input, feedback and support provided by my supervisors. Professor Martha Frederiks has supported me and the research project from the very beginning. Her enthusiasm has encouraged me, and her social engagement as a scholar has inspired me personally and academically. Professor Anne-Marie Korte has always stimulated my thinking by opening new perspectives and intellectual horizons. Her academic mentorship has benefitted me greatly over the past five years. Professor Ezra Chitando from the University of Zimbabwe, who kindly agreed to be involved in the project, has shown a sincere interest in my work and has given valuable feedback on drafts of my texts. I am grateful for having these three scholars as my *Doktoreltern*. I thank the members of the PhD examination committee, Dr David Bos, Professor Rosemarie Buikema, Professor Maaike de Haardt, Professor Birgit Meyer, Dr Fulata Moyo, Professor Volker Küster and Professor Gerald West, for their insightful comments and questions that helped me to revise my dissertation into this book. I wish to extend my thanks to other scholars, colleagues and friends with whom I have collaborated in the past five years and who, in one way or another, have contributed to the project that culminated in this book. They include Dr Masiiwa Ragies Gunda, Professor Beverley Haddad, Professor Björn Krondorfer, Professor Sarojini Nadar, Dr Nyambura Njoroge, Nienke Pruiksma, Professor Burkhard Scherer, Professor Bob Schreiter, my former colleagues at Utrecht University, and the members of the PhD seminar 'Religion, Gender and Multidisciplinarity' of the Netherlands School of Advanced Studies in Theology and Religion. I particularly thank Björn Krondorfer and Anne-Marie Korte for their helpful suggestions to further improve the manuscript of this book in its final stage.

This book was completed in my first year as a postdoctoral research fellow at the School of Oriental and African Studies (SOAS), University of London. I am grateful to the Netherlands Organisation of Scientific Research (NWO), which enabled this fellowship by awarding me a grant through their Rubicon programme. I thank my colleagues in the Department of the Study of Religions, especially

Dr Sîan Hawthorne, and the postgraduate students in the Centre for Gender and Religions Research at SOAS, for providing me with a welcoming and stimulating academic home.

The research presented in this book includes two case studies conducted in church communities in Lusaka, Zambia. I thank Bishop Joshua H.K. Banda, senior pastor of Northmead Assembly of God, and Fr Marc Nsanzurwimo, at the time parish priest in Regiment parish, for allowing me to do research on their congregations, for welcoming me and for participating in the research themselves. I am most grateful to the church members, especially those who were interviewed as part of the study, for sharing their opinions and experiences, often concerning intimate parts of their lives. Zambians often mention the peaceful and friendly atmosphere of their country. Indeed, Zambia has been a wonderful and pleasant place to do research. Thanks to many friends, it has become a place where I feel at home.

My thanks also go to Sarah Lloyd of Ashgate Publishing for supporting the publication of this book and to the Ashgate editorial and production staff for their work in editing and producing this book.

Last but not least, I say thanks to my parents, close friends and relatives, especially to my partner and best friend, Casper Branger, for reminding me that life is more than academic pursuits. Sharing a nice dinner, visiting a museum or theatre, taking a hiking or cycling tour, spending time with my nephews and nieces: activities like these add so much to the quality of my life, and I often wonder why I don't do them more frequently.

List of Abbreviations

AIDS	Acquired Immune Deficiency Syndrome
CC-Z	Catholic Church in Zambia
HIV	Human Immunodeficiency Virus
NAOG	Northmead Assembly of God
NIV	New International Version (Bible translation)
PAOG-Z	Pentecostal Assemblies of God in Zambia
RCC	Roman Catholic Church
SCC	Small Christian Community

Chapter 1
Intersecting Masculinities, Religion and AIDS: An Introduction

'There is a need for men who are circumcised.' This statement was made during a youth meeting in Northmead Assembly of God Church (Lusaka, Zambia), one of the case studies presented in this book. During the meeting the preacher called for a new generation of young people truly committed to the Christian values, a generation of 'men and women of morality'. Then he particularly addressed the young men in the room, stating that the need today is for men who are circumcised. This statement was not intended as a call for a literal circumcision of the male flesh. The preacher employed the image of circumcision to illustrate how a young Christian man is supposed to behave: to control his sexuality and to discipline his body, saying 'no' to temptations and waiting until marriage for sex.

In recent years, male circumcision has been advocated as an adequate prevention strategy with regard to the HIV epidemic in sub-Saharan Africa. The idea is that the removal of the foreskin would efficaciously reduce the sexual transmission of the virus. This prevention strategy is controversial because circumcision, according to critics, violates the integrity of the body. The above quotation of the preacher indicates that, apart from bodily circumcision, there is yet another kind of circumcision: a discursive or spiritual circumcision of men. In the words of the apostle Paul, this is a 'circumcision of the heart' (Rom. 2:29). The case studies presented in this book show that such a metaphorical 'circumcision' of men is practised in some local churches as a religious prevention strategy to respond to the reality of HIV. Although this circumcision is only a discursive practice, it also gives rise to controversy. The question at stake is *what* needs to be circumcised in relation to men in the context of the HIV epidemic and beyond. To elaborate on the metaphor: What needs to be 'cut off'? Broadly speaking, two different answers are provided. The preacher at the youth meeting aims at a circumcision of men's sexual urges and other masculine energies. The strategy here is to teach men certain moral values and self-discipline in order to realise change in their behaviour and lifestyle. This strategy is not specific for the preacher, but is practised, be it in different ways, in many religious communities in Africa (as in other parts of the world). This book presents two case studies of local Zambian churches where men's presumed irresponsible lifestyles and immoral behaviour are considered key factors in the spread of HIV and in other social problems. The book also offers a discussion of the work of a number of African theologians who present a different perspective. In their opinion, men need to be 'cut off' not just from their energies and urges, but also from their patriarchal power and privileges. The theologians present a structural approach where men are analysed as gendered subjects who are positioned in, and benefit from, powered gender relations. For these theologians, gender inequality is one of the fundamental structures underlying the HIV epidemic. Thus, even though the theologians and the churches concur in their perception that something needs to happen with men, they differ in their opinion of what needs to happen, what needs to be 'cut off'.

In addition to the sense of circumcision as a 'cutting-off', the term also means to 'uncover' and 'open'. Developing the metaphor further, this notion can be related to the alternative vision of manhood that is to be realised through the symbolic circumcision. What does the new, ideal man look like, uncovered by the metaphorical circumcision of the foreskin of either immorality or patriarchy? The preacher quoted above, like the case-study churches discussed in this book, targets a new 'generation of men' who are morally upright and who take responsibility for themselves and for others, especially within marriage and the family. The African theologians, on the other hand, express their hope for men who are committed to the ideal of gender justice, who fully respect women as equal human beings and who search for partnership and mutuality in their marriage.

The metaphor of circumcision leads to the subject that is at the heart of the present study: both some theologians and local churches in Africa are more or less explicitly involved in 'masculinity politics', that is, efforts to realise change in male gender practices and identities; but there are significant differences in the understanding of the problems with men and masculinity, and diverging visions of the transformation of masculinities. These convergences and divergences concerning masculinity politics in African Christianity are explored and discussed in this book. Before undertaking this major task, the present chapter introduces some preliminary issues. The first question the reader may grapple with is why men need to be 'circumcised' at all. As suggested above, this has something to do with the HIV epidemic in sub-Saharan Africa.

Gender, Masculinities, and HIV and AIDS

Since its discovery in the early 1980s, HIV has become a global pandemic and has caused a major health and social crisis, particularly in Africa south of the Sahara. Organisations that seek to combat HIV, and academic scholars who seek to explain the spread and impact of HIV, often point to the gendered dimension of the African epidemic. They explain that HIV in sub-Saharan Africa disproportionately affects women and girls – not only in terms of infection rates, but also in terms of the stigmatisation faced by those who are HIV-positive, and the demand for care of relatives as a result of AIDS. The gendered face of HIV is illustrated by a recent UNAIDS (Joint United Nations Programme on HIV/AIDS) report stating that in Africa women account for approximately 60 per cent of HIV infection.[1] Though

---

[1] *Report on the Global AIDS Epidemic 2010* (Geneva, 2010), 25.

physiological aspects play a role, women's vulnerability to HIV is explained predominantly by social, cultural and economic factors. The relations between men and women are said to be embedded in 'structural gender inequalities', both in intimate spheres and in society at large.[2] In view of the sexual transmission of HIV in Africa – which is believed to be predominantly heterosexual[3] – much attention is paid to how these inequalities impact on sexual relations. For example, social scientist Carolyn Baylies points out that women have a 'relative passivity' and 'are often expected to give but not to receive pleasure', while men have the power of 'sexual decision making and initiative' and are allowed 'greater sexual mobility both prior to and after marriage'.[4] More recently, several scholars have criticised the general representation of women as vulnerable and subordinate. They call attention to the differentiation in and variability of sexual and gender relations, and to the agency of women in these relationships.[5] This move is crucial to prevent generalised and simplified understandings of the intersections between gender, sexuality and HIV, as these intersections are more complex than is often suggested.

Men, Masculinities and HIV

If women have a specific vulnerability to HIV, this is related to the behaviour of men that is itself informed by norms related to masculinity that, in the end, also put men themselves at risk.[6] Therefore, from an initial concern with women, studies on gender and HIV have also come to include men and issues of masculinity. Again, there is a tendency towards monolithic representations: where women are said to be powerless, men are associated with domination and control. This easily results in blame discourses about men. For example, in an early publication on

---

[2] J. Boesten and N.K. Poku, 'Gender, Inequalities and HIV/AIDS', in J. Boesten and N.K. Poku (eds), *Gender and HIV/AIDS: Critical Perspectives from the Developing World* (Farnham, 2009), 2.

[3] For a critical discussion of the widespread assumption of an almost exclusively heterosexual transmission of HIV in Africa, see M. Epprecht, *Heterosexual Africa? The History of an Idea from the Age of Exploration to the Age of AIDS* (Athens, 2008).

[4] C. Baylies, 'Perspectives on Gender and AIDS in Africa', in C. Baylies and J. Bujra (eds), *AIDS, Sexuality and Gender in Africa: Collective Strategies and Struggles in Tanzania and Zambia* (London, 2000), 7–8.

[5] E. Kalipeni, J. Oppong and A. Zerai, 'HIV/AIDS, Gender, Agency and Empowerment Issues in Africa', *Social Science and Medicine*, 64/5 (2007): 1015–18; H. Dilger and J. Offe, 'Making the Difference? Structure, Agency and Culture in Anthropological Research on Gender and Aids in Africa', *Curare*, 28/2–3 (2005): 266–80.

[6] Cf. G. Barker and C. Ricardo, *Young Men and the Construction of Masculinity in Sub-Saharan Africa: Implications for HIV/AIDS, Conflict and Violence* (Washington, 2005), 37–42; J. Bujra, 'Targeting Men for a Change: AIDS Discourse and Activism in Africa', in F. Cleaver (ed.), *Masculinities Matter! Men, Gender and Development* (London, 2002), 209–34.

men and HIV, it was stated that 'without men there would be no AIDS epidemic. ... In short, men determine the path of the disease.'[7] Such an account is not only simplistic and generalising; it also does not take into account the social, cultural and economic factors that inform individual men's behaviours.

The concept of masculinity has been employed to investigate the social construction of male gender identity and of men's position in gender relations. However, men are not a homogenous group. In order to account for the variability and differentiation in gender constructions, masculinity is increasingly understood as a plural.[8] Various masculinit*ies* may co-exist in a given context, some of which will be more popular than others. The popular, most influential and prevailing version of masculinity is often referred to as 'hegemonic masculinity'.[9] The hegemonic ideals of masculinity have now become contested because of their implications for HIV. For instance, in his study on men and AIDS in Zambia, anthropologist Anthony Simpson points out:

> At the core of the prevailing hegemonic version of masculinity was the demonstration of male potency in sexual conquest. While there were exceptions, throughout childhood and adolescence (as indeed in adulthood) sexuality for many men was a space to create and restore masculinity.[10]

Apart from sexual conquest and multiple sexual partnerships, hegemonic masculinity is often associated with a reluctance to use condoms, with male domination over women and with violence to women and children.[11] Clearly, these aspects are highly critical, especially in the context of HIV, as they put both men and women at greater risk. Against this background, UNAIDS has stated: 'Given the urgency of curbing HIV rates ... it is important to challenge harmful concepts

---

[7] M. Foreman (ed.), *AIDS and Men: Taking Risks or Taking Responsibility?* (London, 1999), ix.

[8] Cf. R.W. Connell, *Masculinities*, 2nd edn (Berkeley, 2005). Connell's work is influential in the study of masculinities in Africa. See R. Morrell and L. Ouzgane, 'African Masculinities: An Introduction', in L. Ouzgane and R. Morrell (eds), *African Masculinities: Men in Africa from the Late Nineteenth Century to the Present* (New York, 2005), 7–8; S. Miescher and L.A. Lindsay, 'Introduction: Men and Masculinities in Modern Africa', in L.A. Lindsay and S. Miescher (eds), *Men and Masculinities in Modern Africa* (Portsmouth, 2003), 6–7.

[9] The concept of hegemonic masculinity originates from Connell's theory on the hierarchical relations between the various masculinities that coexist in a given society. See Connell, *Masculinities*, 76–81.

[10] A. Simpson, *Boys to Men in the Shadow of AIDS: Masculinities and HIV Risk in Zambia* (New York, 2009), 8.

[11] See T. Shefer, K. Ratele, A. Strebel and N. Shabalala, 'Masculinities in South Africa: A Critical Review of Contemporary Literature on Men's Sexuality', in D. Gibson and A. Hardon (eds), *Rethinking Masculinities, Violence and AIDS* (Amsterdam, 2005), 73–86.

of masculinity, including the way adult men look on risk and sexuality and how boys are socialized to become men.'[12]

Where hegemonic masculinity is thought of as being implicated in the HIV epidemic in various ways, the concept of masculinities as socially constructed and the related notion of differentiation among men suggest that more can be said about men and masculinities. Some crucial issues are raised by Purmina Mane and Peter Aggleton, who state:

> If masculinities are multiple, for example, then some versions may be more useful than others in promoting greater gender equality and improved sexual health. If masculinities are actively constructed, then it may be possible to create more gender-equitable versions of them. Finally, if masculinities are dynamic, over time, shifts away from less helpful versions of masculinity that emphasize dominance and aggression may be possible.[13]

In relation to the HIV epidemic, the constructionist understanding of masculinity brings some important insights. First, it opens up space for active gender politics: what is constructed can also be actively deconstructed and reconstructed. In other words, there is a possibility to realise change among men and to engage in a transformation of masculinities. Indeed, HIV intervention strategies have engaged this space and are 'targeting men for a change', not only for HIV prevention-related purposes but also in a broader project of transforming gender relations.[14] Related to this is a second insight, that being the notion of agency of individual men. The idea that masculinity is not a static, monolithic characteristic naturally defining 'manhood', but that there are several co-existing and competing masculinities, implies that to a certain extent men do have agency to configure and reconfigure their identity and performance as men.[15] Without this agency, it would not make sense to target men for change. Third, when men can change and masculinities can be transformed, at an analytical level attention is to be paid to the changes that actually occur in the configuration of masculinities. Robert Morrell, a scholar of masculinities in southern Africa, points to the challenge of identifying 'what forces operate to effect change in masculinities, when, where and how such changes occur, and what their effects are'.[16] This is an important question with regard to masculinities in Africa in times of AIDS, as the epidemic has mobilised forces that impact on men and masculinities in various ways.

---

[12] *Men and AIDS – A Gendered Approach* (Geneva, 2000), 7.

[13] P. Mane and P. Aggleton, 'Gender and HIV/AIDS: What Do Men Have to Do with It?', *Current Sociology*, 49/6 (2001): 32.

[14] Bujra, *Targeting Men for a Change*, 209–34.

[15] D.S. Gutterman, 'Postmodernism and the Interrogation of Masculinity', in S. Whitehead and F.J. Barrett (eds), *The Masculinities Reader* (Cambridge, 2001), 60–61.

[16] R. Morrell, 'The Times of Change: Men and Masculinity in South Africa', in R. Morrell (ed.), *Changing Men in Southern Africa* (Pietermaritzburg and London, 2001), 7.

These three insights concerning politics, agency and analysis are relevant to the present study and its interest in the intersection of religion, masculinities and HIV. Analytically, the question is how religion is a force operating to effect certain changes in masculinities, and how these changes and their effects can be understood. With regard to active gender politics, the question is whether religious communities, institutions and organisations, as a result of the HIV epidemic, have initiated a strategy to bring about change among men and in masculinities. Applied to the issue of agency, the question is whether and how religion affects and shapes men's agency in relation to hegemonic and alternative ideals of masculinity. These questions underpin this book.

Religion, Masculinities and HIV

The questions raised in the previous section point to the complex intersection of religion, masculinities and HIV. The problematic role of religion with regard to gender, masculinities and HIV is often highlighted. Religion is not considered a force operating to effect constructive change, but rather a force maintaining the status quo of gender inequality and hegemonic conceptions of masculinity. In what follows, I will point out that the role of religion is more complex, because religion – just like gender and masculinity – is not a monolithic but rather a complex and ambiguous phenomenon.

It is widely acknowledged that religion, due to its influence in African societies, is a major factor in the construction of gender in Africa. In view of the above-mentioned gendered face of the HIV epidemic, scholars have pointed to religion as a factor that reinforces the vulnerability of women. A recurring argument is that religions – be they African traditional religion, Christianity or Islam – in their beliefs and practices often reinforce gender inequalities that are critical to the spread of HIV among women and the impact of AIDS on women's lives. For example, two social scientists argue that the problem is with 'male dominance' and with the 'patriarchal construction of marriage and family' upheld by religion, which 'under present circumstances could only lead to female powerlessness and death'.[17] The often repeated criticism is that religious teachings uphold and reinforce male supremacy in gender relations. An example of this is provided by Simpson in his study of a group of Zambian men:

> The young men regularly cited the Book of Genesis where God creates Adam first as evidence of male superiority, explaining that in this instance Christianity and "tradition" were as one. Maleness was automatically deserving of respect.

---

[17] M. Mbilinyi and N. Kaihula, 'Sinners and Outsiders: The Drama of AIDS in Rungwe', in C. Baylies and J. Bujra (eds), *AIDS, Sexuality and Gender in Africa: Collective Strategies and Struggles in Tanzania and Zambia* (London, 2000), 78, 94.

As in so much of everyday Zambian life, precedence was all-important and there was no doubt that Eve, the woman, came second.[18]

The religious support or legitimisation of traditional patriarchal notions of masculinity is often mentioned as a key issue in the intersection of religion, masculinities and HIV. Sometimes it is analysed rather simplistically, as if religious patriarchal ideals of gender directly contribute to the spread of HIV. However, this link can only be indirect. Moreover, the question is what is meant by 'religion': does it refer to formal doctrines and religious teachings or to grassroots religious beliefs and practices, so-called popular or lived religion? It seems that official religion often is used rather eclectically by men. The men in Simpson's study, for example, hardly attend religious services or other religious meetings, but they make use of religious teachings to buttress their claims of male superiority.[19] In this context, Ezra Chitando (whose work will be discussed in the next chapter) speaks about the *abuse* of religious and cultural resources by men.[20] Distinction needs to be made, therefore, between what specific religious traditions teach about the position and roles of men in gender relations, how men involved in these traditions understand and practise this teaching, and how this relates to hegemonic forms of masculinity.

Another issue that is often mentioned is the impact of religion on male sexuality. The idea is that dominant versions of masculinity encourage men to achieve manhood through sexual performance. This would be informed by religious traditions that associate manhood with virility and emphasise the importance for men to transmit 'the vital force of life'.[21] In a context where many religious leaders also discourage the use of condoms, such religiously informed understandings of male sexuality can have destructive effects in the light of HIV. On the other hand, it is likely that Christianity and Islam, and in a certain way also African traditional religions, with their relatively strict sexual moral codes, contest popular ideals of masculinity precisely in the area of sexuality. Religions generally promote chastity, self-control and responsibility rather than unlimited sexual activity. However, the question is whether such religious teachings have any effect upon men's sexual decision-making. Several studies suggest that this effect cannot be presumed, but

---

[18] Simpson, *Boys to Men in the Shadow of AIDS*, 149.

[19] Ibid., 15–16.

[20] E. Chitando, 'Religious Ethics, HIV and AIDS and Masculinities in Southern Africa', in R. Nicolson (ed.), *Persons in Community: African Ethics in a Global Culture* (Scottsville, 2008), 53.

[21] Cf. P. Dover, 'Gender and Embodiment: Expectations of Manliness in a Zambian Village', in L. Ouzgane and R. Morrell (eds), *African Masculinities: Men in Africa from the Late Nineteenth Century to the Present* (New York, 2005), 182–5. The phrase 'the vital force of life' is derived from L. Magesa, *African Religion: The Moral Traditions of Abundant Life* (Maryknoll, 1997), 115–59.

depends on the level of religious involvement and the type of religious affiliation.[22] The men involved in Simpson's study all identify as Christians and are members of Christian churches, yet he found that this was no reliable predictor of sexual activity. He presents Pentecostal men as the only exception: 'They told me that the discipline of regular attendance at church and cell meetings, combined with Bible study, the acknowledgement of their prior sinfulness, and the encouragement of church members sustained them in their decision to forego extramarital sex.'[23] Whether this is specific to Pentecostal men is not clear, as the other participants in Simpson's study do not attend church regularly: they may be church members but are not church-goers.[24]

With regard to the issue of both male supremacy and male sexuality, crucial questions are whether and how religions contest hegemonic ideals of masculinity, what alternative they propose, and how this impacts on men. Engaging these questions, this book does not simply follow the idea of religion as a force that maintains or reinforces a hegemonic type of masculinity that is problematic in the context of HIV. Religion itself is diverse and it interplays with the processes in which masculinities are constructed in multiple and complex ways. Without ignoring the problematic role religious traditions may play with regard to gender, masculinities and HIV, in this book I have a particular interest in the constructive role. Is religion helpful in realising change among men? Do religious institutions actively engage in a transformation of masculinities? How can we understand transformations of masculinity in the sphere of religion? These questions are crucial as in Africa religion is a major factor in processes of personal and social change and transformation.[25]

The Scope and Enquiry of the Study

This book focuses on one major religion in sub-Saharan Africa, Christianity, at two different levels. First, the focus is on local church communities, through case studies in a Catholic and Pentecostal church in Lusaka (Zambia). Comprising a substantial part of the population in many African countries, churches are well

---

[22] J. Trinitapoli and M.D. Regnerus, 'Religion and HIV Risk Behaviors among Married Men: Initial Results from a Study in Rural Sub-Saharan Africa', *Journal for the Scientific Study of Religion*, 45/4 (2006): 505–28; R.C. Garner, 'Safe Sects? Dynamic Religion and AIDS in South Africa', *The Journal of Modern African Studies*, 38/1 (2000): 41–69.

[23] Simpson, *Boys to Men in the Shadow of AIDS*, 169.

[24] Ibid., 3. Considering Simpson's observation that very few men regularly attended church, it is not clear from what evidence he concludes that active church membership is not a predictor of sexual activity except with regard to Pentecostals (cf. 169).

[25] S. Ellis and G. Ter Haar, *Worlds of Power: Religious Thought and Political Practice in Africa* (London, 2004), 163–76.

positioned to influence people's behaviour and to impact on communities. Case studies in local churches enable detailed investigation of the discourses and strategies employed to realise change among men and to transform masculinities. Second, the focus is on African Christian theologians.[26] Issues of gender, HIV and AIDS have been central in discussions among African theologians for the past decade. Recently the issue of masculinities has also been tackled. Thus, some African theologians, such as Ezra Chitando, Musa Dube, Tinyiko Maluleke, Sarojini Nadar and Isabel Phiri, have opened up the field in which this study engages. They not only provide a critical analysis of prevalent masculinities but also present a vision to transform these. The relevance of their work to this book is twofold. On the one hand, these African theologians are academics contributing to the interdisciplinary study of religion and masculinities in Africa, and as such I make use of their work. On the other hand, because African theology understands itself as an engaged Christian reflexive praxis, the African theologians themselves present a specific religious – Christian theological – discourse on masculinity. Therefore their work becomes also object of study. My interest is in the theological dimension in their work: How do they reflect theologically on issues of gender and masculinities in the context of HIV&AIDS? What religious resources are mobilised to envision alternative masculinities? How do they view the role of churches in a transformation of masculinities?

The dual focus on local churches and African theology enables comparison and analysis of the theologians' and churches' approaches to masculinities in relation to each other. The main question of this book is how African theologians and local churches do address and seek to transform men and masculinities in the context of the HIV epidemic. My interest is in the convergences and divergences between the theological scholars and the local church communities, and in the implications these have for the understanding of processes of change in masculinities in African Christianity in the HIV era.

Disciplinary and Methodological Considerations

Written in the field of religious studies, this book particularly contributes to two sub-fields: the study of African Christianity, and the study of men, masculinities and religion.

The Study of African Christianity

Investigating the work of African theologians and the praxis in local Zambian churches, the present study engages in the study of African Christianity as part

---

[26] This refers to scholars trained and mostly working in academic settings who are committed to the project of African (Christian) theology, including scholars in religious and biblical studies whose work reflects a theological engagement.

of the broader examination of world Christianity. The latter seeks to investigate 'the contemporary global configurations of the Christian religion in all their complexities'.[27] The emergence of this field of study is informed by the growing awareness in Western academia of the increasing non-Western character of Christianity in the contemporary world, due to the oft-mentioned shift of Christianity to the global South. The central question is how Christian traditions, identities and practices are (re)shaped in the changing social, cultural and religious contexts in the modern world, and how Christianity is (re)shaping these contexts. Among the key issues is the topic of gender: how are gender identities and gender relations shaped and reshaped by the various types of Christianity worldwide, in relation to the cultural traditions and social challenges in specific contexts? Broadly referring to the regions of Latin America, Africa and Asia, Philip Jenkins observes that 'the rise of Christianity has, in an amazingly short time, effected dramatic changes in gender attitudes. In the long run, the greatest change might be the new emphasis on faithful monogamous marriage and on new concepts of masculinity'.[28] This gender dynamic in world Christianity, particularly the emergence of alternative concepts of masculinity, is the specific interest of the present study.

In the study of world Christianity, Africa is considered an important continent. Not only does Africa accommodate a large proportion of the world's Christian population, but also, as a consequence, it reshapes world Christianity itself. In the words of Andrew Walls, African Christianity can be regarded as 'a major component of contemporary *representative* Christianity, the standard Christianity of the present age, a demonstration model of its character' and even as 'potentially the *representative* Christianity of the twenty-first century' (emphasis original).[29] This means, among other things, that developments in African Christianity are significant to the understanding of world Christianity as a whole. This book presents a study of contemporary African Christianity, or Christianit*ies*,[30] and explores one of the most recent developments and emerging issues, to wit the quest for transformed masculinities that has arisen as a result of the HIV epidemic. Doing so, as mentioned above, the focus is on African Christian theologians and

---

[27] D.T. Irvin, 'World Christianity: An Introduction', *Journal of World Christianity*, 1/1 (2008): 1.

[28] P. Jenkins, *The New Faces of Christianity: Believing the Bible in the Global South* (Oxford, 2006), 165.

[29] A.F. Walls, *The Cross-Cultural Process in Christian History: Studies in the Transmission and Appropriation of Faith* (Maryknoll, 2002), 119, 85.

[30] Because of the diversity of Christian traditions present on the African continent, some scholars prefer to speak of African Christianities as a plural. Cf. P. Kollman, 'Classifying African Christianities: Past, Present and Future: Part One', *Journal of Religion in Africa*, 40/1 (2010): 3–32.

on local church communities. This distinction reveals a critical space between both types of African Christian discourse.[31]

African churches can be considered as primary manifestations of African Christianity in an institutionalised form. Given the plurality of Christianity in Africa, African churches are classified in broad categories such as mainline and independent, Catholic and Protestant, Pentecostal and neo-Pentecostal or Charismatic. The diverse palette reflects the complex ways in which Christianity has developed in (post)colonial African contexts and in our globalising world. The two case studies presented in this book, a Roman Catholic parish and a Pentecostal church, illustrate two of the many positions on this palette: one of a faith community that is part of a worldwide and hierarchically organised church whose administrative centre is in Europe and which in Africa has engaged in a process of 'inculturation', and one of an independent local Zambian church associated with the transnational movement of the Assemblies of God, which has its roots in early twentieth-century North American Pentecostalism.

African theology understands itself as a Christian enterprise. In the words of Kwame Bediako, it is 'an endeavour to demonstrate the true character of African Christian identity'.[32] In doing so, the various strands of African theology seek to engage with African religious and cultural traditions and with the challenges of African societies today. Though a Christian enterprise, African theology gives rise to a particular type of African Christian discourse: an academic, or at least a scholarly reflective discourse.[33] As such, it engages critically with Christianity as practised in African churches. According to Tinyiko Maluleke, African theology has a 'church-enabling task'. He explains that this includes a critical edge: African theology seeks not just to be 'at the service of the church in Africa' but also to enable 'the church to be both prophetic and self critical'.[34] Concretely this means that African theologians themselves often are critical of churches, not at least with

---

[31] One could argue that this is a problematic distinction, first because the pastors and priests in African churches are also theologians and second because the practitioners of 'African theology' often are active church members. However, many African theologians, and certainly the theologians discussed in this book, are rather critical of institutional churches, thus legitimating the comparative approach of this book.

[32] K. Bediako, *Theology and Identity: The Impact of Culture upon Christian Thought in the Second Century and in Modern Africa* (Akropong-Akuapem, 1992), 3.

[33] According to Klaus Hock, African theology is a 'vibrant pulsation of African Christianity in the sphere of academic discourses'. See K. Hock, 'Appropriated Vibrancy: "Immediacy" as a Formative Element in African Theologies', in K. Koschorke (ed.), *African Identities and World Christianity in the Twentieth Century* (Wiesbaden, 2005), 124. However, African theology as a whole is not an academic enterprise in the narrow sense of the word. It is taught at and develops from both state and Christian universities but also emerges from seminaries, and church-related and ecumenical institutions, and so on.

[34] T.S. Maluleke, 'Half a Century of African Christian Theologies: Elements of the Emerging Agenda for the Twenty-First Century', in O.U. Kalu (ed.), *African Christianity: An African Story* (Pretoria, 2005), 474–5.

regard to issues of gender, sexuality and AIDS, and challenge churches to play a more progressive and constructive role. This critical space between African theology on the one hand, and the praxis in local churches on the other, is explored in the present book.

A theological ethnography Methodologically, the study of world Christianity is a diverse field. Scholars employ historical, anthropological and theological perspectives. In this book, I mainly take an analytical theological approach. 'Part of the theological approach to the study of religion', in the words of Frank Whaling, 'is to make available to scholars an accurate and clear account of the conceptual frameworks of different traditions, bearing in mind that the role and purpose of concepts and of theology differs from tradition to tradition.'[35] World Christianity can be understood as a series of local theologies.[36] This notion refers not only to the many contextual theologies that are developed by professional theologians in all parts of the world, but also to the theologies found in local communities of faith that shape Christianity in specific ways within their respective social-cultural contexts. An analytical theological approach to world Christianity, then, is particularly interested in these – often implicit and not systematically articulated – theologies that provide the conceptual framework in which Christian identities and bodies are shaped. It seeks to make explicit and critically analyse the deeply rooted theological concepts and lines of thought in local Christian discourses, and to interpret these in relation to local socio-cultural contexts as well as to wider Christian theological traditions. Concretely, in this study it means that the discourses on masculinity presented by African theologians and found in local churches are analysed as part of the wider theological discourse, and then prove, for example, to be informed by particular understandings of God, Jesus Christ, creation or the relation between gospel and culture.

To be clear, my choice for a theological approach is not informed by a doctrinal interest in Christianity per se, but rather by an anthropological interest in the meaning of Christian beliefs in concrete social contexts and their role in shaping people's lives. In the case studies presented in chapters 3 and 4, theology provides the 'data' for an ethnography of African Christian masculinities. This means that the present study is indebted to the emerging field referred to as the anthropology of Christianity as much as to the recent field of intercultural theology. From intercultural theology I take the basic insight that all theologies are contextually conditioned and, therefore, are involved in ongoing processes of contact, conflict and exchange with their social-cultural environment.[37] Concerning the different functions of intercultural theology distinguished by Volker Küster, the project

---

[35] F. Whaling, 'Theological Approaches', in P. Connolly (ed.), *Approaches to the Study of Religion* (London, 1999), 237.

[36] R.J. Schreiter, *Constructing Local Theologies* (Maryknoll, 1985), 32–3.

[37] See M.J. Cartledge and D. Cheetham, 'Introduction', in M.J. Cartledge and D. Cheetham (eds), *Intercultural Theology: Approaches and Themes* (London, 2011), 2–3.

of this book engages most with the ethical function, specifically in relation to issues of gender transformation. I organise a critical dialogue between different culturally shaped theologies of gender with an 'attitude of respect', opening the way to perspectives for further discussion.[38] The anthropology of Christianity has informed my comparative approach to different African Christian discourses and it had enriched my analytical scope, stimulating me to focus not only on beliefs but also on experiences, performances and bodies – though my main interest here is mainly in religious ideas. Furthermore, I build on discussions in the anthropology of Christianity about questions of modernity, as these are crucial to understand dynamics of gender in African Christianities.[39]

The Study of Masculinities and Religion

With its focus on masculinities in African Christian contexts, this book also contributes to another emerging field, the study of men, masculinities and religion. This field is part of the broader study of religion and gender that critically investigates how sexual difference is interpreted and functions as a principle of social and symbolic ordering in religious discourses, practices and communities. For a long time, the study of religion and gender has focussed almost exclusively on women. This was out of a feminist concern about women being marginalised and subordinated in many religious traditions. In 1995, Ursula King underscored the importance of considering 'not only the construction of femininity but also that of masculinity, especially as far as it is grounded in specific religious teachings, and to analyse it critically'.[40] By now, the study of men and masculinities in the sphere of religion has become a recognised sub-field. It is included in the *Encyclopedia of Religion*, under the lemma 'men's studies in religion', where it is described as follows:

> As a new field of scholarly inquiry, it reflects upon and analyzes the complex connections between men and religion, building upon gender studies, feminist theory and criticism ... Methodologically men's studies in religion is an open field; its object of inquiry is "men" as gendered beings in relation to religion.[41]

---

[38] V. Küster, *Einführung in die Interkulturelle Theologie* (Göttingen, 2011), 116.

[39] F. Cannell, 'The Anthropology of Christianity', in F. Cannell (ed.), *The Anthropology of Christianity* (Durham, 2006), 30–39; B. Meyer, 'Christianity in Africa: From African Independent to Pentecostal-Charismatic Churches', *Annual Review of Anthropology*, 33 (2004), 456–60.

[40] U. King, 'Introduction: Gender and the Study of Religion', in U. King (ed.), *Religion and Gender* (Oxford, 1995), 5.

[41] B. Krondorfer and P. Culbertson, 'Men's Studies in Religion', in L. Jones (ed.), *Encyclopedia of Religion*, 2nd edn (Detroit and New York, 2005), 5861–2.

The latter phrase is important: men are studied as *gendered* beings. Parallel to Simone de Beauvoir's well-known statement that one is not born a woman but becomes one, which has been foundational to feminist analysis and women's studies, the basic insight in academic men's studies is that one is not born a man but is made one. Theoretically this points to the distinction between the categories of sex and gender, which is central to social constructionist approaches to gender. Following this distinction, masculinity is considered a social construction that varies according to culture and history. 'As socio-cultural constructs rather than a biological inevitability, masculinities are inextricably connected with the economic, political, social, psychological, and religious dimensions of human life.'[42]

In the study of men, masculinities and religion, two central questions can be distinguished. As put by Stephen Boyd, one question is 'how men's gender identities shape the religions men create and practice' and the second 'how religions construct and shape men's gender identities'.[43] In this book I mainly take up the latter question: How does religion impact upon and interplay with the ongoing process of the construction of masculinities? Stephen Boyd, Merle Longwood and Mark Muesse identify some areas in which religion – they specifically refer to Christianity and Judaism – may support or resist masculinities: through images of the divine, theological anthropology, ethics, and myth and ritual.[44] In addition also the role of sacred texts can be mentioned. The narratives, beliefs and rituals from religious traditions, which are told, taught and performed in religious communities, may all shape men and masculinities in complex and dynamic ways.

Critical Edges: Patriarchy and Heteronormativity

The study of men, masculinities and religion builds upon gender studies and feminist theory. Its historical precedents are in feminist scholarship in religion and theology. This is illustrated by Björn Krondorfer's reader *Men and Masculinities in Christianity and Judaism*, which opens with a piece from Mary Daly's classic *Beyond God the Father*. Though Krondorfer realises that Daly 'would not want her work to be understood as a stepping-stone toward a study of *men* and religion', in his opinion her trenchant critique of patriarchal religion has challenged men to explain their position and privileges, which has given rise to a (self)critical

---

[42] S.B. Boyd, W.M. Longwood and M.W. Muesse, 'Men, Masculinity and the Study of Religion', in S.B. Boyd, W.M. Longwood and M.W. Muesse (eds), *Redeeming Men: Religion and Masculinities* (Louisville, 1996), xiv.

[43] S.B. Boyd, 'Trajectories in Men's Studies in Religion: Theories, Methodologies, and Issues', *Journal of Men's Studies*, 7/2 (1999): 266.

[44] S.B. Boyd, W.M. Longwood and M.W. Muesse, 'Where Do We Go from Here? Some Concluding Remarks', in S.B. Boyd, W.M. Longwood and M.W. Muesse (eds), *Redeeming Men: Religion and Masculinities* (Louisville, 1996), 286ff.

investigation of men, masculinities and religion.[45] It is for this reason that Krondorfer proposes to define the sub-discipline with the adjective 'critical'. Explaining this, he says:

> By calling the new field "critical men's studies in religion", I wish to emphasize that bringing gender consciousness to the analysis and interpretation of men in relation to all aspects of religion is indispensable; otherwise, we might just slip back into a long tradition of reiterations of male dominance within the sphere of religion. In other words, "critical men's studies in religion" exhibits not only a reflective and empathetic stance toward men as individual and communal beings trying to make sense of their lives within the different demands put upon them by society and religion, but it must also engage these issues with critical sensitivity and scholarly discipline in the context of gender-unjust systems.[46]

The 'gender-unjust systems' mentioned here point first of all to patriarchy as it is subtly or overtly manifested in many religious traditions. To have patriarchy as a major topic under critique implies a critical approach to power in the complex relationships between men and women. This indicates the pro-feminist character of the study of men, masculinities and religion. Garth Kasimu Baker-Fletcher strongly engages with a feminist political agenda when defining the objective of the study field:

> Insofar as the discipline of men's studies in religion does not deal with the historical project of patriarchy as its central and fundamental problematic, it fails as a critical theory. ... As long as men's studies has not taken seriously feminist/womanist/mujerista critiques of male sexism and systematic global patriarchy, it can easily fall prey to the powerful co-opting energies of normative traditionalist ideals of masculinity.[47]

Hence, Baker-Fletcher argues for a critical and deconstructive approach to masculinities, which recognises the equality and rights of women and seeks to liberate women *and men* from patriarchy in order to promote their common humanity.

Apart from patriarchy, heterosexism and homophobia are also mentioned by Krondorfer as part of the gender-unjust systems contested in the critical study of

---

[45] B. Krondorfer, 'The Final Cause: The Cause of Causes – Editor's Introduction', in B. Krondorfer (ed.), *Men and Masculinities in Christianity and Judaism: A Critical Reader* (London, 2009), 3.

[46] B. Krondorfer, 'Introduction', in B. Krondorfer (ed.), *Men and Masculinities in Christianity and Judaism: A Critical Reader* (London, 2009), xvii.

[47] G.K. Baker-Fletcher, 'Critical Theory, Deconstruction and Liberation?', *Journal of Men's Studies*, 7/2 (1999): 277.

men, masculinities and religion.[48] In his perception, scholars in this field generally agree 'that a critique of the heterosexual-normative framing of religious and theological issues is necessary, and that a vision of full equality of all humans is desired'.[49] This critical edge is captured by Michael Clark's saying that the sub-discipline is not only pro-feminist but also gay-affirmative.[50] The critical sensitivities to patriarchy and heteronormativity clearly set the parameters and define the analytical framework as well as the political commitments of the study of religion and masculinities.

In the present study I follow the definition of men's studies in religion as a critical activity. My approach to the African Christian discourses on men and masculinity is informed by a critical sensitivity. This primarily concerns patriarchy. However, the concept of patriarchy, originating from classic Western feminist theory, has been problematised in recent years. An important criticism is that the classic feminist understanding of patriarchy is monolithic and does not take into account the different ways in which gender relations are shaped in cross-cultural contexts.[51] Furthermore, postcolonial criticism shows that the concept of patriarchy, when used to analyse gender in African contexts, runs the risk of reinforcing and reproducing colonial and essentialist representations of African men as dominant and oppressive, and of African women as powerless and subordinate.[52] Additionally, it is not clear how the massive concept of patriarchy relates to the conceptualisation of multiple masculinities. Against this background I am somewhat reticent to employ patriarchy as a central concept in my analysis, as I will further explain in Chapter 6. However, I have a critical interest in the various and complex ways in which gender is ordered and power is distributed in discourses on masculinity. In this study I also adopt a critical sensitivity to heteronormativity. Investigating the discourses on masculinity of African theologians and in the local churches, I am sensitive to how masculinities are defined in terms of sexuality: are there explicit or implicit assumptions of heterosexuality, significant silences on homosexuality and/or overt expressions of homophobia?

The Western Scholar and the Study of African Christianity

Doing the research and writing this book, as a European male scholar I have been aware of the burden of history of Western academic engagement with the

---

[48] Krondorfer, 'Editor's Introduction', xvii.

[49] B. Krondorfer, 'Who's Afraid of Gay Theology? Men's Studies, Gay Scholars, and Heterosexual Silence', *Theology and Sexuality*, 13/3 (2007): 264.

[50] J.M. Clark, 'A Gay Man's Wish List for the Future of Men's Studies in Religion', *Journal of Men's Studies*, 7/2 (1999): 270

[51] Cf. J. Butler, *Gender Trouble: Feminism and the Subversion of Identity*, 2nd edn (London, 2006), 48.

[52] See S. Arnfred, 'Re-thinking Sexualities in Africa: Introduction', in S. Arnfred (ed.), *Re-thinking Sexualities in Africa* (Uppsala, 2004), 11–12.

African continent in general and with the study of religion in Africa in particular. Postcolonial critics have denounced the cultural hegemony from 'the West' in the production of knowledge about the oriental 'other' and the representation of the 'other' in the colonial period. Referring to Edward Said, who is just such a critic, postcolonial feminist theologian Kwok Pui-Lan states that Said's work 'issues a clarion call to [Western] Christian theologians and scholars in Christianity' because it was the Christian West that was implicated with the production and reproduction of negative images of colonial subjects.[53] Africa is no exception here: not only the history but also the study of Christianity in Africa have been characterised by Western hegemony and negative representations of the African 'other'.[54]

From the realisation of Western hegemony in the production of knowledge about 'non-Western' subjects, it would be highly problematic to write a book about masculinities in African Christianity without taking into account the pioneering work of African theologians in this area. At the same time, I am aware that I am not a participant in their project of African theology. My subject position is different and consequently so are my academic perspective and approach. In serious acknowledgement of this, in Chapter 2 I will first examine the work of African theologians on issues of gender, masculinities and HIV, as much as possible *on their own terms*. Only at a second stage, mainly in Chapter 6, will I engage critically with their work, based on my observations of the issues which have our shared concern. Here I will bring in my academic perspective more explicitly and provide some criticism of the way African theological scholars analyse and reflect on religion and masculinities.

With regard to the case studies in local churches, a critical postcolonial sensitivity makes one aware of the problem of 'seeing self through others'. This points to the phenomenon denounced by postcolonial critics, that the other is only conceived in terms of the self – generally as a counter-image of the self. Applying this to the study of African Christianity, Jane Soothill comments that 'in analyses of non-Western expressions of Christianity there is a tendency to assess the beliefs and practices of "others" in terms of their similarity to or difference from the beliefs and practices of our Western Christian "selves"'.[55] Though the study of world Christianity is fully aware of Christianity not being a Western religion but having multiple faces, and though it realises that this raises challenges for the Western scholar studying other types of Christianity, there is little methodological reflection on doing cross-cultural research. Cultural anthropologists have reflected

---

[53] P.-L. Kwok, *Postcolonial Imagination and Feminist Theology* (Louisville, 2005), 3.

[54] Cf. E.P. Antonio, 'Introduction: Inculturation and Postcolonial Discourse', in E.P. Antonio (ed.), *Inculturation and Postcolonial Discourse in African Theology* (New York, 2006), 9–11; M.W. Dube, 'Postcoloniality, Feminist Spaces, and Religion', in L.E. Donaldson and P.-L. Kwok (eds), *Postcolonialism, Feminism and Religious Discourse* (New York, 2002), 100–120.

[55] J.E. Soothill, *Gender, Social Change and Spiritual Power: Charismatic Christianity in Ghana* (Leiden, 2007), 24.

on this issue far more explicitly. For example, Soothill, herself an anthropologist studying gender in Charismatic churches in Ghana, mentions the imperative of examining these churches 'on their own terms and within a local context that takes seriously the religious world-views of believers; rather, that is, than with reference to a normative, Western-derived construction of what Christianity is or ought to be'.[56] This sounds very sympathetic and it is an approach I can identify with. The suggestion of analysing discourses 'on their own terms' may, however, neglect the role of the researcher. It is the researcher who introduces the analytical tools and a specific sensitivity to certain issues. It is also the researcher who, simply by his or her presence and his or her specific interests and questions, will trigger certain responses in fieldwork, especially when conducting interviews. Therefore, rather than claiming objectivity, the researcher is to account for his or her subjectivity. In other words, being aware of the risk of seeing self through others, it has also to be acknowledged that the other cannot be seen otherwise than through one's own eyes. In this book I do not intend to evaluate the case-study churches from any normative point of view, either theologically or theoretically. Yet when examining and analysing the discourses in these churches, specifically with regard to the issues of gender and masculinities that are central to this study, I make use of my own theoretical perspectives, analytical tools and critical sensitivities. Inescapably this affects the way the material presented in this book is analysed and organised.

Case Studies in Local Churches in Zambia

The Context of Zambia

This book presents case studies in two local churches in Lusaka, the capital city of Zambia, in Southern-Central Africa. Since independence in 1964, Zambia has been faced with many socio-economic problems, such as economic decline, inflation, unemployment and poverty. In contrast to several other African countries, politically Zambia has remained relatively stable and peaceful. Apparently, the post-independence politics of mixing the various ethnic groups and creating a national Zambian identity has been successful, helped by urbanisation and the promotion of English as the official language.[57]

---

[56] Ibid.

[57] The Zambian government uses a classification which counts 73 ethnic groups. For a brief survey of these groups, see G.C. Bond, 'Zambia: Peoples and Cultures', in J. Middleton (ed.), *Encyclopedia of Africa South of the Sahara. Part IV* (New York, 1997), 414–17. Anthropologists indicate that ethnicity is a factor of decreasing importance for personal identity and the organisation of social life. See J. Davison, *Gender, Lineage, and Ethnicity* in *Southern Africa* (Boulder, 1997), 153–5; K.T. Hansen, *Keeping House in Lusaka* (New York, 1997), 114ff.

One of the major challenges faced by Zambia is the HIV epidemic. With an overall HIV prevalence rate of about 14 per cent, AIDS is said to be 'the most serious threat to the development agenda in Zambia'.[58] The sociologists and AIDS researchers Carolyn Baylies and Janet Bujra observe a shift in the focus of the Zambian HIV prevention policy in the 1990s, from a narrow focus on risky sexual behaviour to a broader focus on 'vulnerability as situated in relations of power and access to resources'.[59] As part of this shift, gender became highlighted as a factor of major importance. Currently the National AIDS Council, which coordinates the Zambian response to the epidemic, advocates a multi-sectoral approach to HIV, and one of its guiding principles is that gender and HIV are co-related. This relation is understood as follows:

> Gender issues that perpetuate the dominance of male interests and lack of self assertiveness on the part of women in sexual relations put both men and women at risk. Women are taught to never refuse their husbands sex regardless of the number of extra-marital partners he may have or his non-willingness to use condoms.[60]

The quotation indicates quite a generalising understanding of gender with monolithic representations of men and women respectively. In reality, however, gender is a more complex phenomenon in Zambia.

Historically, there is not one traditional Zambian configuration of gender. Zambia has a rich ethnic-cultural diversity, and historically the various groups have different kinship systems: matrilineal, patrilineal or mixed. The traditional gendered organisation of kinship, marriage and family life in the various groups is a question for ethnographic research. What matters here is the diversity in this area. Furthermore, colonial history, missionary Christianity, the money economy, urbanisation, modernisation and suchlike have all impacted on traditional configurations of gender in communities that are part of modern Zambia.[61] Nowadays the Zambian government and numerous non-governmental organisations seek to promote gender equality, and these efforts have been reinforced in response to the HIV epidemic. Thus, rather than something static and monolithic, gender in present-day Zambia is dynamic and diverse. Both progressive and reactionary forces are involved in the complex processes in which gender identities and gender relations are constantly (re)shaped.

---

[58] *Zambia – Country Situation* (Geneva, 2008), 1.

[59] J. Bujra and C. Baylies, 'Responses to the AIDS Epidemic in Tanzania and Zambia', in C. Baylies and J. Bujra (eds), *AIDS, Sexuality and Gender in Africa: Collective Strategies and Struggles in Tanzania and Zambia* (London, 2000), 32.

[60] *National HIV and AIDS Strategic Framework 2006–2010* (Lusaka, 2006), 14.

[61] Cf. T. Rasing, *The Bush Burnt, the Stones Remain: Female Initiation Rites in Urban Zambia* (Münster, 2002), esp. 78–125; Hansen, *Keeping House in Lusaka*, 16–17 and 98–103.

What is said about gender in general, of course also applies to masculinities in particular. The traditional roles of men in marriage, the family and the community, as well as the cultural-religious meanings attached to manhood, in modern times are subjected to change. Among others developments, the HIV epidemic has put major challenges to men and masculinities in Zambia.[62] The case studies presented in this book will show how Christianity interplays with the current dynamics of gender and masculinities in present-day Zambia.

Christianity in Zambia

As a result of colonial government and missionary activity, Christianity from the second half of the nineteenth century onwards has become a major religion in Zambia. Though indigenous religion remains a relevant force and though Islam is slowly increasing its popularity, Zambians predominantly identify as Christian.[63] From independence the general idea has grown that 'to be Zambian means to be a Christian'.[64] Apparently, in the postcolonial era Christianity has become an integral part of the Zambian identity – something that even is recorded in the constitutional preamble, which presents Zambia as 'a Christian nation'.[65]

Present-day Zambian Christianity knows great diversity. The Christian churches in the country often are categorised by the three so-called 'mother bodies' that bring churches together and represent them in public affairs. These umbrella organisations are the Council of Churches in Zambia (mainly for the mainline Protestant churches), the Zambia Episcopal Conference (representing the Roman Catholic Church in Zambia), and the Evangelical Fellowship of Zambia (in which Evangelical and some Pentecostal churches collaborate). These organisations collaborate on several issues concerning Zambian society. In 2001 a fourth 'mother body' joined the scene, the Independent Churches Organisation of Zambia, which represents a number of Charismatic or neo-Pentecostal churches. This illustrates a development in recent decades, in which Pentecostal and Charismatic churches have gained ground in Zambia, as all over the African continent.[66] These churches

---

[62] Cf. Simpson, *Boys to Men in the Shadow of AIDS*; P. Dover, 'Gender and Embodiment: Expectations of Manliness in a Zambian Village', in L. Ouzgane and R. Morrell (eds), *African Masculinities: Men in Africa from the Late Nineteenth Century to the Present* (New York, 2005), 173–88.

[63] Austin Cheyeka, in 'Towards a History of the Charismatic Churches in Post-Colonial Zambia', in J.B. Gewald, M. Hinfelaar and G. Macola (eds), *One Zambia, Many Histories: Towards a History of Post-Colonial Zambia* (Leiden, 2008), 146, gives a percentage of 87 per cent, based on the 2000 nation-wide census.

[64] E. Colson, *Tonga Religious Life in the Twentieth Century* (Lusaka, 2006), 249.

[65] For the background to this declaration, see P. Gifford, 'Chiluba's Christian Nation: Christianity as a Factor in Zambian Politics 1991–1996', *Journal of Contemporary Religion*, 13/3 (1998), 363–81.

[66] Cf. Cheyeka, *Towards a History*, 144–63.

are prominently present in the media and in the public sphere in a city like Lusaka. At the same time, the influence and vitality of the so-called mainline churches should not be underestimated.

Case Studies

The question of how men and masculinities are addressed, contested and transformed in local churches calls for in-depth qualitative research, such as through case studies. Case-study research does not aim to give a representative account of the issues under investigation, but to provide detailed understanding of these issues from a few cases. The hope is that this sheds new light on the subject in general. The two case studies presented in this book can never be representative of the churches in Zambia, and certainly not of African Christianity at large. However, they demonstrate some of the diversity of Christianity in Zambia and in Africa in general. The first case study, Regiment parish, is part of the largest denomination in Zambia, the Roman Catholic Church. The second case study, Northmead Assembly of God, belongs to the rapidly growing and diverse movement of Pentecostal and Charismatic churches. Both churches turned out to be rich empirical cases for the purpose of this study.

The actual fieldwork was conducted over more than five months, spread over two periods (September–November 2008 and June–August 2009). In both churches I regularly attended Sunday services, youth meetings, men's fellowship meetings, wedding services, meetings for married couples, workshops on HIV and AIDS, Bible studies, prayer meetings and other events. Apart from attending the formal church activities, I spent a substantial amount of time at church, informally socialising and conversing with church members and pastors. As people got to know me, I was invited by some to their homes or spent time with them elsewhere. The collected materials, then, include fieldwork notes, recorded sermons and speeches, newsletters, booklets, magazines, and – in case of Northmead Assembly of God – DVDs with sermons on specific themes. Another body of collected data consists of interviews. About 45 semi-structured, explorative interviews were conducted, with church members of various ages, predominantly with men but also with some women. Also, a number of pastors and priests in the churches were interviewed, as well as a few officials in organisations related to the churches. All interviewees are referred to in this book with fictive names, except those interviewed in their function as pastor or priest in the church who gave permission to be quoted by name.

The interviews and the other materials collected during the fieldwork form the body of data on which the case studies are based. The case studies thus include both formal and informal discourses in the churches.[67] The formal discourse, such

---

[67] I understand 'discourse' in Foucauldian terms, as not only expressing and reflecting but also constituting and constructing social realities through language. Discourses contain powerful messages that form and shape and make sense of the social world, and enable the

as sermons, gives an idea of the churches' ideals of masculinity. By including the voices of men about their own male identities and experiences, it becomes clear how male church members understand and evaluate themselves in relation to these ideals. It is important to include the voices of women about men and masculinity, and therefore I have conducted some interviews with women.[68] Yet I have opted to interview mainly men. The reason is that in the literature on religion, gender and HIV a lot is said *about* men and the problems associated with masculinities, often in generalising and blaming ways, while the voices of men themselves are hardly included and the diversity and complexity of masculinities are hardly taken into account.

Overview

The structure of this book corresponds with the research questions formulated above. Following this introduction, in Chapter 2 the focus is on the groundbreaking work of a group of African theologians. The question is how they analyse, reflect upon, and envision masculinities in the context of the HIV epidemic. In order to put this question in a wider context, the chapter does not simply focus on the recent debate on masculinities among some African theologians but investigates broader discussions about gender and HIV in African theology. The following two chapters focus on African Christianity as manifested in local churches. Two case studies are presented: the Roman Catholic Regiment parish (Chapter 3) and the Pentecostal Northmead Assembly of God (Chapter 4). These chapters offer a detailed theological ethnographic account of Catholic and Pentecostal masculinities in contemporary Zambia as constructed in local faith communities. Chapter 5 brings the lines of the previous chapters together and further explores them through a comparative approach. The chapter discusses the convergences and divergences by looking at the ways in which the case-study churches and the theologians work towards a transformation of masculinities. First, the case studies are critically compared with each other and are discussed in relation to broader scholarly literature on Catholicism and Pentecostalism in Africa. Second, the transformations of masculinity in the case-study churches are compared with the account of African theologians on the transformation of masculinities. This gives

---

subject (individual) to position and identify himself/herself in and in relation to this world. Hence, theories of gender and discourse focus on the discursive construction of gender, or on gender as discourse. With regard to masculinities, Stephen Whitehead and Frank Barrett state that 'masculinities exists as discourse – dominant and subordinated ways of thinking, talking and acting as males, and as such provide the very means by which males "become" men"'. See S. Whitehead and F.J. Barrett, 'The Sociology of Masculinity', in S. Whitehead and F.J. Barrett (eds), *The Masculinities Reader* (Cambridge, 2001), 21.

[68] Cf. M.C. Gutmann, 'Trafficking in Men: The Anthropology of Masculinity', *Annual Review of Anthropology*, 26 (1997): 400.

critical insight into the different trajectories and theologies surrounding the change of men and masculinities in African Christianity. The comparison in Chapter 5 raises some crucial theoretical questions about the analysis and understanding of transformations of masculinity in religious contexts such as the case study churches. Chapter 6 explores these questions by discussing some conceptual frames to understand religious discourse on masculinity and by introducing the concept of male agency that is more sensitive to the transformative dimension of discourse that is, at first sight, rather traditional or patriarchal. This concluding chapter explores in an original way how the critical scholar of men, masculinities and religion can understand transformations of masculinities at a grassroots level in all their complexities as contributing to a vision of gender justice.

Chapter 2
Transforming Masculinities towards Gender Justice: African Theologians

'African men are what they are because of their socialization into patriarchy, a sense of being the dominant sex and persons to whom service is owned.'[1] This statement of Mercy Oduyoye, one of the most prominent women in African theology, illustrates the tone of the discussion about men and masculinities among African theologians. Though Oduyoye made this statement in 1997, the issue of masculinities has only recently become an explicit theme in African theological scholarship. The topic has emerged as a result of the engagement in African theology with issues of gender, HIV and AIDS in the first decade of the twenty-first century. This chapter analyses the current debate on masculinities in African theological scholarship. The aims are to contextualise this debate in the broader field of African theology, to identify the central theoretical and theological concepts in this debate, and to understand how African theologians envision a transformation of masculinities in the context of the HIV epidemic. The chapter is based on an analysis of a wide range of publications by African theologians. These theologians come from different parts of the continent (though mainly from Southern Africa) and from different Christian traditions (though most of them have a mainstream Protestant background). They correspond in their commitment to take African social and cultural realities as the starting point of their theological analysis and reflection.

The Study of Gender in African Theology

African Women's Theology

Issues of gender entered the scene of African theology thanks to the efforts of African women theologians. African theology emerged in the 1960s as an enterprise almost exclusively of male theologians. They intended to develop a theology with an African face. However, as Mercy Oduyoye comments, they did not speak about women's issues and actually presented a theology with an African

---

[1] M.A. Oduyoye, 'Acting to Construct Africa: The Agency by Women', in R. van Eijk and J. van Lin (eds), *Africans Reconstructing Africa* (Nijmegen, 1997), 38.

male face.[2] Therefore Oduyoye has been in the forefront of developing African women's theology.[3] In 1989 the Circle of Concerned African Women Theologians was founded, uniting women from all over the African continent and from several religious traditions (but predominantly Christian), and creating a space to theologise from women's experiences.[4] Thanks to the Circle, women theologians have become a major voice, and are even considered 'the most vibrant trend', in African theology today.[5]

When African women theologians seek to bring women's experiences into theology, what then are the particular experiences of women, in their opinion? Oduyoye gives a clear answer to this question, saying: '[T]he reality is that there are many Africas – the Africa of the rich and the Africa of the poor; the Africa of men who command and that of women who obey is experienced differently.'[6] The difference in men's and women's experience is understood as a difference in social position and power: men are in command, and women are to obey. This, of course, is a generalised picture. African women theologians acknowledge that the experiences of women in Africa vary according to their specific location in terms of class, race, culture, nationality and religion. However, it is believed that women generally experience, in one way or another, sexism and patriarchal oppression. Therefore, as Isabel Phiri says, 'African women theologians are united in voicing their views against patriarchy.'[7] The major concern of these theologians is that the humanity of women is not fully respected but rather threatened by the patriarchal traditions in African societies, cultures and religions. African women theologians do not only address but also seek to transform the critical realities that

---

[2] M.A. Oduyoye, 'The Roots of African Christian Feminism', in J.S. Pobee and C.F. Hallencreutz (eds), *Variations in Christian Theology in Africa* (Nairobi, 1979), 33.

[3] Among African women theologians there is an ongoing debate on naming their work. In her early publications Oduyoye used the term 'feminist theology', and some other women theologians still use this term. Others, however, have shown a reticence to label their work as feminist because of the association of feminism with Western white middle-class women's issues. Several alternative names have been suggested, but the most common one is simply African women's theology (or theologies). Cf. I.A. Phiri and S. Nadar, 'Introduction: "Treading Softly but Firmly"', in I.A. Phiri and S. Nadar (eds), *African Women, Religion and Health: Essays in Honor of Mercy Amba Ewudziwa Oduyoye* (Maryknoll, 2006), 3–4.

[4] Cf. M.A. Oduyoye, 'The Circle', in M.A. Oduyoye and M.R.A. Kanyoro (eds), *Talitha, Qumi! Proceedings of the Convocation of African Women Theologians* (Ibadan, 1990), 1–26.

[5] E. Chitando, *Troubled but not Destroyed* (Geneva, 2009), 31.

[6] M.A. Oduyoye, 'The Search for a Two-Winged Theology. Women's Participation in the Development of Theology in Africa: The Inaugural Address', in M.A. Oduyoye and M.R.A. Kanyoro (eds), *Talitha, Qumi! Proceedings of the Convocation of African Women Theologians* (Ibadan, 1990), 41.

[7] I.A. Phiri, 'Major Challenges for African Women Theologians in Theological Education (1989–2008)', *International Review of Mission*, 98/1 (2009): 106.

are oppressing to women. For them, the study of gender in religion and culture 'is not just a new line in the academic industry, but a perspective that requires analysis leading to action that will orientate people and communities toward justice'.[8] Overviewing the work of the Circle, Sarojini Nadar and Isabel Phiri point out that 'our work is framed by an ideology and concern for the liberation of women'.[9] This project of women's liberation is not a goal in itself but aims at the fullness of life for all of humanity, women and men together.

Criticism of African (Male) Theology

African women theologians relate critically to the two major strands in African (male) theology: liberation and inculturation theology.[10] First, they point out that liberation theology, in its analysis of structures of injustice, systematically ignores gender issues.[11] According to this criticism, African male liberation theologians are concerned with poverty and economic oppression in postcolonial Africa, and – in South Africa during Apartheid – with oppression in terms of colour, but they ignore that women are 'at the bottom of the heap when it comes to oppression and exploitation'.[12] Therefore it is the so-called 'trilogy of race, class and gender' that is central in African women's liberation theology.[13] Second, with regard to inculturation theology, African women theologians point out that here culture is approached rather uncritically. Seeking to reclaim and affirm African culture, inculturation theologians would overlook cultural traditions of patriarchy that marginalise and oppress women.[14] African women theologians employ a gender-sensitive hermeneutics and call for a 'critical solidarity' with African cultural traditions.[15] As Musimbi Kanyoro puts it: '[W]e make the claim that inculturation is not sufficient unless the cultures we reclaim are analyzed and are deemed worthy in terms of justice and support for life and the dignity of women is ascertained.'[16]

---

[8] M.A. Oduyoye, *Daughters of Anowa: African Women and Patriarchy* (Maryknoll, 1995), 89.

[9] Phiri and Nadar, 'Introduction: "Treading Softly but Firmly"', 5.

[10] For an introduction to both types of African theology, see E. Martey, *African Theology: Inculturation and Liberation* (Maryknoll, 1993).

[11] Oduyoye, *Daughters of Anowa*, 180.

[12] N.J. Njoroge, *Kiama Kia Ngo: An African Christian Feminist Ethic of Resistance and Transformation* (Accra, 2000), 130.

[13] Phiri and Nadar, 'Introduction: "Treading Softly but Firmly"', 4–6.

[14] M. Mutambara, 'African Women Theologies Critique Inculturation', in E.P. Antonio (ed.), *Inculturation and Postcolonial Discourse in African Theology* (New York, 2006), 173–91.

[15] Phiri and Nadar, 'Introduction: "Treading Softly but Firmly"', 8.

[16] M.R.A. Kanyoro, *Introducing Feminist Cultural Hermeneutics: An African Perspective* (London, 2002), 26.

African women theologians have challenged male colleagues to take women's experience in African cultures, religions and societies seriously and to develop a theology that is liberating to men and women together. However, according to Philomena Mwaura, male theologians demonstrate a 'theological unwillingness to deal with women's issues and concerns'.[17] This view is supported by Tinyiko Maluleke, one of the few African men in theology who engage in dialogue and collaboration with women theologians. According to his assessment, African male theology is so 'bewildered and confused' by the new developments in its own context, such as the end of Apartheid, globalisation, and the emergence of gender and human rights questions, that it is unable to engage with the issues raised by women theologians.[18] However, Maluleke also points to an unwillingness to do so:

> [B]y and large African Theology has been at peace with the patriarchy inherited from both Western and African cultures. The logic of patriarchy has been so internalized that even when dealing with similar issues of dehumanization, oppression and exclusion, African theologians have not been able to make the connections. Ideologically and spiritually, therefore, African theology has remained largely beholden to the supremacist ideas when it comes to gender relations.[19]

Yet a number of African male theologians have taken up the challenge put by women's theology. They share the concern about the oppression of women and have committed themselves to the ideal of a new community of women and men together. Examples are Simon Maimela, who struggles to be a Christian in a patriarchal society,[20] Laurenti Magesa, who calls for the full inclusion of women in the church's ministry and who supports the theological project of women's liberation and gender justice,[21] the late John Mary Walligo, who sought to promote the equality of women and men,[22] and Maluleke, who denounces violence against

---

[17] P.N. Mwaura, 'Gender Mainstreaming in African Theology: An African Women's Perspective', *Voices from the Third World*, 24/1 (2001): 166.

[18] T.S. Maluleke, 'African "Ruths", Ruthless Africas: Reflections of an African Mordechai', in M.W. Dube (ed.), *Other Ways of Reading: African Women and the Bible* (Atlanta, 2001), 237–8.

[19] T.S. Maluleke, 'An African Theology Perspective on Patriarchy', in *The Evil of Patriarchy in Church, Society and Politics* (Cape Town, 2009), 33.

[20] S. Maimela, 'Seeking to be Christian in Patriarchal Society', *Journal of Black Theology in South Africa*, 9/2 (1995): 27–42.

[21] L. Magesa, 'The Challenge of African Woman Defined Theology for the 21st Century', in N.W. Ndung'u and P.N. Mwaura (eds), *Challenges and Prospects of the Church in Africa. Theological Reflections of the 21st Century* (Nairobi, 2005), 88–101; L. Magesa, 'Christology, African Women and Ministry', *African Ecclesial Review*, 38/2 (1996): 66–88.

[22] J.M. Walligo, *Struggle for Equality: Women and Empowerment in Uganda* (Eldoret, 2002).

women and seeks to overcome patriarchy.[23] Referring to these and some other names, Phiri, in her evaluative account of 30 years of African women's theology, observes that now there is a 'serious and deliberate critical engagement' from a number of African male theologians with the issues raised by women theologians.[24]

Apparently, gender issues are being mainstreamed slowly but surely in African theology. However, the engagement of the above-mentioned male theologians with gender is actually an engagement with *women's* issues, arising from their sensitivity to the concerns expressed by African women theologians. Thus, nowadays, issues such as sexual and domestic violence against women and other overt manifestations of gender injustice are critically addressed by several male theologians. But a thorough and self-critical analysis of patriarchy, with a focus on the position of men and the construction of masculinities in patriarchal gender systems, has hardly been provided. Maluleke stated in 1997 that male theologians cannot simply join African women theologians but must first become 'born again'. By this he meant that male theologians 'have yet to consciously problematize, deeply reflect and *agonize* over their role and status both as perpetrators and beneficiaries of patriarchy'.[25] Up to the present, however, the in-depth reflection he calls for is still in its infancy. It is a very recent development that issues concerning men and masculinities are discussed openly and critically by some male theologians, and an HIV epidemic was needed to initiate this.

Gender, Patriarchy and Gender Justice

Central to the discussions in African theology initiated by women theologians are three major concepts: gender, patriarchy and gender justice. As will become clear later in this chapter, these concepts are also crucial to the current discussions of masculinities in the context of the HIV epidemic. How, then, are these concepts understood theoretically and theologically?

Gender African women theologians have adopted gender as a major analytical tool. The concept enables them to analyse and understand women's experiences of oppression not just as *women's* issues but as an issue in the relationship between men and women. This relationship is understood in terms of power, and it is exactly the powered dimension of the relation between men and women that is central to gender studies in African theology. For example, Musa Dube points out that '[a]t the centre of gender relations is the concept of power and powerlessness.

---

[23] T.S. Maluleke and S. Nadar, 'Breaking the Covenant of Violence against Women', *Journal of Theology for Southern Africa*, 114 (2002): 5–17.

[24] Phiri, *Major Challenges for African Women Theologians*, 116.

[25] T.S. Maluleke, 'The "Smoke Screens" Called Black and African Liberation Theologies – the Challenge of African Women Theology', *Journal of Constructive Theology*, 3/2 (1997): 42.

The problem is that gender disempowers half of humanity – women.'[26] From this perception, African women theologians have developed a critical hermeneutics to analyse the powered processes that construe the identities of and relations between men and women. They employ and apply this hermeneutics to African culture and biblical scripture and to the social, political, economical and religious realities of today's world. According to Musimbi Kanyoro,

> Gender analysis takes into account ways in which roles, attitudes, values and relationships regarding women and men are constructed by societies all over the world. The concepts and practices of equality and discrimination determined by social, economic, religious and cultural factors lie at the heart of gender-sensitive perspectives. Theological engagement with gender issues seeks to expose harm and injustices that are in society and are extended to Scripture and the teachings and practices of the Church through culture.[27]

This quotation clearly reflects a social constructionist understanding of gender. Musa Dube highlights the political advantage of this perspective when she says that 'gender (1) is not natural, (2) is not divine, (3) has to do with social relationships of women and men, and (4) can be reconstructed and transformed by the society, for since it is culturally constructed it can be socially deconstructed'.[28] A constructivist understanding enables African women theologians to criticise those who consider the roles of men and women in gender relations as fixed because of biology, creation or tradition. It also opens up the possibility of change. If gender is a construct, it can be not only deconstructed but also reconstructed. African theologians involved in the study of gender engage in this theoretical space for social transformation. In Oduyoye's words: 'Recognizing and becoming sensitive to gender in theology leads to a theology that is liberative, that does not remain theoretical but demands ethical choices that will empower the transformation of relationships that have been damaged by sexism and misogynistic attitudes.'[29]

Patriarchy As gender is understood as a concept of power, the concern of African women theologians and some male colleagues is that power is unequally distributed in gender relations, with women generally excluded from and subjected to the power held by men. It is this reality of asymmetry in gender relations, manifested and maintained in numerous practices and beliefs, which is captured by the theologians with the concept of patriarchy. Etymologically, 'patriarchy'

---

[26] M.W. Dube, 'Culture, Gender and HIV/AIDS: Understanding and Acting on the Issues', in M.W. Dube (ed.), *HIV/AIDS and the Curriculum: Methods of Integrating HIV/AIDS in Theological Programmes* (Geneva, 2003), 88.

[27] Kanyoro, *Introducing Feminist Cultural Hermeneutics*, 17.

[28] Dube, *Culture, Gender and HIV/AIDS*, 86.

[29] M.A. Oduyoye, 'Gender and Theology in Africa Today', *Journal of Constructive Theology*, 8/2 (2002): 43.

means the rule of the father. Hence, Phiri defines it as 'a father-ruled structure where all power and authority rests in the hands of the male head of the family'.[30] Kanyoro indicates a broader understanding, as in her opinion patriarchy refers to 'an unjust hierarchical and dualistic ordering of life which discriminates against women'.[31] The primary concern of the theologians is with patriarchy as a cultural and religious ideology that assigns power and authority to men and creates a hierarchy in gender relations. In the words of Maluleke, patriarchy is an ideology that 'speaks of the supremacy of the male.'[32] The major concern of African women theologians is that the ideology of patriarchy is materialised in social, economic and political structures which benefit men and do not respect women as equal human beings. Though it is recognised that women's experiences vary within patriarchal settings and that some women may have some privilege and power, it is believed that ultimately 'women in all patriarchal cultures are perceived to have inferior status compared to men'.[33]

Investigating the ideological basis of patriarchy, the theologians generally consider African cultures and traditional religions as patriarchal. However, a central thesis in their work is that Western colonial government and missionary Christianity have introduced a far more 'monolithic patriarchy' in which 'male and female are rigidly opposed to each other'.[34] At best, Christianity came as a mixed blessing for African women, as Phiri points out: on the one hand Christianity opposed some cultural practices that were harmful to women, but on the other hand it imposed other oppressions and denied women's full humanity.[35] Writing about patriarchal gender ideology, Oduyoye states that 'the church in Africa continues to use the Hebrew Scriptures and the Epistles of St. Paul to reinforce the norms of traditional religion and culture'.[36] A concrete example is the idea of male headship in marriage and the family, which is often legitimated with reference to African culture and the Bible, but which is rejected by women theologians because it symbolises and reaffirms the asymmetry in gender relations.[37]

Clearly, patriarchy is firmly opposed by African women theologians and those male theologians who have joined their endeavours. It is considered the root cause of the many evils African women are faced with in the home, the church and the community. Patriarchal ideology has been rejected in firm

---

[30] I.A. Phiri, *Women, Presbyterianism and Patriarchy: Religious Experience of Chewa Women in Central Malawi* (Blantyre, 1997), 12.

[31] Kanyoro, *Introducing Feminist Cultural Hermeneutics*, 17, note 10.

[32] Maluleke, *An African Theology Perspective on Patriarchy*, 31.

[33] Mwaura, *Gender Mainstreaming in African Theology*, 171.

[34] Oduyoye, *Daughters of Anowa*, 157.

[35] Phiri, *Women, Presbyterianism and Patriarchy*, 80.

[36] Oduyoye, *Daughters of Anowa*, 174.

[37] Cf. R.N. Uchem, *Overcoming Women's Subordination: An Igbo African and Christian Perspective. Envisioning an Inclusive Theology with Reference to Women* (Enugu, 2001), 144–5.

theological language. For instance, Mwaura refers to patriarchy as a sin, and Maimela declares it to be an 'idolatrous god' because it contradicts the 'central message of the Christian faith', being the dignity of life of all humanity.[38] Hence these theologians call for a transformation of gender relations beyond patriarchy, towards a reality called gender justice.

Gender justice Gender-sensitive African theologians do not accept patriarchy as a given but envisage a new kind of gender relations to be realised in the family, the church, the community and society at large. They use different concepts to describe the new gender arrangement that is to be realised. Writing specifically about marriage, Rosemary Uchem proposes 'an equal-partnership model' of gender relations, which in practice would mean that leadership is shared rather than hierarchical.[39] Likewise, Fulata Moyo qualifies the marital relationship with the notions of mutuality and companionship.[40] Two other theologians, Isabel Phiri and Nyambura Njoroge, envision a new and liberated community of men and women in the church and the society.[41] They understand this community as fully recognising the human dignity of women, allowing the full participation of women, and as sharing authority between men and women. Sharing authority assumes a sense of equality of men and women, and indeed the concept of gender equality often appears in publications and is central, for example, in the work of Musa Dube and John Mary Walligo.[42] The meaning of proposed concepts such as equality, partnership, mutuality and others is hardly elaborated upon. It is difficult, therefore, to compare them and to see whether the theologians share exactly the same vision for a transformation of gender relations. There are some indications of differences of opinion on the issue of what equality of the sexes exactly means and how radical a transformation of gender relations should be. For example, Catholic theologian Laurenti Magesa expresses his concern that African women theologians in their arguments for gender equality tend to neglect the differences between the sexes. According to Magesa, gender equality means that woman and man share an 'equal human dignity', but he emphasises that this does not eradicate the 'innate sexual qualities which God has endowed each sex'. For a project of gender transformation this means, in his opinion, that 'the true meaning

---

[38] Mwaura, *Gender Mainstreaming in African Theology*, 175; Maimela, *Seeking to be Christian*, 31.

[39] Uchem, *Overcoming Women's Subordination*, 228.

[40] F.L. Moyo, 'Sex, Gender, Power and HIV/AIDS in Malawi: Threats and Challenges to Women Being Church', in I.A. Phiri and S. Nadar (eds), *On Being Church: African Women's Voices and Visions* (Geneva, 2005), 134–5.

[41] Njoroge, *Kiama Kia Ngo*, 155–6; Phiri, *Women, Presbyterianism and Patriarchy*, chapter 6.

[42] See Walligo, *Struggle for Equality*; M.W. Dube, 'Grant Me Justice: Female and Male Equality in the New Testament', *Journal of Religion and Theology in Namibia*, 3 (2001): 82–115.

of motherhood', which 'lies in the ability to nurture life' should not be jettisoned 'in the name of woman's liberation'.[43] Apparently, Magesa considers African women theologians to be too radically feminist in their transformative vision of gender relations. Though Magesa and the women theologians he criticises have a shared concern about the oppression and marginalisation of women, and a shared commitment to realise more balanced relations between the sexes, they differ in their understanding of what transformed relations between men and women should look like.

In spite of these differences, theologically it is important that gender-critical African theologians correspond in their understanding that gender is an issue of justice. Though the precise meaning of the concept of 'gender justice' for the social relations between men and women remains somewhat vague, it clearly has a strong ethical-theological connotation. As Phiri puts it:

> Gender justice means promoting the humanity of both women and men in the church and using their gifts as revealed by God. Any form of discrimination and oppression mars the image of God in creation and humanity, for God is a God of justice and the practice of Christianity is supposed to reflect the justice of God.[44]

In this argument, gender justice is based theologically on the understanding of God. Indeed, Phiri says that gender justice 'has its origins in our concept of God'.[45] This makes the quest for gender justice so urgent for these theologians and, in their opinion, also for the church. Because of the deeply theological connotations, in the words of Magesa, justice in gender relations is 'a Christian imperative' and an 'in integral part of living the gospel'.[46] The vision of gender justice, so passionately advocated by these theologians, is informed by several theological notions.

In the quotation above, Phiri states that 'God is a God of justice'. This is in line with the broader movement of liberation theology that African women theologians associate themselves with. As much as God, according to classic Latin American liberation theology, has a preferential option for the poor, in the view of gender-sensitive African theologians God opts for women because they are oppressed and marginalised.[47] Mwaura puts forwards this understanding with a reference to Gal. 3:28 when she states that God is depicted in the Bible 'as not the creator or validator of existing hierarchical and oppressive social order, but [as] one who liberates us from it, the one who opens up a community of equals where there is no slave, nor

---

[43] Magesa, *The Challenge of African Woman Defined Theology*, 99–100.

[44] I.A. Phiri, 'Life in Fullness: Gender Justice. A Perspective from Africa', *Journal of Constructive Theology*, 8/2 (2002): 77.

[45] Ibid., 79.

[46] Magesa, *The Challenge of African Woman Defined Theology*, 101.

[47] See Maimela, *Seeking to be Christian*, 27–42, who for his argument against patriarchy explicitly adopts the typical discourse of liberation theology.

free, no Jew or Gentile, but all are one in Christ Jesus'.[48] This understanding of God inspires the rejection of patriarchy and a commitment to women's liberation. Additionally, African women theologians have developed a more particular line of thought on God and gender justice that starts from the concept of God in African traditional religions. The explicit female, gender-neutral and inclusive images of God in these religions and its myths are reclaimed.[49] Hence the patriarchal God who, in Oduyoye's words, is 'enthroned' in Africa under the influence of Christianity and Islam, is replaced by images of God that affirm the equality and dignity of women and men together.[50]

Alongside the traditional African creation myths, the biblical creation accounts are used to develop a theology of gender justice.[51] African women theologians re-read and re-visit the Genesis creation stories with a critical hermeneutic in order to overcome the traditional patriarchal interpretation that women are second in the order of creation.[52] A notion that is recovered and affirmed in this reading is that humankind is equally created in the image of God as male and female (Genesis 1:27). On this basis, African women theologians claim the full humanity, dignity and equality of women in relation to men. The concept of gender justice, then, is based theologically not only on the understanding of God but also on the anthropological notion that men and women are created in the image of God. Actually, both lines of thought are closely related, as is apparent from Kanyoro's statement: 'Women, as well as men, are made in the divine image of God and therefore any pattern of discrimination, domination or oppression is contrary to God's justice and sovereignty.'[53]

Gender justice, in the work of the gender-critical African theologians, also has a Christological basis. First, reference is made to the historical Jesus of Nazareth. Several scholars point out how Jesus, according to the gospels, dealt with women in a liberating and de-stigmatising way, including them in the circle of his disciples and breaking with the patriarchal status quo of his day. For Dube, 'it is clear that Jesus came to a world of gender imbalance, a world that sentenced many women to violence and to the disease of gender injustice. However, he undertook to announce liberation, to undermine gender inequality and to begin charting the path of gender justice.'[54] Precisely because of his counter-cultural, liberating

---

[48] Mwaura, *Gender Mainstreaming in African Theology*, 176.

[49] R. Teteki Abbey, 'Rediscovering Ataa Naa Nyonmo – the Father Mother God', in N.J. Njoroge and M.W. Dube (eds), *Talitha Cum! Theologies of African Women* (Pietermaritzburg, 2001), 140–57; Oduyoye, *Daughters of Anowa*, 21–35, 178–80.

[50] Cf. M.A. Oduyoye, *Introducing African Women's Theology* (Cleveland, 2001), 43.

[51] Uchem, *Overcoming Women's Subordination*, 179–90; M.A. Oduyoye, *Hearing and Knowing: Theological Reflections on Christianity in Africa* (Maryknoll, 1986), 90–96, 130–31.

[52] Cf. Phiri, *Women, Presbyterianism and Patriarchy*, 155.

[53] Kanyoro, *Introducing Feminist Cultural Hermeneutics*, 17.

[54] M.W. Dube, 'Who do You Say that I Am?', *Feminist Theology*, 15/3 (2007): 361.

relationships to women, Jesus 'has become for us the Christ', Oduyoye and Amoah write, using an inclusive 'us' of African women.[55] According to Nasimiyu-Wasike, not only the practice of Jesus' ministry, but also the event of incarnation itself underpins gender justice. In the incarnation, she says, 'the humanity of Jesus is united to every other human being, granting everyone dignity, which mandates justice for all'.[56] Second, though Jesus is crucified, as the risen Christ and Lord he is believed to continue bringing liberation to women and realising gender justice. For example, Uchem observes a growing commitment in our contemporary world to change the situation of women's subordination and she explains this as 'a sign of the active presence and activity of the Spirit of Jesus'.[57] A third Christological argument for gender justice is the idea that through baptism in Christ one enters a new community established by Christ. A popular verse is Gal. 3:28, which states that there is 'neither Jew or Greek, slave or free, male or female for all are one in Christ'. This is not understood in terms of an eradication of sexual difference but rather in terms of 'a life of partnership between men and women' that arises from the new creation in Christ.[58]

The latter points to the eschatological foundation of gender justice, which is central in the work of Oduyoye and Phiri. As they make clear, the engagement of African theologians with a transformation of gender relations is actually an anticipation of their hope for the realisation of the biblical vision of a new earth and a new human community. This vision tells them that 'the tyranny of patriarchy is bound to end'.[59] Though this is said to be a 'utopian vision', at the same time the eschatological hope functions as a 'midwife for new beginning' which, according to Moyo, is foretasted in every marital relationship that is characterised by partnership and mutual sexual pleasure.[60] Phiri even indicates that a transformation

---

[55] M.A. Oduyoye and E. Amoah, 'The Christ for African Women', in M.A. Oduyoye and V. Fabella (eds), *With Passion and Compassion: Third World Women Doing Theology* (Maryknoll, 1988), 43.

[56] A. Nasimiyu-Wasike, 'Imagining Jesus Christ in the African Context at the Dawn of a New Millennium', in N.W. Ndung'u and P.N. Mwaura (eds), *Challenges and Prospects of the Church in Africa: Theological Reflections of the 21st Century* (Nairobi, 2005), 112.

[57] Uchem, *Overcoming Women's Subordination*, 209.

[58] Ibid., 208–9. See also Phiri, *Women, Presbyterianism and Patriarchy*, 156; Oduyoye, *Hearing and Knowing*, 137.

[59] Oduyoye, *Introducing African Women's Theology*, 119. See also I.A. Phiri, 'A Theological Analysis of the Voices of Teenage Girls on Men's Role in the Fight against HIV/AIDS in KwaZulu-Natal, South Africa', *Journal of Theology for Southern Africa*, 120 (2004): 43–5; Phiri, *Life in Fullness*, 78–9.

[60] F.L. Moyo, 'A Quest for Women's Sexual Empowerment through Education in an HIV and AIDS Context. The Case of Kukonzekera Chinkhoswe Chachikhristu (KCC) among aMang'Anja and aYao Christians of t/a Mwambo in Rural Zomba, Malawi' (PhD thesis, University of KwaZulu-Natal, 2009), 6–7. The phrase 'utopian vision' comes from Phiri, *Life in Fullness*, 79, while the phrase 'midwife of new beginnings' is used by F.L. Moyo, 'Navigating Experiences of Healing: A Narrative Theology of Eschatological Hope

of gender relations towards gender justice is not only a foretaste of, but even a precondition for the eschatological future to come: 'Justice for all humanity is not only important but it is necessary for the realization of the presence of God on earth.'[61]

Gender justice thus is a deeply theological concept. Though its concrete meaning remains somewhat vague, it is a key notion underlying the opposition to patriarchy and motivating the quest for a new arrangement of male–female relationships. On the basis of their theology of gender justice, gender-critical African theologians label patriarchy as a sin and call upon churches to transform oppressive gender structures and ideologies in their own midst and in society more broadly.

Gender, Transformation and the Role of the Church

African women theologians are very critical of Christian churches for maintaining and reinforcing patriarchy. Concretely, they point for example to women's exclusion from the full ministry in many churches, to the general silence of churches on issues such as domestic and sexual violence against women, to churches' legitimisation of male dominance in marital and gender relations, to the literalist and women-oppressive interpretations of scripture that prevail in churches, and so on.[62] The general feeling is expressed by Oduyoye when she states: 'There is a myth in Christian circles that the church brought liberation to the African woman. Indeed, this is a myth, a claim glibly made and difficult to illustrate with concrete or continuing examples.'[63] From this critical appraisal, the theologians are calling upon churches for transformation. Magesa identifies three challenges raised by women theologians to churches in Africa:

> They lie in the anthropological sphere where the task is to re-imagine cultural perceptions with regard to the feminine and masculine. Then there is the theological sphere, strictly so called, in which the concern is about predominant theological language and images and liturgical symbols. And, finally, there is the ethical sphere where questions about sexuality, the beginning of human life itself, arise.[64]

It is believed that when churches indeed transform their teaching and structures in line with the vision of gender justice, they can become instruments for the

---

as Healing', in I.A. Phiri and S. Nadar (eds), *African Women, Religion and Health: Essays in Honor of Mercy Amba Ewudziwa Oduyoye* (Maryknoll, 2006), 250.

[61] Phiri, *A Theological Analysis of the Voices of Teenage Girls*, 45.

[62] For example, see the various essays collected in I.A. Phiri and S. Nadar (eds), *On Being Church: African Women's Voices and Visions* (Geneva, 2005).

[63] Oduyoye, *Daughters of Anowa*, 172.

[64] Magesa, *The Challenge of African Woman Defined Theology*, 93.

transformation of gender relations in society. As Oduyoye says: 'Women hope for a transformed Church, because in Africa, the Church remains an institution with a potential for contributing to bringing in the new life that women struggle for.'[65] African women theologians develop an ecclesiology in which the pursuit of gender justice is a central part of the church's mission.[66] The church's mission of gender justice is mainly understood as something in relation to women. Women have to be fully included in the structures of the church; the church has to respect women's full dignity and to promote equality in marriage and so on. However, recently the scope of work towards gender justice has been widened: it includes not only the liberation of women, but also the transformation of men and masculinities. This development is a direct result of the HIV epidemic.

HIV and AIDS and the Need for Gender Justice

Since their appearance in the mid 1980s HIV and AIDS have had a major impact on communities and societies in Africa. Initially, African theologians, with a few exceptions, kept silent on HIV and AIDS. Only with the turn of the new millennium did it become a trend to reflect on issues related to the epidemic.[67] This change is marked, for example, by the statement of Tinyiko Maluleke that the HIV epidemic is the new *kairos* to the church and theology in Africa.[68] However, although quite a number of African theologians, particularly women theologians, are addressing issues of HIV and AIDS in their work, Ezra Chitando still observes 'a worrying lull' in the response to the epidemic in African theology at large.[69] His conclusion is that 'African theology prides itself as a contextual theology, [but] its inability to tackle the HIV epidemic signals that this is more a claim than a fact'.[70]

The reticence in African theology to respond to the epidemic has been explained by the link between HIV and sexuality, specifically the association of HIV with 'promiscuous' sexual behaviours. As Fulata Moyo points out, when European missionary Christianity came to Africa it did not deal with issues of sexuality, and

---

[65] Oduyoye, *Introducing African Women's Theology*, 116.

[66] Cf. S. Nadar, 'Towards a Feminist Missiological Agenda: A Case Study on the Jacob Zuma Rape Trial', *Missionalia*, 37/1 (2009): 85–102; Phiri, *Life in Fullness*, 73–81.

[67] See M.T. Frederiks, 'HIV and Aids: Mapping Theological Responses in Africa', *Exchange*, 37/1 (2008): 4–23 and A.S. van Klinken, 'The Ongoing Challenge of HIV and AIDS to African Theology: A Review Article', *Exchange*, 40/1 (2011): 89–107.

[68] T.S. Maluleke, 'The Challenge of HIV/AIDS for Theological Education in Africa. Towards an HIV/AIDS Sensitive Curriculum', *Missionalia*, 29/2 (2001): 130. The word 'kairos' is an allusion to the renowned Kairos Document (1985) that addressed Apartheid in South Africa. Maluleke thus suggests that HIV/AIDS is as urgent for the contemporary African theological agenda as Apartheid was in the 1980s.

[69] See Chitando, *Troubled but not Destroyed*, 6.

[70] Ibid., 63.

hence sexuality has been a taboo issue in African churches and among African theologians.[71] Because of this taboo, Moyo argues, sexuality is hardly discussed, and if so, only in a negative and moralising way. Thus, when the HIV epidemic emerged in the 1980s and 1990s, the popular belief among many Christians and church leaders was that AIDS was a punishment from God for one's immoral sexual behaviour. This theological perception, and the resulting stigmatisation of people living with HIV and AIDS, in churches and communities has been critically addressed by some African theologians.[72] They challenge churches to respond to the epidemic constructively, and they provide churches with theologies of compassion and solidarity.[73]

The perception of HIV as a divine punishment for sexual sin is explained by Gerald West on the basis of the 'theology of retribution' that, in his opinion, prevails in Christianity and African traditional religions.[74] In African theological responses to the epidemic, this paradigm is increasingly criticised and is replaced by a different perspective. A so-called HIV liberation theology has evolved. Maluleke was one of the first to suggest that an African liberation theology nowadays should engage with HIV and AIDS.[75] His call was based on the link he observed between poverty levels and the impact and spread of HIV in Africa. From then on, several other African theologians have engaged in the paradigm of liberation theology to address the HIV epidemic. Pointing to poverty and global economic exploitation, migration labour, unequal access to health care and unequal distribution of medicine, gender inequality, and so on, it is argued that HIV 'is a social injustice driven epidemic'[76] embedded in 'structural sins'.[77] Different from popular Christian understandings of HIV and AIDS, the primary concern of these theologians is not with individual morality but with structural injustice. Musa Dube articulates the implications of this paradigm for the church and theology in view of the epidemic as follows:

> Clearly, the challenge confronting the church and its mission in the HIV/ AIDS and globalization era is the need to address structural sins with an equal commitment with which individual sin is addressed. Members of society/church

---

[71] F.L. Moyo, 'The AIDS Crisis: A Challenge to the Integrity of the Church in Malawi', in K.R. Ross (ed.), *Faith at the Frontiers of Knowledge* (Blantyre, 1998), 100–104.

[72] Cf. E. Chitando and M.R. Gunda, 'HIV and AIDS, Stigma and Liberation', *Exchange*, 36/2 (2007): 184–97; I.A. Phiri, 'HIV/AIDS: An African Theological Response in Mission', *The Ecumenical Review*, 56/4 (2004): 422–31.

[73] Cf. M.W. Dube, *The HIV & AIDS Bible: Selected Essays* (Scranton, 2008); B. Bujo and M. Czerny (eds), *AIDS in Africa: Theological Reflections* (Nairobi, 2007).

[74] G. West and B. Zengele, 'Reading Job "Positively" in the Context of HIV/AIDS in South Africa', *Concilium*, 4 (2004): 114.

[75] Maluleke, *The Challenge of HIV/AIDS for Theological Education in Africa*, 134.

[76] Dube, *The HIV & AIDS Bible*, 47–53.

[77] Phiri, *HIV/AIDS: An African Theological Response in Mission*, 428.

may very well know and believe in the values of abstinence and faithfulness, but social injustice does not always allow them to live by these values. Theological strategies of confronting structural sin are therefore vital, for HIV/AIDS is not just about individual lack of morality, but also an individual's lack of social justice in their lives.[78]

Dube herself is a major representative of an African HIV liberation theology. Under the name of 'prophecy' she has proposed a theological strategy of confronting the unjust structures that underlie the HIV epidemic.[79] In her opinion, the method of prophecy is informed by 'the divine imperative to respond to the violation of life, as a violation of God's creation, God's image, God's dignity – God's body'.[80] This quotation indicates that the emerging liberation theology of HIV is fundamentally rooted in the understanding of God. Rather than a God who punishes people for (sexual or other) sin, this theology believes in a God siding with the oppressed and marginalised, meaning that nowadays 'God is on the side of those affected and infected with HIV/AIDS'.[81] Hence, the theologians call upon churches to show solidarity, to promote life and justice, and to transform relationships and structures at a global, communal and individual level.

African Women Theologians on HIV&AIDS and Gender

A substantial, if not the major, part of the theological response to the HIV epidemic in Africa is provided by African women theologians. From the early 2000s the Circle has made HIV and AIDS its top priority issue. As Phiri explains, 'African women theologians have felt the need to use their communal power to challenge the HIV/AIDS pandemic from the perspectives of religion, culture and social practice in order to save life.'[82] Indeed the Circle has mobilised the communal power of its members, resulting in a significant body of literature being published on issues related to HIV and AIDS.

In their response to the epidemic, African women theologians by and large engage in the paradigm of an HIV liberation theology. The option for this paradigm is understandable from the background of African women's theology as part of the tradition of liberation theologies. However, there is also a more specific reason.

---

[78] M.W. Dube, 'Theological Challenges: Proclaiming the Fullness of Life in the HIV/AIDS & Global Economic Era', *International Review of Mission*, 91/363 (2002): 542.

[79] M.W. Dube, 'The Prophetic Method in the New Testament', in M.W. Dube (ed.), *HIV/AIDS and the Curriculum: Methods of Integrating HIV/AIDS in Theological Programmes* (Geneva, 2003), 43–58.

[80] Dube, *The HIV & AIDS Bible*, 13.

[81] Phiri, *HIV/AIDS: An African Theological Response in Mission*, 430.

[82] I.A. Phiri, 'African Women of Faith Speak Out in an HIV/AIDS Era', in I.A. Phiri, B. Haddad and M. Masenya (eds), *African Women, HIV/AIDS and Faith Communities* (Pietermaritzburg, 2003), 8.

Responding to the challenges raised by the epidemic, the Circle has opted for a 'gender-based response'.[83] This was informed by the growing awareness that HIV is a gendered epidemic. As Njoroge formulates it, AIDS is 'a disease with a woman's face' and the epidemic shows the 'destructive nature of gender inequality and injustice'.[84] It is for this reason that the HIV epidemic has become a major challenge to African women theologians: their engagement with the issue is a way of being faithful to their original mission. Understanding HIV as embedded in social injustices, they pay particular attention to gender injustice as a major structure in society that facilitates the epidemic to thrive. As Dube puts it,

> In this HIV&AIDS era, however, gender inequalities are second only to poverty in being a major driving force behind the spread of HIV&AIDS. Many economically, culturally, politically, and religiously powerless women find that abstaining, being faithful, or having a condom or femidom [female condom] will not save them from HIV&AIDS infection.[85]

As this quotation indicates, the HIV epidemic has reinforced African women theologians' critical analysis of gender inequalities and their commitment to gender transformation. It is argued that the struggle for gender justice should be at the centre of the church's response to the HIV epidemic, because 'as long as there is gender injustice in Africa, HIV/AIDS will continue unabated'.[86]

When it comes to gender and HIV, the theologians are first and foremost concerned with women. This concern is threefold. First, it is said that socialisation, cultural practices, economic factors and prevalent religious beliefs enhance women's susceptibility to HIV infection.[87] Second, the concern is that women in particular suffer from the stigmatisation of people living with HIV, because HIV-related stigma is a gendered phenomenon.[88] Third, it is said that women

---

[83] Phiri, *African Women of Faith Speak Out in an HIV/AIDS Era*, 8–17.

[84] N.J. Njoroge, 'AIDS: The Disease that Speaks Multiple Languages and Thrives on Other Pandemics', *Journal of Constructive Theology*, 10/2 (2004): 4 and 8.

[85] Dube, *The HIV & AIDS Bible*, 50.

[86] Phiri, *Life in Fullness*, 79.

[87] Cf. N. Kamau, 'African Cultures and Gender in the Context of HIV and AIDS: Probing these Practices', in B. Haddad (ed.), *Religion and HIV and AIDS: Charting the Terrain* (Scottsville, 2011), 257–72; S. Chirongoma, 'Women, Poverty, and HIV in Zimbabwe: An Exploration of Inequalities in Health Care', in I.A. Phiri and S. Nadar (eds), *African Women, Religion, and Health: Essays in Honor of Mercy Amba Ewudziwa Oduyoye* (Maryknoll, 2006), 173–86; C.R.A. Shisanya, 'The Impact of HIV/AIDS on Women in Kenya', in M.N. Getui and M.M. Theuri (eds), *Quests for Abundant Life in Africa* (Nairobi, 2002), 48–54.

[88] C.R.A. Shisanya, 'Today's Lepers: Experiences of Women Living with HIV/AIDS in Kenya', in T.M. Hinga et al. (eds), *Women, Religion and HIV/AIDS in Africa: Responding to Ethical and Theological Challenges* (Pietermaritzburg, 2008), 144–66; P.N.

are disproportionately affected by some of the outcomes of the epidemic: they are burdened with the care of people who suffer from AIDS-related diseases, and they are faced with the economic/financial consequences, such as the costs of medicine and a loss of household income.[89] Thus, gender as it is constructed in African societies today, is believed to increase in several ways the impact of the epidemic on women's lives. Succinctly put, women are 'at the centre of the storm of the HIV/AIDS pandemic'.[90] This is explained by gender inequalities. Referring to the high HIV rates among women, Constance Shisanya argues that 'power imbalance between genders considerably explains why women are more vulnerable to HIV/AIDS than men to a large extent'.[91] Because sexual contact in heterosexual relations takes place within the gender relations between men and women, a gender imbalance directly impacts upon sexual relations and thus can be critical in view of the sexual transmission of HIV. This is precisely the major concern of the theologians. Having argued that gender relations are defined by power and powerlessness, Dube points out:

> This serious discrepancy in the distribution of power is our unmaking in the HIV/AIDS era. It is the fertile soil upon which the virus thrives. Women who have been constructed as powerless cannot insist on safer sex. They can hardly abstain, nor does faithfulness to their partners help.[92]

This quotation hints at the issue of sexual decision-making. It is believed that a woman – either as a wife in the marital relationship, or as a girl in relation to a boyfriend or 'sugar daddy', or as a sex worker in relation to a client – is hardly in the position to have control over her own body and sexuality and to protect herself from HIV. As Moyo puts it: 'Sexuality is about power for those who determine the what, when, where and how of sex, be it socio-economic and/or religio-cultural. In heterosexual relationships, those who have this power are men.'[93] That sexual and gender relations are a power game is particularly demonstrated in the phenomenon of violence against women and children. This is another issue the theologians are concerned about, and they point out that sexual violence increases women's

---

Mwaura, 'Stigmatization and Discrimination of HIV/AIDS Women in Kenya: A Violation of Human Rights and its Theological Implications', *Exchange*, 37/1 (2008): 35–51.

[89] E.g., M.W. Dube, 'Grant Me Justice: Towards Gender-Sensitive Multi-Sectoral HIV/AIDS Readings of the Bible', in M.W. Dube and M.R.A. Kanyoro (eds), *Grant Me Justice! HIV/AIDS & Gender Readings of the Bible* (Pietermaritzburg, 2004), 10–11; Shisanya, *The Impact of HIV/AIDS*, 55–8.

[90] Phiri, *African Women of Faith Speak Out in an HIV/AIDS Era*, 15.

[91] Shisanya, *The Impact of HIV/AIDS*, 61.

[92] Dube, *Culture, Gender and HIV/AIDS*, 88.

[93] F.L. Moyo, 'Religion, Spirituality and being a Woman in Africa: Gender Construction within the African Religio-Cultural Experiences', *Agenda*, 61 (2004): 73.

vulnerability to HIV.⁹⁴ Gender-based violence is considered 'a demonstration of who is in power' and as the ultimate result and worst manifestation of gender inequality.⁹⁵

Remarkably, while discussing issues of gender, sexuality and HIV, the theologians hardly pay attention to homosexuality or same-sex practices. It is simply not considered a relevant issue. According to Phiri, 'in Europe and America the spread of HIV is mainly through homosexual relationships, [but] in Africa it is predominantly through heterosexual multiple relationships'.⁹⁶ Similar statements can be found in many other publications, but are hardly substantiated. The silence of most African theologians on homosexuality in relation to HIV corresponds with the wider perception of HIV in Africa as being a heterosexual epidemic.⁹⁷ Because homosexuality and heterosexuality are often understood as exclusive categories, the possibility that same-sex practices may contribute even to the heterosexual transmission of the virus is generally ignored.⁹⁸ Additionally, African theologians may also have strategic considerations to keep silent about homosexuality in their response to the HIV epidemic: the issue is so controversial that it may complicate the fight against HIV and AIDS-related stigma.⁹⁹ Chitando touches cautiously on the issue when he states that the epidemic provides churches in Africa with an opportunity to discuss sexuality in an 'open and liberating way',¹⁰⁰ mentioning in particular 'the need to interact with men who have sex with men'.¹⁰¹ However, he does not explore the issue. On the contrary, by saying that 'heterosexual transmission lies behind the rapid spread of HIV in Africa', the discussion is

---

[94] Cf. B. Haddad, 'Choosing to Remain Silent: Links between Gender Violence, HIV/AIDS and the South African Church', in I.A. Phiri, B. Haddad and M. Masenya (eds), *African Women, HIV/AIDS and Faith Communities* (Pietermaritzburg, 2003), 149–67; I.A. Phiri, 'Why does God Allow our Husbands to Hurt Us? Overcoming Violence against Women', *Journal of Theology for Southern Africa*, 114 (2002): 19–30.

[95] Phiri, *African Women of Faith Speak Out in an HIV/AIDS Era*, 14.

[96] Phiri, *HIV/AIDS: An African Theological Response in Mission*, 424.

[97] See M. Epprecht, *Heterosexual Africa? The History of an Idea from the Age of Exploration to the Age of AIDS* (Athens, 2008), 1–33.

[98] An exception is Kenyan woman theologian Constance Shisanya, who points out that the 'homosexual tendencies of some married men in Kenya equally make their wives to be vulnerable to HIV/AIDS' (Shisanya, *The Impact of HIV/AIDS*, 51). However, for Shisanya this is a reason to emphasise the norm of heterosexuality and to underline the 'prophetic role' of the church to condemn homosexuality (ibid., 62), which only reinforces the taboo.

[99] See A.S. van Klinken and M.R. Gunda, 'Taking Up the Cudgels against Gay Rights? Trends and Trajectories in African Christian Theologies on Homosexuality', *Journal of Homosexuality*, 59/1 (2012): 122–3.

[100] E. Chitando, *Living with Hope: African Churches and HIV/AIDS 1* (Geneva, 2007), 33.

[101] Ibid., 24. See also Chitando, *Acting in Hope: African Churches and HIV/AIDS 2* (Geneva, 2007), 50, 53 and 90.

limited to heterosexuality again.¹⁰² Recently, some women theologians such as Dube and Njoroge have tried to open up the debate. According to Njoroge, the reality of AIDS forces African theologians 'to make a U-turn in their teaching and theologizing', meaning that theologians have to discuss and reflect on topics they dared not study before, including homosexuality.¹⁰³ Dube makes homosexuality part of her HIV and AIDS liberation theology; she considers homophobia as one of the structures of injustice underlying the epidemic that need to be addressed.¹⁰⁴ Clearly, the silence on homosexuality in African theology has been broken, but the topic and its intersection with issues of gender and HIV are yet to be explored.¹⁰⁵

The Critical Role of Religion and Culture

Analysing women's observed lack of power in sexual and gender relations, and women's subsequent vulnerability to HIV, the theologians particularly address cultural and religious practices and teachings. These would maintain and reinforce the harmful realities women live in. According to Madipoane Masenya, African women are 'trapped between two canons' of African culture and Christianity, both of which put them at risk of HIV.¹⁰⁶ In relation to gender-related violence, Maluleke and Nadar speak about an 'unholy trinity' of religion, culture and gender socialisation that underwrites sexual and physical violence against women.¹⁰⁷

With regard to 'African culture', several cultural practices that expose women to HIV are identified.¹⁰⁸ Examples are the payment of dowry, female circumcision, polygamy, dry sex, widow cleansing and widow inheritance.¹⁰⁹ These practices

---

¹⁰² Chitando, *Living with Hope*, 33.

¹⁰³ N.J. Njoroge, 'Beyond Suffering and Lament: Theology of Hope and Life', in D.C. Marks (ed.), *Shaping a Global Theological Mind* (Aldershot, 2008), 119.

¹⁰⁴ Dube, *The HIV & AIDS Bible*, 5, 33, 47, 162, 173, 182; M.W. Dube, 'Service for/on Homosexuals', in M.W. Dube (ed.), *Africa Praying: A Handbook on HIV/AIDS Sensitive Sermon Guidelines and Liturgy* (Geneva, 2003), 209–14.

¹⁰⁵ For a more detailed discussion, see Van Klinken and Gunda, *Taking Up the Cudgels against Gay Rights?*, 128–32. See also the special issue on same-sex relationships of *Journal of Gender and Religion in Africa*, 17/2 (2011), edited by Sarojini Nadar and Isabel Phiri. This volume includes groundbreaking articles, but strangely enough they hardly relate same-sex sexuality to issues of HIV/AIDS.

¹⁰⁶ M. Masenya, 'Trapped between Two "Canons": African-South African Christian Women in the HIV/AIDS Era', in I.A. Phiri, B. Haddad and M. Masenya (eds), *African Women, HIV/AIDS and Faith Communities* (Pietermaritzburg, 2003), 113–27.

¹⁰⁷ Maluleke and Nadar, *Breaking the Covenant*, 14–15.

¹⁰⁸ 'African culture' is often referred to in a generalising way, as is critically observed in M.W. Dube, 'HIV and AIDS Research and Writing in the Circle of African Concerned African Women Theologians 2002–2006', in E. Chitando and N. Hadebe (eds), *Compassionate Circles: African Women Theologians Facing HIV* (Geneva, 2009), 184.

¹⁰⁹ E.g. C. Ambasa-Shisanya, 'Widowhood and HIV Transmission in Siaya District, Kenya', in E. Chitando and N. Hadebe (eds), *Compassionate Circles: African Women*

are considered as illustrations of African cultures being harmful to women; they demonstrate that women cannot take control over their sexuality or their bodies, as this control is assigned to men. Therefore, according to Dube, problematic cultural practices should not be understood as isolated cases but as symptoms of the patriarchal system in African cultures.[110]

The control and domination of men over women and women's sexuality is linked by several theologians to the concept of male headship, which is central to prevailing cultural and Christian perceptions of marriage. In view of HIV, the criticism of this concept is threefold. First, headship is said to be a major symbol empowering men and disempowering women when it comes to sexual decision-making. As Masenya points out:

> The view that the headship of men is viewed as God-ordained assigns all authority and power to control to men. This includes the control of women's bodies. The understanding that a wife must be subject to her husband in everything would thus also be understood to entail that she must always be willing to avail her body for her husband's sexual gratification.[111]

In addition to this criticism, Moyo adds a second issue. According to her assessment, the concept of headship and other teachings, taught to girls during traditional and Christianised initiation rites, not only subordinate women's sexuality to that of men, but also insist upon women to always respect and protect the dignity of the husband. She denounces 'the immense concern to protect the dignity of the head of the families' even in cases of abuse and violence, which 'does not take into account the whole question of the woman's dignity'.[112] Third, Hinga indicates that the notion of male headship functions as a justification of domestic violence against women and may keep a woman locked up in a marriage with a husband who is sleeping around or abuses her.[113] Against this background the theologians

---

Theologians Facing HIV (Geneva, 2009), 53–70; F.L. Moyo, 'The Making of Vulnerable, Gyrating and Dangerous Menstruating Women through *Chinamwali* Socialization', in E. Chitando and N. Hadebe (eds), *Compassionate Circles: African Women Theologians Facing HIV* (Geneva, 2009), 35–52; H. Ayanga, 'Religio-cultural Challenges in Women's Fight against HIV/AIDS in Africa', in T.M. Hinga et al. (eds), *Women, Religion and HIV/AIDS in Africa: Responding to Ethical and Theological Challenges* (Pietermaritzburg, 2008), 34–48.

[110] M.W. Dube, 'In the Circle of Life: African Women Theologians' Engagement with HIV and AIDS', in E. Chitando and N. Hadebe (eds), *Compassionate Circles: African Women Theologians Facing HIV* (Geneva, 2009), 215.

[111] Masenya, 'Trapped between Two "Canons"', 119.

[112] Moyo, *Sex, Gender, Power and HIV/AIDS in Malawi*, 133.

[113] T.M. Hinga, 'AIDS, Religion and Women in Africa: Theo-Ethical Challenges and Imperatives', in T.M. Hinga and others (eds), *Women, Religion and HIV/AIDS in Africa: Responding to Ethical and Theological Challenges* (Pietermaritzburg, 2008), 91–2.

call for a revision of theologies of marriage and gender, because 'if nothing is done to change the status of married women, the HIV/AIDS pandemic will go on wiping out communities'.[114]

Regarding the critical role of religion in gender and HIV, another issue addressed is the role of religious institutions, in particular Christian churches and church leaders. Apart from the more general critique of churches adhering to patriarchal ideology, several specific aspects are mentioned. It is argued that churches, rather than liberating women from harmful cultural practices, accept or at least tolerate these practices such as dowry, virginity testing, widow inheritance, and so on. According to Moyo, though some churches have Christianised traditional initiation rites for girls, they have not made use of this opportunity to empower women in the area of sexual decision-making. The same is true, she says, for many pastors, who in their premarital and marital counselling teach women to subordinate their sexuality to that of men. Hence, Moyo concludes that 'the Church inadvertently reinforces women's vulnerability to HIV/AIDS'.[115] This view is supported by Maluleke and Nadar, who found pastors justifying gender-based violence and insisting that women stay in abusive relationships.[116] Furthermore, Moyo has revealed that some churches are deeply implicated in practices that violate women's bodies, for example by demanding that women show 'hospitality' to their pastors.[117] These and other issues are taken as an illustration that African churches generally continue to be insensitive to gender issues and remain 'the bastion of patriarchy', and thus are indifferent to the widespread argument that gender inequality is a major factor driving the epidemic.[118]

As appears from the account above, a wide range of issues concerning culture and religion are addressed by theologians working on gender and HIV. Whatever particular issue is addressed, almost all publications finally point to patriarchy as the root problem. As a cultural and religious ideology and a deeply rooted social structure, patriarchy is said to give rise to various practices and beliefs that facilitate the spread and impact of HIV and that increase the vulnerability of women. Hence the general perception among the theologians is that HIV cannot be dealt with without dealing with patriarchy. As Njoroge states,

> Reductionist ways of understanding gender inequality demonstrate either naivety or a deep-seated ignorance of the oppressive and dehumanising nature of patriarchy and sexism in our families, societies and religious communities. It is of great importance that when we engage in gender discourse in theology,

---

[114] Phiri, *African Women of Faith Speak Out in an HIV/AIDS Era*, 10.

[115] Moyo, *Sex, Gender, Power and HIV/AIDS in Malawi*, 131.

[116] Maluleke and Nadar, *Breaking the Covenant*, 9, 11, 14.

[117] F.L. Moyo, '"When the Telling itself is a Taboo": The Phoebe Practice', in I.A. Phiri and S. Nadar (eds), *On Being Church: African Women's Voices and Visions* (Geneva, 2005), 184–202.

[118] Chitando, *Living with Hope*, 26.

in the search for recognition, reconciliation, healing, justice and fullness of life, that we confront the fundamental problems of patriarchy and sexism in the face of the pandemic.[119]

Whatever is meant by 'reductionist' understandings of gender inequality, it is clear that Njoroge, like her colleagues in the Circle and sympathising male theologians such as Chitando and Maluleke, radically opposes all forms of gender inequality. They principally consider gender inequality an injustice, and therefore aim at a deconstruction of patriarchy and embark on the transformation of gender relations towards gender justice.

The Imperative of Transformation

For gender-critical African theologians, the HIV epidemic has clearly shown that patriarchy is a dangerous and life-threatening ideology, especially to women but, consequently, also to men. Out of this realisation they have insisted even more on the need to transform gender relations. As mentioned above, the understanding of gender as a social construct opens up the possibility of change. Elaborating on this notion, Musa Dube states:

> Any theologian, lecturer, leader or worker who lives in the human-rights era – who believes in democracy, and wants to contribute positively to the fight against HIV/AIDS which is turning our dark-peopled continent into a red fire-inflamed continent of death – must not only seek to understand fully how gender is socially and culturally constructed, how it disempowers half of humanity, how it fuels the spread of HIV/AIDS, but also [seek] to change gender constructions so that they empower men and women. It is up to the society to be instrumental to change and transformation. The present set-up benefits no one – men or women.[120]

Central to this call for change of gender constructions is the concept of empowerment. Gender is to empower men *and* women, Dube says, and she considers this particularly crucial in the context of HIV. Hence, African women theologians underline the need for women's sexual empowerment. They not only consider it an intervention and prevention strategy in the face of HIV, but also a way for women to regain their dignity. The most elaborate account in this area is provided by Moyo, who creatively employs cultural, biblical and theological resources in order to develop an empowering 'barefoot women's theology of sexuality'.[121] Though Moyo's primary quest is for sexual empowerment, she

---

[119] N.J. Njoroge, *Gender Justice, Ministry and Healing: A Christian Response to the HIV Pandemic* (London, 2009), 3.

[120] Dube, *Culture, Gender and HIV/AIDS*, 95.

[121] Moyo, *A Quest for Women's Sexual Empowerment*, see esp. chapter 7.

insists upon a wider change of gender relations, especially in marriage. She presents the notions of mutuality and companionship as qualifications of marital-sexual relationships, building these notions upon the anthropological concept of the equality of men and women as co-bearers of the image of God. According to Moyo, the empowerment of women along these lines will 'help women to realize that they are not sexual objects at the mercy of men's sexual prowess, but that they are companions and partners in this sexual act which is a holy and pleasant gift from God' and will 'enhance mutual love, and thus contribute to the mutuality of sexual fulfilment, faithfulness and healing in heterosexual relationships, culminating in HIV/AIDS prevention'.[122]

The empowerment of women and the transformation of gender relations are considered key to the church's mission in times of HIV and AIDS. In the words of Chitando, challenging patriarchy and building communities of gender justice are major characteristics of 'AIDS-competent churches'.[123] This is remarkable because churches, as mentioned above, are strongly criticised for maintaining and reinforcing gender inequalities that expose women to HIV. For gender-critical African theologians, Dube explains, the church is a 'beloved problem child' which is both critically spoken to and of which much is demanded.[124]

In the context of the HIV epidemic, the quest for gender justice and the call upon churches to align with this vision and to engage in a transformation of gender relations have been further specified. More explicit than before, gender transformation now aims to realise an equal share of power between women and men in order to guarantee autonomy and mutuality in sexual and wider gender relations. Against this background of what has been called 'HIV+ feminism',[125] the topic of masculinities has become an emerging issue.

The Quest for Liberating and Redemptive Masculinities

It is a very recent development that men are more explicitly addressed and that the concept of masculinities has appeared in debates about gender in African theology. This is a direct result of the above-outlined gender-based response to the HIV epidemic under the leadership of African women theologians. In 2007, the Circle of Concerned African Women Theologians, for the very first time, invited male theologians to its Pan-African conference in Yaoundé, Cameroon. The general theme was gender and HIV, but the conference had a particular focus on masculinities. As Phiri explains, this focus was informed by 'the realization

---

[122] Moyo, *Sex, Gender, Power and HIV/AIDS in Malawi*, 135.
[123] Chitando, *Acting in Hope*, 8.
[124] Dube, *HIV and AIDS Research and Writing in the Circle*, 190.
[125] M.W. Dube, 'HIV+ Feminisms, Postcoloniality and the Global AIDS Crisis', in D.N. Hopkins and M. Lewis (eds), *Another World is Possible: Spiritualities and Religions of Global Darker People* (London, 2009), 157.

that women alone cannot stop the spread of HIV in Africa'.[126] Hence, the quest of the conference was for 'liberating masculinities' that are helpful to combat HIV.[127] This conference was a milestone, both for the collaboration of African men and women theologians on issues of gender, and for the introduction of the theme of masculinities into African theological debates. According to Chitando, it is a major challenge to the various strands of African theology 'to take the theme of reconstructing and liberating masculinities seriously in the time of HIV'.[128] Clearly, Chitando himself has set the trend in the emerging field of studies on religion, masculinities and HIV in African theology, with other scholars engaging in the field more or less actively. What, then, are the critical issues that are addressed concerning men and masculinities, what alternative type of masculinity is envisioned and what are the instruments to bring about a transformation of masculinities?

Contesting HIV-critical African Masculinities

The concern of African theologians with hegemonic forms of masculinity is informed by their gender-critical analysis of the structures underlying the HIV epidemic and by their trenchant critique of patriarchy. Additionally, it is informed by the concern about gender-based violence, which seems to be a major issue especially in South Africa.[129] Against this background, masculinities are referred to by adjectives such as 'aggressive',[130] 'destructive',[131] 'dangerous and deadly',[132] and men are said to be characterised by a 'machismo of sexual aggressiveness'.[133] Though the plural of masculinities is used more and more in order to prevent essentialism and to account for the different ways men perform their manhood,[134] it is believed that these adjectives generally apply to popular forms of masculinity

---

[126] Phiri, *Major Challenges for African Women Theologians*, 107.

[127] Ibid., 116.

[128] Chitando, *Troubled but not Destroyed*, 89.

[129] E.g., G. West, 'The Contribution of Tamar's Story to the Construction of Alternative African Masculinities', in S.T. Kamionkowski and W. Kim (eds), *Bodies, Embodiment and Theology of the Hebrew Bible* (New York, 2010), 184–200; S. Nadar, 'Palatable Patriarchy and Violence against Wo/men in South Africa – Angus Buchan's Mighty Men's Conference as a Case Study on Masculinism', *Scriptura*, 102/3 (2009): 551–61.

[130] Chitando, *Living with Hope*, 31.

[131] E. Chitando and S. Chirongoma, 'Challenging Masculinities: Religious Studies, Men and HIV in Africa', *Journal of Constructive Theology*, 14/1 (2008): 65.

[132] R. Gabaitse, 'Searching for Contextual Relevance: The Department of Theology and Religious Studies, University of Botswana's Response to HIV and AIDS', in E. Chitando (ed.), *Mainstreaming HIV and AIDS in Theological Education: Experiences and Explorations* (Geneva, 2008), 43.

[133] Moyo, *Sex, Gender, Power and HIV/AIDS in Malawi*, 131.

[134] Chitando and Chirongoma, *Challenging Masculinities*, 56–8.

in African societies today. There are several reasons why these masculinities are considered to be dangerous, destructive and even deadly in the context of the HIV epidemic.

First, the issue that is addressed most often concerns male sexuality, which is not surprising in view of HIV being a sexually transmitted disease. As already mentioned above, the theologians perceive sexuality as being embedded in the wider and unequal gender relations between men and women. According to Moyo, 'sexuality is a power issue at the mercy of those who have the decision-making power – in this case, men'.[135] This is critical, in particular when men misuse their power. The concern is that men use sexuality to demonstrate their manhood. For example, men are said to engage in unprotected sex in order 'to prove to their friends that they are real men, and real men take risks'.[136] Chitando points to widespread cultural notions of men as 'sexual predators' that make men preoccupied with virility: they consider themselves as having 'uncontrollable sexual urges' and therefore easily engage in multiple sexual relationships.[137] Kä Mana explains this from the background of patriarchy: in traditional African patriarchal and polygamous cultures masculinity is defined in terms of power, potency and fertility.[138] This is the reason, he says, why HIV-prevention messages focusing on abstinence, fidelity and/or condom use are hardly effective: these prevention methods are experienced by men as a demasculinisation, castration and loss of erotic power. It is this socio-cultural and religious construct of male sexuality, sometimes captured in the concept of machismo,[139] which is considered particularly dangerous and indeed potentially deadly in the context of HIV.

Inherent to machismo is also a sense of aggressiveness. Indeed, another major concern about prevalent masculinities regards the violent behaviour of men in domestic settings and sexual relations. For the theologians, domestic and sexual violence is a direct consequence of patriarchy, as patriarchy puts men on top of the gender order and gives men power that can easily be abused. Rosinah Gabaitse, for example, explains 'passion killing', where women are killed by former lovers, as 'a consequence of a destructive system', that being patriarchy, and as a 'result of the patriarchal construction of masculinity, where men are given enormous power,

---

[135] Moyo, *Sex, Gender, Power and HIV/AIDS in Malawi*, 130.

[136] Gabaitse, *Searching for Contextual Relevance*, 42.

[137] E. Chitando, 'Religious Ethics, HIV and AIDS and Masculinities in Southern Africa', in R. Nicolson (ed.), *Persons in Community: African Ethics in a Global Culture* (Scottsville, 2008), 52–3.

[138] Kä Mana, 'Culture, Societé et Sciences Humaines Dans la Lutte Contre le VIH-SIDA en Afrique', in Kä Mana, J.-B. Kenmogne and H. Yinda (eds), *Religion, Culture et VIH-SIDA en Afrique: un Hommage au Docteur Jaap Breetvelt* (Yaoundé, 2004), 67–72.

[139] Though originating from Latin America, the term 'machismo' is used by some theologians to capture the construct of male sexuality in African contexts (cf. Chitando and Chirongoma, *Challenging Masculinities*, 58; Moyo, *Sex, Gender, Power and HIV/AIDS in Malawi*, 131).

sense of entitlement and privilege over women by their political and socio-cultural systems'.[140] Likewise, Nadar in her analysis of sexual violence in South Africa, points out that patriarchy provides an ideological framework 'which tells men that it is okay to rape because society does not really see it as rape'.[141] In addition to discussion around passion killings and rape, reference is made to the many other subtle and overt forms of violence of men against women and children through which men maintain and reaffirm their position in the patriarchal order.[142] For the theologians, all this illustrates the dangerous and destructive side of hegemonic versions of masculinity.

Apart from the major issues of sexuality and violence, some other critical issues with regard to masculinities are mentioned but are less elaborated upon. Chitando and Chirongoma address the lack of men's leadership in the face of HIV. They critically observe that, though patriarchy puts men in the position of leaders at family, community and national level, men generally are absent in the response to HIV and AIDS, when it comes to prevention, care and support programmes.[143] One explanation given is that patriarchal masculinities do not allow men to engage in care, but rather demand that men are cared for by women. Furthermore, Chitando relates dominant masculinities to the stigmatisation of women living with HIV.[144] What is noteworthy here is that the various problematic aspects of popular masculinities are all related to and explained from the root problem of patriarchy. This is important, as it points to the level of analysis. Though the behaviour of individual men is taken into account and is critically addressed, this behaviour is explained from deeply rooted structures and ideologies of gender and the subsequent masculinities. This structural approach, as will be explored below, has direct implications for the political project of a transformation of masculinities. This project does not just focus on the behavioural change of individual men, but also on deconstructing the patriarchal basis of masculinities and on promoting 'liberative' and 'redemptive' types of masculinity. As Maluleke puts it, 'the myriad challenges brought about by the HIV pandemic cannot be dealt with without dealing with patriarchy and masculinity issues'.[145]

---

[140] R. Gabaitse, 'Passion Killings in Botswana: Masculinity at Crossroads', in E. Chitando and S. Chirongoma (eds), *Redemptive Masculinities: Men, HIV and Religion* (Geneva, 2012), 307.

[141] Nadar, *Towards a Feminist Missiological Agenda*, 97. See also K. Owino, '"Maleness" and its Possible Influence on Abuse and Domestic Violence in South Africa: A Critique of Some Expressions of Evangelical Theology', *Journal of Constructive Theology*, 16:2 (2010), 146–68.

[142] Chitando and Chirongoma, *Challenging Masculinities*, 61.

[143] Ibid., 63–4.

[144] Chitando, *Religious Ethics, HIV and AIDS and Masculinities in Southern Africa*, 54–5.

[145] Maluleke, *An African Theology Perspective on Patriarchy*, 34.

Envisioning Alternative Masculinities

The critical examination of popular masculinities and their impact in the context of HIV leads the African theologians into a quest to transform masculinities. Theoretically, this is possible because of the social constructionist understanding of gender, which, as mentioned above, opens up the possibility of change and reconstruction. Chitando and Chirongoma explicitly locate their call to transform masculinities within this theoretical perspective:

> Having accepted the value of the concept of masculinities, it becomes possible to embrace the idea that men can be transformed. There is no single fixed identity for men. Men can, do, and must change, as experience indicates. ... It has become clear that the social construction of manhood needs to be interrogated. Too often, men have imbibed cultural values that threaten the well-being of women and children. ... There is therefore need to work with men to enable them to appreciate that they can express themselves in ways that are not harmful to women, children and themselves. This has become particularly urgent in the context of the HIV epidemic.[146]

Though the urgency to work with men and change masculinities might be clear, the question arises as to the direction of this transformation. 'What transformed definitions of masculinity do we need to develop?' Fulata Moyo wonders.[147] Elaborate answers to this recent question have not yet been provided, but the few theological publications on the subject certainly give an indication. In these publications, theologians follow different strategies to develop a vision of transformative masculinities. For example, Lovemore Togarasei investigates Pauline masculinity in the New Testament, in the hope that a 'biblically centred masculinity' will be attractive to African Christian men and will be effective in the response to HIV and AIDS.[148] Where Togarasei looks to the Bible, Julius Gathogo revitalises traditional perceptions of manhood in Kikuyu culture to develop a vision for masculinity today.[149] In spite of the different resources that are employed, the contours of the ideal of masculinity that is envisioned largely correspond. This vision is in line with the wider theological vision for gender relations that has been outlined above. Masculinities are intended to move from patriarchy to gender justice. In the words of Chitando, 'Men must be challenged to

---

[146] Chitando and Chirongoma, *Challenging Masculinities*, 57–8.

[147] Moyo, *Sex, Gender, Power and HIV/AIDS in Malawi*, 131.

[148] L. Togarasei, 'Paul and Masculinity: Implications for HIV and AIDS Responses among African Christians', in E. Chitando and S. Chirongoma (eds), *Redemptive Masculinities: Men, HIV and Religion* (Geneva, 2012), 245.

[149] J.M. Gathogo, 'Chasing a Leopard Out of the Homestead: Mundurume's Task in the Era of HIV and AIDS', in E. Chitando and S. Chirongoma (eds), *Redemptive Masculinities: Men, HIV and Religion* (Geneva, 2012), 447–70.

give up their privileges in pursuit of gender justice. This will provide a formidable line of defence against HIV.'[150] Masculinities that meet the criterion of gender justice are believed to be liberating and redemptive.

Liberating masculinities 'Liberating' is one of the adjectives that appear in the theological discourse as a qualification of the new type of masculinity that is envisioned. The term 'liberating masculinities' was used, for example, during the 2007 Circle conference.[151] It appears that 'liberation' here actually has two subjects: it concerns women as well as men, both of whom need to be liberated from patriarchy in order to foster the humanity of all. Chitando understands this two-sided impact of 'liberation' in the line of liberation theology and its key insight that 'the oppressor is also a victim of his/her oppression'.[152] On the one hand, the new type of masculinity is thought of as supporting the liberation of women in African churches, cultures and societies.[153] Though the word is not used, it is a kind of pro-feminist masculinity that, as Chitando and Chirongoma say, encourages men willingly to 'forgo the patriarchal dividend', 'to identify with women and children, and to work towards gender justice'.[154] On the other hand, the concept of liberating masculinities also points to the liberation of men.[155] The deconstruction of patriarchy and the eradication of gender inequalities are considered to be liberative for men, because these realities also limit men. For example, Dube states that in the end nobody benefits from patriarchy, especially not in the present HIV era, and that patriarchy is a threat to humanity in general.[156] The idea is that prevalent masculinities are based on 'falsehood and lies about manhood',[157] and men need to be liberated from this in order to realise their human potential. This line of thought is also expressed by Oduoye in the above-mentioned statement about the liberation of men: 'To educate men means to bring them to the realization that if all they have is their maleness, then they do not count for much. Herein lies the need for the liberation of men.'[158] It is believed that only when patriarchy is abandoned, and power is shared, can men live up to the full humanity they share with women.

---

[150] E. Chitando, 'A New Man for a New Era? Zimbabwean Pentecostalism, Masculinities and the HIV Epidemic', *Missionalia*, 35/3 (2007): 122.

[151] Phiri, *Major Challenges for African Women Theologians*, 107 and 116.

[152] Chitando, *Troubled but not Destroyed*, 93.

[153] Chitando, *Acting in Hope*, 47.

[154] Chitando and Chirongoma, *Challenging Masculinities*, 66.

[155] Chitando, *Troubled but not Destroyed*, 92.

[156] Dube, *The HIV & AIDS Bible*, 139–40.

[157] *The Girl Child, Women, Religion and HIV/AIDS in Africa: Gender Perspectives. Report of the 4th Pan African Conference of the Circle of Concerned African Women Theologians Yaoundé, Cameroun*, 2–8 September 2007, 7.

[158] Oduyoye, *Acting to Construct Africa*, 38.

Redemptive masculinities The second concept proposed is that of 'redemptive masculinities'. This term is used by Gerald West in his activist-academic project of doing contextual Bible study with men on issues related to masculinity. Rather than defining the meaning of redemptive masculinities, West, in a section entitled 'In search of redemptive masculinities', reads the Bible story about Tamar being raped by her brother Amnon, looks through the eyes of Tamar, and then says:

> Tamar summons forth, anticipates, hopes for, a man who understands "No," who understands what it means to be in relationship as a "brother," who is able to resist using force, who respects the socio-cultural traditions of his community, who is able to discern and desist from doing what is disgraceful, who considers the situation of the other, who considers the consequences of his actions for himself, who is willing to pause and examine other options, who is willing to listen to rational argument.[159]

Apparently, such a man as described here is considered as embodying a redemptive kind of masculinity. Where the emphasis in this quotation is on the ability to control the self and to think before acting, Chitando, in a reference to redemptive masculinities, associates it with men's concern about others, their affirmation of life and of the community.[160] The latter aspect is also emphasised by Dube, who presents the African traditional religious concept of *setho/ubuntu* as a criterion for masculinities, meaning that these masculinities are constantly questioned as to whether they enhance the community, the relationships with others.[161] Concretely this would mean, she suggests, that harmful behaviours are renounced and that men engage in care and become loving and compassionate. As Chitando says: 'Macho attitudes must be replaced with those that show sensitivity and solidarity.'[162] This would not only imply that men adopt safer sexual practices and no longer violate women and children, but also that they start to give care to people with HIV and help to overcome stigmatisation and discrimination.[163] In this way, masculinities are thought of as becoming redemptive to the community, especially to those community members who suffer the most under the pressure of hegemonic masculinities. Chitando and Chirongoma acknowledge the soteriological connotation of the notion of 'redemptive masculinities', though they want to avoid the image of the male saviour. They say that they embrace and employ the concept because of the 'spiritual dimension' it evokes and the related

---

[159] West, *The Contribution of Tamar's Story*, 194.
[160] Chitando, *Troubled but not Destroyed*, 98.
[161] M.W. Dube, 'Adinkra! Four Hearts Joined Together on Becoming Healer-Teachers of African Indigenous Religion/s in HIV & AIDS Prevention', in I.A. Phiri and S. Nadar (eds), *African Women, Religion, and Health: Essays in Honor of Mercy Amba Ewudziwa Oduyoye* (Maryknoll, 2006), 141, 151, 152.
[162] Chitando, *Acting in Hope*, 49.
[163] Cf. Chitando and Chirongoma, *Challenging Masculinities*, 56–61.

hope for masculinities 'that are life-giving in a world reeling from the effects of violence and the HIV and AIDS epidemic'.[164]

A constructive use of power   In line with the notion of redemptive masculinities is the call for a constructive use of men's power. As mentioned above, hegemonic masculinities are associated by the theologians with dominating and aggressive behaviours of men. They explain this by considering the way in which patriarchy attaches power disproportionately to men, and men's abuse of this power. The project of transforming gender relations and masculinities first and foremost insists upon a redistribution of power in order to realise equal gender relations and to overcome patriarchy. However, at the same time the meaning of power is redefined in order that men can use their power constructively, that is, to the benefit of their families and the community. For example, from a Bible study on 'the graveyard man' in Mark 5, Maluleke first points out how the power and strength of this man are symptoms of his sickness, and then comments that 'one of the fundamental challenges that lies before us is a thorough examination of the understanding and uses of power and strength in various areas of life. ... Are there more positive, more life and community affirming notions and practices of power?'[165] This question is even more urgent, as Chitando makes clear, because due to patriarchy men actually hold most positions of leadership at various levels in society, from the family up to the government. Therefore, 'men must re-define power and leadership so that they work towards the good of all'.[166]

The figure of Jesus is frequently presented as a model for men to look to in order to redefine their sense of power. Having raised the question of life- and community-affirming notions and practices of power, Maluleke points to Jesus as the one who gave us 'more than clues to such practices of power'[167] because he related to people 'in life-affirming rather than violent ways'.[168] In a similar way, Cheryl Dibeela says that Jesus demonstrates alternative types of power, those being the 'power to care, love and embrace those who are different'.[169] Hence

---

[164] E. Chitando and S. Chirongoma, 'Introduction', in E. Chitando and S. Chirongoma (eds), *Redemptive Masculinities: Men, HIV and Religion* (Geneva, 2012), 2.

[165] T.S. Maluleke, 'The Graveyardman, the "Escaped Convict" and the Girl-Child: A Mission of Awakening, an Awakening of Mission', *International Review of Mission*, 91/363 (2002): 552.

[166] Chitando and Chirongoma, *Challenging Masculinities*, 64.

[167] Maluleke, 'The Graveyardman', 552.

[168] T.S. Maluleke, 'Men and their Role in Community', in M.W. Dube (ed.), *Africa Praying: A Handbook on HIV/AIDS Sensitive Sermon Guidelines and Liturgy* (Geneva, 2003), 192.

[169] C. Dibeela, 'Men and the use of Power', in M.W. Dube (ed.), *Africa Praying: A Handbook on HIV/AIDS Sensitive Sermon Guidelines and Liturgy* (Geneva, 2003), 194. See also Chitando, *Religious Ethics, HIV and AIDS and Masculinities in Southern Africa*, 60.

she calls upon men in the current HIV era to use their power to love and care for their wives and children, and to protect them from HIV infection. Dube, from a re-reading of the Bible story about Jesus healing the daughter of Jairus (Mark 5), acknowledges that both Jairus and Jesus appear in this story as powerful men, but emphasises that they use their power to empower others who are vulnerable. She presents this as an example for men nowadays: 'I believe that this model highlights that the powerful men in our families, churches, academy and society, do have a role in building gender empowerment and in fighting against the forces of death that globalization and HIV/AIDS unleash against the girl-child of today.'[170]

The arguments for a constructive use of men's power are not to be understood as part of a restorative project such as the 'reinvention of African patriarchy'.[171] It will be clear by now that the theologians discussed in this chapter are very suspicious of the very idea of men's power. However, realising that many men actually hold positions of power, they insist upon men's responsibilities to apply this power in a constructive way.

Strategies to Transform Masculinities towards Gender Justice

With the need to transform masculinities and the broad direction of this transformation being clear, the remaining question is how this project is to be undertaken – how to get men involved in an alternative type of masculinity, one that is liberating, redemptive and constructive. It is acknowledged that this demands, in the words of Paul Leshota, a profound personal conversion (*metanoia*) of men.[172] But how can such a conversion be brought about?

Several suggestions have been made, though these are yet to be developed in more concrete strategies of transformation. First, an academic strategy in theology and religious studies has been proposed. Chitando has underscored the need for African theologies of inculturation, liberation and reconstruction to engage constructively with the quest for alternative masculinities in order to make true

---

[170] M.W. Dube, 'Talitha Cum! Calling the Girl-Child and Women to Life in the HIV/AIDS & Globalization Era', in M. Degiglio-Bellemare and G.M. Garcia (eds), *Talitha Cum! The Grace of Solidarity in a Globalized World* (Geneva, 2004), 88.

[171] See C. Isike and U.O. Uzodike, 'Modernizing without Westernizing: Reinventing African Patriarchies to Combat the HIV and AIDS Epidemic in Africa', *Journal of Constructive Theology*, 14/1 (2008): 3–20. Both authors are scholars in political studies. Though their article does not deal with religion or theology it was published in a special issue of *Journal of Constructive Theology* dealing with masculinities, HIV and AIDS. The reinvention of patriarchy they propose is defined by the terms 'modernizing without westernizing', meaning that they want to avoid western (pro-feminist) views that tend to depict patriarchy as something negative, and aim to recover the values of traditional, pre-colonial African patriarchy.

[172] P. Leshota, 'The Spell of Discrete Islands of Consciousness: My Journey with Masculinities in the Context of HIV and AIDS', in E. Chitando and S. Chirongoma (eds), *Redemptive Masculinities: Men, HIV and Religion* (Geneva, 2012), 165.

their claim to be contextually relevant.[173] Together with Chirongoma, he has also highlighted the role that could be played by academic departments of religious studies.[174] In their view, these are places where critical masculinities are to be deconstructed and where alternative masculinities could be formulated, drawing on notions derived from the different religions in Africa. Also, students can be trained to become gender activists, mobilising religious resources and communities in the quest for gender justice and transformed masculinities.

Second, Gerald West and others have proposed a community-based strategy to construct alternative masculinities through the use of contextual Bible study. This method has been used to address, among other things, issues of gender violence and HIV in communities. Recently the method has also been applied to involve men in the transformation of masculinities.[175] According to West, a Bible study such as on the story of Amnon raping Tamar produces a social space where dominant masculinities are disrupted and contradicted, and where alternative masculinities can be articulated, which may lead to social transformation.[176]

Third, an important strategy is to involve local churches in the transformation of masculinities. This is developed in particular by Chitando, but it is in line with the wider vision for a transformation of gender relations. Clearly, gender-critical African theologians are very critical of Christian churches for maintaining and reinforcing patriarchal ideology and practices. However, they seize the HIV epidemic as an opportunity to get churches committed to the vision of gender justice and to make this part of their mission. What is at issue here, in their opinion, is the reliability of churches. Beverley Haddad puts this poignantly, saying: 'The church can no longer assert to being the moral watchdog of society without challenging men to take responsibility for their sexual behaviour. ... One cannot theologise nor moralise while patriarchy continues unabated.'[177] Thus, addressing critical male behaviours in areas of sexuality and gender violence is considered a major task of churches. Even further, the ideology and structures informing these behaviours – i.e. patriarchy – need to be contested by churches and church leaders, according to Haddad and others. Chitando draws the argument more specifically to masculinities when he says:

---

[173] Chitando, *Troubled but not Destroyed*, 88–9, 125

[174] Chitando and Chirongoma, *Challenging Masculinities*, 55–69.

[175] See G.O. West and P. Zondi-Mabizela, 'The Bible Story that Became a Campaign: The Tamar Campaign in South Africa (and Beyond)', *Ministerial Formation*, July (2004): 5–13.

[176] West, *The Contribution of Tamar's Story*, 184–200. As the director of the Ujaama Centre for Biblical and Theological Community Development and Research (University of KwaZulu-Natal, South Africa), West has initiated the Tamar Campaign. In this campaign, the Bible story on the rape of Tamar (2 Samuel 13:1–22) is used to address issues of gender-based violence among women and young girls, and recently also among men.

[177] Haddad, *Choosing to Remain Silent*, 155.

> The HIV epidemic challenges African churches to rethink their mission towards men. Yes, many denominations do have active men's groups but how many members do they have? More crucially, are such groups promoting gender equality? Are they challenging conventional forms of masculinity? How can hegemonic masculinities be deconstructed among Christian youth and men? Such questions are critical as African churches strive towards AIDS competence.[178]

It is clear from this quotation that to address, challenge and transform masculinities are central tasks for churches that seek to be 'AIDS competent'. Chitando gives many concrete suggestions for how churches could engage in this task, for example through preaching in Sunday services, the curriculum of Sunday schools, and activities for the youths', women's and men's groups. Furthermore, he says that mission has to be reconceptualised because of HIV, and that churches therefore have to engage in a 'creative evangelism' of reaching out to men in the so-called worldly places. Thus, through a wide range of church activities, men are to be sensitised to the harmful aspects of prevalent masculinities, and are to be challenged to develop more constructive understandings of themselves as men. It is believed that when churches are fully committed to the vision of gender justice, and when all church departments are actively involved in the shaping of new ideals of manhood, not only masculinities but subsequently society as a whole will be transformed in a radical way.

Conclusion

The topic of men and masculinities has only recently emerged in African theological scholarship as a result of the concern with issues related to gender, HIV and AIDS. However, the discussion of this subject is deeply influenced by the tradition of African women's theology, which is characterised by a feminist theological commitment. Though the immediate reason for the current engagement with masculinities is the HIV epidemic, the fundamental concern is with patriarchy as an ideology and a social structure that is oppressive to women. Consequently, hegemonic forms of masculinity are problematised in terms of their patriarchal character, suggesting that patriarchal masculinities directly contribute to male irresponsibility, violence against women, the spread of HIV, etcetera. In line with the vision of gender justice that is central to African women's theology, the theologians call for a transformation towards redemptive and liberating masculinities – that is, masculinities that are non-patriarchal and promote equality, mutuality and partnership in gender relations.

With their critique of patriarchal forms of masculinity and their structural approach to a transformation of masculinities, the African theologians discussed in this chapter are in the tradition of gender-critical scholarship in theology and

---

[178] Chitando, *Acting in Hope*, 40–41.

religious studies. Feminist theologians all over the world have explained women's experiences of oppression from within the framework of patriarchy and have criticised its religious underpinnings and expressions.[179] As already mentioned in Chapter 1, the emerging study of men, masculinities and religion in Western academia is clearly pro-feminist, out of the conviction that

> Without a thorough and succinct investigation of masculinities and masculine experiences in all their complexity under patriarchy and a study of alternatives to patriarchy ... the effort of feminist/*mujerista*/womanist scholars of religion would remain only partially successful in bringing forth a sophisticated model of the construction of gender and in understanding its impact on religion.[180]

In the words of Garth Kasimu Baker-Fletcher, 'the historical project of patriarchy' is the 'central and fundamental problematic' that scholars of masculinities and religion should deal with.[181] More recently, Joseph Gelfer has firmly stated that there is 'an obvious and profound ethical impetus for resisting patriarchy' in the study of men, masculinities and religion – a study field whose theoretical and hermeneutical foundations he defines as 'explicitly feminist'.[182] The point I would like to make here is not that these authors, as well as the African theologians, conceptualise patriarchy in a rather monolithic way. I will come back to this in Chapter 6, pointing out that the monolithic concept of patriarchy hinders a detailed and nuanced analysis of religious discourse on masculinity that often is quite complex and ambiguous. At this place I want to attend briefly to another problem.

The theologians discussed in this chapter present themselves as *African* theologians and intend to develop *African* contextual theologies. Clearly, in their work they address issues that are relevant and important in local African contexts and their theological proposals are constructive in these contexts. In developing their theology, they also make use of resources from African cultural and religious traditions, if it serves their quest for social transformation. However, this does not conceal the fact that these African theologians are part of a global (pro)feminist academic discourse that is embedded in Western Enlightenment thought, with central values such as equality, freedom and autonomy. Carrie Pemberton in her study of the Circle has critically discussed the idea that 'the voiced elite' of African women theologians can develop a theology and do political advocacy for 'the

---

[179] R.R. Ruether, 'Patriarchy', in L.M. Russell and J.S. Clarkson (eds), *Feminist Dictionary of Feminist Theologies* (Louisville, 1996), 205–7.

[180] S.B. Boyd, 'Trajectories in Men's Studies in Religion: Theories, Methodologies, and Issues', *Journal of Men's Studies*, 7/2 (1999): 266.

[181] G.K. Baker-Fletcher, 'Critical Theory, Deconstruction and Liberation?', *Journal of Men's Studies*, 7/2 (1999): 277.

[182] J. Gelfer, *Numen, Old Men: Contemporary Masculine Spiritualities and the Problem of Patriarchy* (London, 2009), 11, 15.

mute majority' of grassroots African women.[183] This problem of representation is also relevant to the discussion about (the transformation of) masculinities. For example, in her analysis of teenage girls' contributions to an essay competition about men's role in the fight against HIV and AIDS, Isabel Phiri found that these girls considered the notion of male headship as a potentially constructive resource: 'They saw this headship as coming with responsibility to reduce the spread of HIV/AIDS. ... This position was viewed as positive because it can be connected to authority in stopping gender-based violence and the spread of HIV/AIDS.'[184] Phiri does not further reflect on the significance of this finding and the questions it raises. She may explain the girls' suggestion as an example of the internalisation of patriarchy.[185] However, such an explanation would indicate a superior position of the feminist theologian over the women she speaks for. I think that the girls' suggestion raises a crucial question for Phiri and her fellow theologians working on issues of gender and masculinities. If these girls – and perhaps many other women in Africa – consider male headship acceptable and even useful because it can help men to behave responsibly, on what basis then is this notion criticised and categorically rejected by African women theologians? Of course, it is because of the obvious patriarchal connotation of male headship that these scholars, out of their feminist commitments, reject the concept. However, this raises complex questions about African women theologians' relationship to, and representation of, grassroots African women who do not share their feminist commitment and do not necessarily experience patriarchal ideas as oppressive. For gender-critical scholars more generally, it raises the question of whether a notion such as male headship can be rejected before carefully analysing how it operates in specific religious discourses and in socio-cultural contexts. To be clear, I am not raising these questions to advocate male headship, but to underline the need for African gender-critical theologians – and for scholars in the critical study of men, masculinities and religion – to reflect on the role of normative theological and political ideals in the analysis of gender and masculinities in the sphere of religion.[186] The complex issues I briefly raise here will appear to be crucial in view of the case studies presented in the following chapters. Both case-study churches, as one can imagine, present a trajectory and theology to transform masculinities that clearly conflict with the vision of the theologians to transform masculinities from patriarchy towards gender justice.

---

[183] C. Pemberton, *Circle Thinking: African Women Theologians in Dialogue with the West* (Leiden, 2003), 166–8.

[184] Phiri, *A Theological Analysis of the Voices of Teenage Girls*, 38 and 40.

[185] Cf. Phiri, *Life in Fullness: Gender Justice*, 76.

[186] Exemplary of the type of reflection I have in mind here is the work of feminist anthropologist Saba Mahmood, *Politics of Piety: The Islamic Revival and the Feminist Subject* (Princeton, 2005).

Chapter 3

Shaping Responsible Family Men: Masculinities in a Catholic Parish

'Joachim is the model of every catholic husband and father. He was a model of love, faithfulness, obedience, devotion, diligence, goodness, openness of husband and wife to one another. He is still a model of catholic men.'[1] This quotation from the constitution of the St Joachim Catholic Men's Organization in Zambia presents St Joachim as a model of Catholic manhood and gives a clear insight in how an ideal Catholic manhood is envisioned. Conducting a case study in Regiment parish in Lusaka, I found a local group of Joachims, as the members of the organisation are known, modelling themselves after this religious ideal of masculinity represented by an ancient saint figure. The promotion of such an ideal in a contemporary Zambian setting, and the resulting imitative practice among Catholic men, is an interesting example of a 'transformation of masculinities' at a grassroots level in African Christianity. The present and the next chapter explore such transformations through case studies in local church communities in Zambia, beginning with Regiment parish. In addition to the promotion of St Joachim as a model of Catholic manhood, this Catholic parish works with men and addresses issues of masculinity in various ways, not at least out of a concern about the HIV epidemic.[2]

Regiment Parish

Regiment parish, located in the south-eastern part of Lusaka, covers a large area with mainly high-density compounds but also some low-density areas. This difference is reflected in the membership: a minority of the parishioners belong to urban Zambia's middle class, but the majority are in the lower class. The parish is organised into 27 geographical sections, so-called Small Christian Communities (SCCs). During the period in which this research was conducted, Fr Marc Nswanzurwimo was the priest in charge. He originates from Burundi and is a member of the Missionaries of Africa. In 2009 this missionary society handed over the pastoral responsibility to the diocese. The priest is assisted by the parish

---

[1] *Constitution of St Joachim Catholic Men's Organization* (Lusaka, 2001), 1.

[2] This chapter is partly based on interviews. All names of interviewees mentioned in the footnotes are fictive except when referring to members of church officials (the parish priest and a diocesan staff member) who were interviewed in their professional role.

pastoral council, the main administrative body. As a Catholic parish, Regiment is part of the Archdiocese of Lusaka. The different dioceses in the country are related through the Zambia Episcopal Conference, which is the governing body of the Catholic Church in Zambia (CC-Z). Finally, the Archdiocese of Lusaka is under the Catholic hierarchy in Rome. Though Rome is far away from Lusaka, Regiment parish is clearly part of a world church. Therefore this case study includes some documents from the higher echelons in the church as far as relevant for the understanding of certain beliefs and practices in the parish.

Central to parish life is Mass, which is celebrated daily. On Sundays there are three Masses (one in English and two in a vernacular language), attended by about 2,000 people. Once every two weeks people are supposed to meet on Sunday afternoon in their SCC, and the young people in their SCC's youth section. The SCCs are called 'the arteries of the church', which indicates that they are considered crucial for the life of the parish.[3] Several lay groups are active in the parish, including Aktio, Legio and Marriage Encounter, women's groups such as St Anne and Nazareth, and also a men's organisation named St Joachim. These groups are part of regional, national or global Catholic lay movements that aim to contribute to the life, spirituality and mission of the church.

In line with the policy of the Zambian Catholic bishops, who want the church to be 'a caring family' for those in need, Regiment parish is involved in community work.[4] For example, in the early 1990s, a home-based care programme was established as a response to the increasing numbers of people in the community infected with HIV. The programme is run by a group called Caring Women. There is also a group, Caring Youth, who assist in home-based care and organise workshops on HIV and AIDS for their fellow youths. Other examples of social involvement are the community school and the youth skill training centre established by the parish. It is believed that through education young people's chances of employment will increase, the cycle of poverty will be broken and the HIV epidemic can be slowed and one day stopped. This indicates an awareness of the social factors underlying the epidemic, such as poverty, unemployment and broken families. Regiment parish is a typical example of the African Catholic ecclesiology of the church as 'the Family of God'.[5] Here, the church is understood

---

[3] 'Let Your Light Shine', *Diamond Jubilee: Regiment Catholic Church 1939–1999* (Lusaka, 1999), 17.

[4] Catholic Bishops of Zambia, 'The Church as a Caring Family: A Pastoral Letter to all Catholics by the Bishops of Zambia on the 1997 Theme for the Synod Implementation' (21 March 1997), in J. Komakoma (ed.), *The Social Teaching of the Catholic Bishops and Other Christian Leaders in Zambia: Major Pastoral Letters and Statements 1953–2001* (Ndola, 2003), 353–67.

[5] This ecclesiology was adopted by the First African Synod (meeting of the African Catholic bishops in Rome) in 1994, and has also been embraced by the Zambian Episcopal Conference. See Catholic Bishops of Zambia, 'Called to be the Family of God: A Pastoral Letter from the Catholic Bishops of Zambia to Launch the Five Year African Synod

in an open and inclusive way, standing in the middle of the community, being in solidarity with the weak and the poor, and promoting justice in society. As it was stated in a sermon, 'there are no boundaries; there is no fence; because the church is open to anybody who is in need; they are part of our community and we will share with them'.[6] Clearly, this has resulted in the church responding actively to HIV and AIDS and other social challenges.

Where are Men and Masculinities Addressed?

At various places and in different ways men and issues related to masculinity are discussed in Regiment parish. It is not that the parish has an explicit policy to actively embark on a transformation of masculinities. Rather, there is a concern about men, and hence some efforts are made to effect change in men's behaviour and to promote alternative understandings of manhood. What, then, are the places where, and the means by which, these efforts are made?

Youth Activities

The parish has an active youth programme in which over a hundred young people between the ages of 15 to 25 participate. They attend the weekly youth Mass, participate in the SCC youth sections, and/or attend the activities for the youth organised at parish level. The objective of the youth programme is twofold. First, it provides young people with an alternative place to spend their leisure time. The church wants to keep youths away from the bars, to prevent them from drinking and having sexual relationships. Therefore a youth hall has been established on the parish ground. According to a youth leader, this provides the youth with 'a second home' where they can take refuge from the problems they may have at home.[7] Second, the youth programme aims to familiarise young people with the Catholic faith. The activities include Bible study and prayer, study of religious and cultural issues, and workshops on topics such as employment and HIV and AIDS. In these activities, issues related to moral behaviour are often discussed, such as sexuality and relationships. Clearly, the parish seeks to raise young people's interest in and commitment to the Catholic faith and its moral values. Yet a youth leader complained that this is difficult because most youths 'are just traditional Catholics' and the church has little impact on their lives.[8] Interestingly, this youth leader commented that it is particularly difficult to work with male

---

Programme' (May 1996), in J. Komakoma (ed.), *The Social Teaching of the Catholic Bishops and Other Christian Leaders in Zambia: Major Pastoral Letters and Statements 1953–2001* (Ndola, 2003), 341–6.

[6] Sermon in the English Mass, Regiment parish Lusaka, 26 July 2009.
[7] Interview with Bensson Mbuzi, Lusaka, 11 November 2008.
[8] Ibid.

youths, as they are faced with peer pressure and with social-cultural norms that contrast with the church's moral teaching. This suggests, however, that the youth programme is a place where young men are more or less explicitly targeted for change. My interviews with some of the male youths actively participating in the programme indeed show that their participation affects their sense of morality and their religious and male identity.

Marriage Teaching and Counselling

Regiment parish has several groups and programmes concerned with marriage. Before a marriage is blessed in the church, a couple receives premarital teaching: a course of twelve sessions dealing with issues such as communication, sexuality, male–female roles, spirituality, budgeting and the upbringing of children. The parish has assigned this task to the local section of Marriage Encounter, an international and originally Catholic movement aiming at the renewal of 'the extraordinary vocation of marriage'.[9] Apart from this compulsory course for the couple, the bride and the groom may also receive individual teaching from members of the women's groups Nazareth or St Anne (for the bride) or from members of St Joachim (for the groom). Here, spouses-to-be are prepared in the traditional way, though the teaching is said to be Christianised.[10] Once married, problems may arise in the marital relationship. In that case the church offers assistance, such as through the SCC to which the couple belongs, through groups like Nazareth, St Anne, St Joachim and Marriage Encounter, or through the parish priest. As divorce is never an option according to Catholic teaching, marital counselling always aims to keep the couple together. Because it is better to prevent than to cure, Marriage Encounter also organises weekends for married couples. These weekends aim to increase so-called 'couple power', that is, the level of intimacy and communication in marriage.[11]

The enormous concern with marital life corresponds with the policy of the CC-Z at large. The bishops have declared 'the evangelisation of the family' to be a priority, and marriage is considered the key to building strong families.[12] Out

---

[9] 'Sacramental Marriage', World Wide Marriage Encounter, accessed 27 December 2011, www.wwme.org/sacramental-marriage.html.

[10] As one member of the Nazareth group explained to me, the difference between the teaching they provide and the teaching provided by Marriage Encounter is 'the cultural dimension': Marriage Encounter, in her opinion, bases its teaching on the Bible and the Christian tradition, while the other groups also bring in traditional Zambian teachings.

[11] Interview with John and Anne Machechali, Lusaka, 3 November 2008.

[12] Catholic Bishops of Zambia, 'The Missionary Family: A Pastoral Letter to all Catholics from the Bishops of Zambia on the 1999 Theme for the Implementation of the African Synod' (25 March 1999), in J. Komakoma (ed.), *The Social Teaching of the Catholic Bishops and Other Christian Leaders in Zambia: Major Pastoral Letters and Statements 1953–2001* (Ndola, 2003), 405.

of an awareness that urbanisation, modernisation and Zambia's fragile economic situation pose many problems and difficulties to marriages and families, the church

> calls for the promotion of family values and the support of families through intensified marriage preparation, enrichment courses, and family life education especially directed at young people. It further urges Christians to ground their marriages and family life.[13]

In the activities concerned with marriage, the role of the male partner is made subject of discussion. The position of the husband in marriage, his duties in the family, the family values he has to respect and promote – all these and other issues are often raised and discussed. Therefore, according to the parish priest, the (pre) marital teaching and counselling programme is the most important means the church has to address men and issues related to masculinity.[14]

St Joachim Men's Organisation

St Joachim is the name of a Catholic men's organisation in Zambia that also has a local section in Regiment parish. In the late 1990s, this lay movement was established as the first men's organisation in the Archdiocese of Lusaka, aiming to get men more involved in the church and more committed to the Catholic faith. According to the constitution,

> the aim of the organization is to promote unity, spiritual growth and matrimonial well-being of its members. To do works of charity, to actively participate in small Christian communities, to promote baptism vows and to promote the catholic doctrine as well as promote the dignity of the family.[15]

In order to realise this objective, the organisation promotes its patron Saint Joachim as 'the model of every Catholic husband and father'.[16]

According to an apocryphal gospel, the *Protoevangelium of James*, Joachim was the father of Mary and thus the grandfather of Jesus. The story has it that Joachim and his wife Anne were childless into old age. On one particular day, Joachim's temple offering is refused because he has 'not made seed in Israel'. He then retires to the desert to pray and fast for 40 days and nights. An angel visits Anne, who is at home lamenting, as she believes her husband has left her; the angel also visits Joachim in the desert, telling him that he and his wife will

---

[13] D. Musonda, 'General Introduction: Moral and Pastoral Issues', in J. Komakoma (ed.), *The Social Teaching of the Catholic Bishops and Other Christian Leaders in Zambia: Major Pastoral Letters and Statements 1953–2001* (Ndola, 2003), 14–15.

[14] Interview with Fr Marc Nsanzurwimo, Lusaka, 28 July 2009.

[15] *Constitution of St Joachim Catholic Men's Organization*, 8.

[16] Ibid., 1.

have a child. After Joachim and Anne are re-united, Mary is born. In the history of Christianity there is a popular devotion to St Anne and, to a lesser extent, to St Joachim. This popularity has been accredited to its close connection with the cult of the Virgin Mary, and the fact that 'Christian married couples find in the parents of Mary a model of conjugal life such as they do not find in Joseph and Mary, at least not on the level of conjugal relationships'.[17] The case of the St Joachim men's organisation (and its women's counterpart, St Anne) in Zambia shows that this tradition continues to date. It is even renewed, since Joachim now is explicitly promoted as an ideal model of Catholic manhood.[18]

The section of St Joachim in Regiment parish has about 40 members of middle and older age. The group gathers officially once a month, but almost every Sunday informally. Issues concerning the parish and the SCCs are discussed, and personal, matrimonial and family problems are shared. Members are supposed to participate actively in the SCCs and in the parish. Furthermore, they provide practical services at parish and diocese level. Clearly, to be a member of St Joachim is demanding in terms of time. This seems to be a deliberate strategy of the organisation. As one of the committee members explained, when men are occupied with church affairs they have no time left for 'earthly things'.[19] The organisation has a strict disciplinary code of conduct, and in cases of misconduct members may be expelled. Some Joachim members indicated that the high moral demands discourage other men from joining the group. Yet the members themselves testify that the demands are worth it. Membership seems to provide them with a certain status and they earn respect in the community.

The St Joachim group is a very interesting organisation in terms of the construction of Catholic masculinity, not just because the members seriously try to remodel themselves as men after the example of their patron saint, but also because these members are considered exemplary by other men in the community. As a diocesan staff member commented, Joachim members are an 'elite of Catholic men' and therefore are a means of the church in the evangelisation of society.[20]

Sermons at Mass

Sunday Mass is the largest gathering of men in the parish. Even though there is complaint about men's low attendance at Mass, still hundreds of men assemble there. This could be an excellent opportunity to address men, but in fact this is not done actively. When it does happen, it is rather by the way, through jokes, small

---

[17] J.P. Asselin, 'Anne and Joachim, SS.', in B.L. Marthaler et al. (ed.), *New Catholic Encyclopedia*, 2nd edn (Detroit, 2003), 469.

[18] For a more detailed account, see A.S. van Klinken, 'St. Joachim as a Model of Catholic Manhood in Times of AIDS: A Case Study on Masculinity in an African Christian Context', *CrossCurrents*, 61/4 (2011): 467–79.

[19] Interview with Marc Bwali, Lusaka, 9 November 2008.

[20] Interview with Gerald Tembo (Archdiocese of Lusaka), Lusaka, 11 November 2008.

stories and examples. For instance, once in a sermon a comment was made that men are often better acquainted with the names of players in the football team than with the names of their children. On one occasion, men were more explicitly addressed, when the archdiocese had dedicated a special Sunday for men under the theme 'Men, Take Up the Challenge!' In the sermon men were called to take responsibility in the church and in the community, and a similar message from the archbishop, T.G. Mpundu, was read.[21]

The fact that generally issues of men and masculinity are not addressed explicitly is explained by Fr Nsanzurwimo with reference to the fact that sermons in the Catholic Church follow the lectionary and are relatively short. In his opinion, Protestant pastors 'can preach about what they want' but for priests that is not possible.[22] This is not to say that sermons are not relevant to the formation of Catholic masculinity. Values such as love, responsibility, forgiveness and solidarity are often underlined in preaching and are related to people's life in the family and the community. In one way or another, this may have impact on men's perceptions of the Christian faith and of themselves as Christian men.

Small Christian Communities

What has been said about Mass also largely applies to the SCC meetings. Generally speaking, men's participation in the SCCs is considered insufficient. However, a number of men are actively involved in their SCC and in the parish at large, and they also try to involve fellow men in their sections. Discussions in the SCC meetings are about a variety of topics, including issues concerning marriage, family life, the community, and HIV and AIDS. Such discussions may touch on the role of men and on issues concerning masculinity, but there is no explicit policy to do so.

Pastoral Letters of the Bishops

The Catholic bishops of Zambia frequently publish pastoral letters and statements on social, economic, political and moral issues affecting the nation. In these documents, men and issues related to masculinity are hardly ever mentioned explicitly. However, the bishops appear to be very much concerned with women's issues. They frequently express their concern about the oppression of women in families, the grabbing of widows' property, women's lack of decision-making power, the sexual exploitation of women and violence against women. The bishops address these realities critically, for example saying that 'these are signs of denial of basic human rights, an injustice which cries out to our Creator'.[23]

---

[21] T.G. Mpundu, 'Men, Take Up the Challenge!', Parish newsletter, 254 (19 July 2009).
[22] Interview with Fr Marc Nsanzurwimo, Lusaka, 4 November 2008.
[23] Catholic Bishops of Zambia, 'You Shall be My Witnesses: Pastoral Letter of the Catholic Bishops of Zambia to Mark 100 Years of Catholic Faith in Zambia' (9 July 1991),

They further underline the rights of women and emphasise the need to respect women's dignity. In a 2009 letter they directly call upon the government 'to take immediate measures to domesticate protocols and enact laws that promote gender equality and empower women'.[24] In view of the concern of the bishops about women's issues, it is striking that they hardly address the role of men. The only time they briefly do so is in their letter *Choose Life*, which is about abortion. Here a critical reference is made to young men and to the so-called sugar daddies who – according to the bishops – perceive girls as no more than objects of pleasure and who cause pregnancies without taking responsibility.[25] The fact that men and aspects of masculinity are not very explicitly addressed indicates that the concern about women's issues has not yet led the bishops to a critical analysis of masculinities or to a strategy to promote an alternative ideal of manhood.

Critical Issues Concerning Men and Masculinities

Clearly, at various places and in different ways, men and issues related to masculinity are addressed, although not always explicitly and actively. The next and more interesting questions are: Which issues are addressed critically among men and what type of masculinity is contested? The reconstruction offered in this section gives a good insight in the general perception of men and popular forms of masculinity in the parish and broader Catholic circles.

Sexuality

One of the major issues the church is concerned about is sexual behaviour. Of course this is a broader concern that relates to both men and women. The Roman Catholic Church (RCC) teaches that sexual relationships have to be an expression of marital love and have to be open to procreation.[26] Therefore the church only advocates abstinence before and fidelity in marriage as preventive measures against HIV transmission; it rejects the use of condoms. In Regiment parish, the

---

in J. Komakoma (ed.), *The Social Teaching of the Catholic Bishops and Other Christian Leaders in Zambia: Major Pastoral Letters and Statements 1953–2001* (Ndola, 2003), 254.

[24] Catholic Bishops of Zambia, *A Call to Integrity: A Pastoral Letter from the Zambia Episcopal Conference on the Role of all Zambians to Work for the Common Good of our Nation* (Lusaka, 2009), 6.

[25] Catholic Bishops of Zambia, 'Choose Life: The Sacred Value of Human Life and the Evil of Promoting Abortion: A Pastoral Letter from the Catholic Bishops' (30 November 1997), in J. Komakoma (ed.), *The Social Teaching of the Catholic Bishops and Other Christian Leaders in Zambia: Major Pastoral Letters and Statements 1953–2001* (Ndola, 2003), 379 and 386.

[26] See *The Truth and Meaning of Human Sexuality: Guidelines for Education within the Family* (Rome, 1995), nos 14 and 15.

HIV epidemic has reinforced the emphasis on the church's moral teachings on sexuality. In 1995 a behavioural change programme was established, targeting the youth 'to help them see the Christian path in the whole area of sexuality and human development'.[27] To date, workshops where issues of sexuality and HIV are discussed are frequently organised for youth. Also the Zambian Catholic youth magazine *Speak Out!* and various booklets distributed in the parish often pay attention to these issues.[28] Furthermore, the place of sexuality in marriage, and the importance of marital fidelity, is discussed in the pre-marital teaching sessions. This emphasis on the moral norms regarding sexuality corresponds with the understanding of the Zambian bishops that the HIV epidemic is largely a result of immoral sexual behaviour.[29] The bishops call for a revaluation of 'the true meaning of the sexual act as an expression of love between a man and a woman in marriage and open to the transmission of life', which in their opinion is part of 'our Zambian and Christian heritage'.[30]

Interestingly, in the discussions about sexuality specific reference is sometimes made to men. The main concern is with popular understandings of sexuality as a way to prove manhood. For instance, a youth leader pointed out that 'the social and cultural system' tells young men 'that if you are able to sleep with ten or eleven women you are a champion'.[31] He explained that the parish youth programme seeks to correct popular perceptions like these through mentoring and teaching. Young men's sexual behaviour is also addressed in the youth magazine *Speak Out!* The magazine has published 'A letter to my future husband' in which a young woman writes:

> Apparently, manhood doesn't come automatically for males. Some guys seem to spend their entire lives trying to "prove their manhood" – by hunting, playing sports, driving fast, and, unfortunately, by having sex. It seems rather strange to us women that guys think having sex proves they're a man. ... I want more from you. I want you to respect your sexuality as much as I respect mine.[32]

---

[27] 'Let Your Light Shine', 14.

[28] The Catholic publishing house Pauline Publications (Nairobi, Kenya) has a series of booklets with titles such as *About AIDS*, *About Boys and Girls*, *About Sex* and *About True Love Waits*. These booklets are available for reading in the youth hall, are on sale in the parish bookshops, and are used in youth activities.

[29] Catholic Bishops of Zambia, 'Have Life to the Full. A Pastoral Letter from the Catholic Bishops of Zambia on HIV/AIDS' (24 November 2002), in African Jesuit AIDS Network (ed.), *Catholic Bishops of Africa and Madagascar Speak Out on HIV & AIDS* (Nairobi, 2004), 93.

[30] Catholic Bishops of Zambia, 'The Church as a Caring Family', 357.

[31] Interview with Bensson Mbuzi, Lusaka, 11 November 2008.

[32] M. Mugala-Ng'Ambi, 'An Open Letter to My Future Husband', *Speak Out!*, 26/2 (2009): 8.

Clearly, popular perceptions of masculinity and sexuality are addressed here, and young men are challenged – by their imaginative future wife! – to change their ways.

Sexual behaviour is discussed among adult married men. One parishioner told me about a recent men's meeting where the question was raised of why men, even if they are Christian, are more promiscuous than women. The conclusion of the resulting discussion, as he narrated it, was that men's difficulty with marital fidelity needs to be understood from the traditional practice of polygamy. Traditionally a man was allowed to have more than one wife, in order for him 'to be satisfied in terms of sex' and to demonstrate economic status.[33] The church has banned polygamy, but this has not eradicated the popular idea that to be a real man one needs to have more than one woman. Regardless of whether this explanation is correct or not, some female parishioners involved in marital counselling have argued that men are far more likely than women to engage in extramarital affairs. Infidelity on the man's part is one of the most common marital problems women say they are faced with. Moreover, a male parishioner undergoing marital counselling commented that when women engage in sexual relationships outside marriage it is often out of poverty, while men are simply driven by 'lust for other women'.[34] Perhaps it is because of these reasons that the bishops, in one of the few references to men in their pastoral letters, explicitly address male sexuality. They specifically point to the objectification of girls and the female body: 'Boys frequently perceive girls as mere objects for pleasure and abuse the meaning of "love" in order to obtain the satisfaction of their desires. ... This attitude is not uncommon among men also.'[35] All this does not provide any empirical evidence that men indeed have 'indiscriminate sex' and that they are more 'promiscuous' than women, but it does show that male sexuality is a major concern in the church.

While the popular perception of manhood as being performed through sexuality is addressed critically, strangely enough, at the same time it is also reinforced by the literature on offer in the church. Several booklets for youth explain that it is a natural urge of boys and men to be preoccupied with sex, as this is part of their biological make-up. For example, the booklet *Boys Growing Up* reads:

> A boy has different carnal desires than a girl. He may feel the need to sleep with a girl, just to satisfy his sexual drive. A girl for her part will sleep with a boy in order to feel specially chosen by him, or to have a child. It is rare that a girl will do so for the pleasure of sex alone.[36]

The suggestion here is that the emotional aspect of sexuality is less developed among boys compared to girls. For a boy it would be normal to want to sleep

---

[33] Interview with Haggai Mwansa, Lusaka, 6 July 2009.
[34] Interview with Marc Bwali, Lusaka, 9 November 2008.
[35] Catholic Bishops of Zambia, 'Choose Life', 386.
[36] C.N. Nganda, *Boys Growing Up*, 5th reprint (Nairobi, 2007), 57.

with a girl just for sexual satisfaction. The 'carnal desire' of boys is presented in the book as part of the 'masculine pattern'. This pattern is explained from the natural hormones that arouse the need in boys to give new life and hence urge them to engage in sexual relationships. Theologically it is explained from the sexual instinct that God has given to men in order for the human race to multiply. The essentialist idea that men's sexuality is naturally 'unrestrained' may have the unintentional effect of making it more acceptable, or at least understandable, when a man engages in sexual affairs before or outside marriage.[37] Trying to counteract this effect, the church puts a strong emphasis on the control of the sexual urges. As will be explored below, men are not supposed to follow the desires of the flesh – even though these are natural – but have to master them spiritually.

Alcoholism

Unlike some other churches in Zambia, the Catholic Church does not reject the use of alcohol. Alcohol as such is not considered a moral issue: 'Nowhere in the Bible it is said: "Thou shalt not drink."'[38] However, the church is definitely concerned about the excessive drinking of alcohol, because this makes people 'guilty of undisciplined conduct'.[39] In Regiment parish, drinking is considered a major problem in the community, especially among men. Parish youths explained to me that boys generally start drinking in their teenage years. Several women pointed out that their husbands often hang around in bars during the day. This is explained by the lack of recreational facilities in the compounds: 'The only thing people can do is to go to a pub and have a beer.'[40] Peer pressure is also said to play a critical role. The parish leadership realises that alcoholism has a negative impact on families and the community. As Nsanzurwimo explained:

> So like in a family, when a man is a drunkard or a womaniser it has a consequence for the economy of the family, the communication of the family, relationships in the family, even in the neighbourhood. And sometimes it is carried over in the children. It is very difficult to recover from the drinking or womanising habit of your father. These are the most critical areas for men, drinking and womanising.[41]

---

[37] Cf. M. Mayblin, *Gender, Catholicism, and Morality in Brazil: Virtuous Husbands, Powerful Wives* (New York, 2010), 136–7, where a similar observation is made about male sexuality in a Brazilian Catholic context. There 'a man's sexual appetite is said to be naturally *quente* (hot), which justifies, in an unspoken way, his extramarital affairs'.
[38] N.O. Oloo, *About Drinking*, rev. edn (Nairobi, 2007), 15.
[39] Ibid., 9.
[40] Interview with Raymond Malambo, Lusaka, 27 July 2009.
[41] Interview with Fr Marc Nsanzurwimo, Lusaka, 28 July 2009.

The concern here is not only about the economic consequences of alcoholism for the family, but also about the bad example drinking fathers set for their sons. Some of the youths also demonstrated an awareness of the consequences of drinking they observe among their peers: it affects the results at school and it costs a great deal of money. Besides, many realise that alcohol can have extremely grave consequences in the current era of HIV. As a young man said: 'Most of the people of my age die because of AIDS. There is too much freedom: they drink alcohol, lose their senses and have sex.'[42] The link between drinking alcohol and contracting HIV is also made in booklets with suggestive titles such as *I bought AIDS in a Bar*.[43]

Clearly, there is a concern about excessive drinking, specifically in relation to men. Yet the approach is nuanced, as drinking alcohol is not simply prohibited; rather, men are sensitised to the negative consequences and are encouraged to limit their intake. Interestingly, some interviewees argued that there is need to take a more radical stance towards alcohol than does the church leadership. They told me that they have decided, maybe under the influence of Pentecostal peers,[44] to abstain from alcohol completely, or at least to limit themselves very strictly. Often they came to this decision after having observed the impact that alcoholism has or has had on the life of a close friend or relative.

Irresponsibility in Marriage and Family Life

As mentioned above, in Regiment parish and the broader CC-Z there is a strong concern with marriage and family life. This is informed by the awareness of the many problems faced by families nowadays, such as poverty and disease. However, there is also an awareness of the disruption of families from inside out. In this context, men and their role in marriage and family life are specifically singled out. According to Nsanzurwimo,

> If there is a member of the family [who] causes most problems in the family, it is the man. Not the man as gender but as the head of the family and as the husband. It is like in a community or organisation: if the head is rotten the whole organisation collapses.[45]

What, then, are the problems that would be caused by men in their families? In short, the problem is said to be with the irresponsibility of men: they do not live

---

[42] Interview with William Kunda, Lusaka, 11 November 2008.

[43] *I Bought AIDS in a Bar, and Other True Stories* (Nairobi, 2002).

[44] Pentecostal churches in Africa categorically oppose the drinking of alcohol and have made it a major issue; this lies in contrast to mainstream churches such as the Catholic Church. See R. van Dijk, 'Modernity's Limits: Pentecostalism and the Moral Rejection of Alcohol in Malawi', in D.F. Bryceson (ed.), *Alcohol in Africa: Mixing Business, Pleasure, and Politics* (Portsmouth, 2002), 261.

[45] Interview with Fr Marc Nsanzurwimo, Lusaka, 28 July 2009.

up to the responsibilities they have as head of the family. As Nsanzurwimo puts it: 'The problem is [that] the man does not match up to what is expected from him.'[46] This overall irresponsibility is illustrated with several examples.

It is generally believed that a man has the role to provide for the family. Of course, it is realised that it may be difficult for men to fulfil this task because of the economic situation. However, it is also said that men often simply neglect this responsibility, as they would prefer to spend their money in bars rather than bringing it into the home. In the words of a female marital counsellor: 'They [men] keep their salaries for themselves, and the woman has to ask always for money when she wants to buy something.'[47]

Men's tendency to engage in extramarital affairs is also cited as a major cause of problems in marriages and families. This behaviour is considered problematic, not only from a moral perspective but also from the perspective of the household finances. As a parishioner explained, 'the more unfaithful you become, the more resources you deny your family just because you have to womanise'.[48] In other words, a married man who is dating will take financial resources that are supposed to be put into the home and spend them on girlfriends.

Another critical issue in this context is men's irresponsibility towards, and absence from, the family. In a meeting with a parish women's group, the members complained that their husbands hardly spend any time at home, because they prefer to hang around with friends in bars. As one of them described:

> [S]ome go very early in the morning for drinking. They are from home for the whole day. Come back when the children are sleeping. They think that is life. Sometimes they even don't know what grades their own children are in; even the names they don't know.[49]

Parallel to this criticism, it is said that husbands spend too little time with their wives. 'From the moment they are married, his wife is no longer an outing partner for him', an instructor said in a Marriage Encounter workshop.[50]

Last but not least, there is a concern about 'the dictatorial behaviour of men' in their marriage and family. This points to autocratic ways of decision-making and to men's attitudes of superiority towards their wives. Several interviewees explained this behaviour with a reference to 'African tradition' where the notion of male headship, in their opinion, is understood in terms of domination.

All these criticisms exemplify the general idea in the parish that men do not take seriously the responsibility they have as husbands in marriage and as fathers

---

[46] Interview with Fr Marc Nsanzurwimo, Lusaka, 4 November 2008.
[47] Interview with Rosalyn Banda, Lusaka, 28 October 2008.
[48] Interview with Bensson Mbuzi, 11 November 2008.
[49] Interview with members of the Nazareth group in Regiment Parish, Lusaka, 27 October 2008.
[50] Marriage Encounter workshop in Regiment parish, Lusaka, 25 July 2009.

in their families. This is believed to affect the wellbeing of women and children negatively, and it is therefore a major concern of the church.

Injustices to Women

As noted above, the Catholic bishops of Zambia often express a concern in their writings about 'injustices to women'.[51] Examples are grabbing the property of widows, sexual and domestic violence against women, sexual exploitation of women, high poverty and illiteracy levels among women, women's huge burden of taking care of children and the sick, and the oppression of women in the family and in society. These issues are often addressed in a discourse of human rights and justice. The bishops say, for example, that 'in many instances women are treated in ways which deny our fundamental Christian belief in the basic equality of human beings, a belief founded in the biblical revelation that all persons are created in the image and likeness of God (Genesis 1:27)'.[52] Remarkably, though the injustices done to women are often addressed, the documents hardly mention the initiators and perpetrators who, in many cases, will be men. Only with regard to sexual issues is explicit reference made to the role of men:

> Boys frequently perceive girls as mere objects for pleasure and abuse the meaning of "love" in order to obtain the satisfaction of their desires. ... We also note that the portrayal of violence and of the domination over women by men in books and on the screen cannot be dissociated from an increase in the sexual exploitation of women.[53]

Here boys and men are explicitly mentioned in relation to sexual violence, domination over women and the sexual exploitation of women. This behaviour is explained with a brief reference to external influences, such as the media, but it is not further analysed or reflected upon.

In light of the injustices to women mentioned by the bishops, it is noteworthy that the constitution of the St Joachim men's organisation says among other things that the group aims to help men 'to cultivate positive attitudes towards women'.[54] Explaining this, the executives of the Regiment section of St Joachim pointed to phenomena such as wife-beating, domestic violence and oppressive attitudes

---

[51] Catholic Bishops of Zambia, 'You Shall be My Witness', 254–5; idem, 'The Church as a Caring Family', 359; idem, 'Choose Life', 379–80.
[52] Catholic Bishops of Zambia, 'You Shall Be My Witness', 254.
[53] Catholic Bishops of Zambia, 'Choose Life', 386–7.
[54] *Constitution of St Joachim Catholic Men's Organization*, 9.

of men towards women.⁵⁵ They consider it a major task of their organisation to address these practices and to promote positive attitudes to women among men.

Low Commitment to Church and Faith

A major concern in the parish and more broadly in the CC-Z is men's lack of involvement in the church and their lack of commitment to the faith. Several active parishioners made statements to the effect that most men are only 'Sunday worshippers' and have 'apathy towards church matters'. It is believed that men, even if they come to Mass on Sunday, often forget about church for the rest of the week. Moreover, it is observed that fewer men than women attend Mass, and men participate only marginally in the SCCs. Referring to the ecclesiology of the church as the family of God, a diocesan staff member explained why the low participation of men is a major concern: 'When we talk of the church as a family, the church is not complete without the men, the fathers.'⁵⁶

Asked for explanations of men's low participation, various reasons were given. It is commonly believed that most men are simply not interested in issues related to the church and faith. Their interest would be diverted to 'the things of this world', such as watching football, hanging around in bars, and enjoying themselves with women.⁵⁷ It was also suggested that some men are so occupied with their task of being the provider of the family that they are always working to make money and do not have time for church activities. Another interesting explanation was that men shy away from SCC meetings because their wives are present and may disclose how things are at home. Yet another explanation I heard was that Catholic men lack self-confidence with regard to church activities because most of them know so little about the Bible and the Christian faith.

Whatever the reasons for their low involvement in the church, men are challenged to become more committed. Members of St Joachim told me that they try to evangelise fellow men in their communities, and likewise women told me that they encourage their husbands to go to Mass and to attend the SCC meetings. The youth activities and the (pre)-marital counselling attempt to make boys and men familiar with the Catholic faith and to increase their participation in church. Out of the concern about men's lack of involvement, at one time the archdiocese dedicated a special Sunday to men. Under the title 'Men – take up the challenge' a message was spread in all parishes, which stated:

> What a wonderful opportunity for Catholic men in our Archdiocese to realize and
> take up the challenge of getting involved in the mission of Christ. Most Catholic

---

⁵⁵ Interview with the executive committee members of St Joachim in Regiment Parish, Lusaka, 11 October 2008.
⁵⁶ Interview with Gerald Tembo (Archdiocese of Lusaka), Lusaka, 11 November 2008.
⁵⁷ Interview with John Kabonde, Lusaka, 14 July 2009.

men do not participate in a number of activities taking place in the parish. ... [I]t is indeed true that men are usually fewer during Church celebrations and less involved compared to women. Through the intercession of St Paul, we pray that the Lord may slowly bring them to the true and intimate knowledge of the Gospel of Christ and, in turn to communicate it to others including their households.[58]

That particular Sunday, a similar message was also preached during Mass. Referring to faithful men like Stephen, Timothy and Titus who, according to the New Testament epistles, assisted Paul and engaged in the mission of the early church, the officiating priest emphasised that the church today is in great need for such men truly committed to the service of God.

Though men are criticised for their lack of involvement with church and faith affairs, the church leadership realises that the impact of this is small. According to Nsanzurwimo, more creative ways of evangelisation are needed to reach men: 'You have to minister to them in the pubs or wherever they are.'[59] Apparently this is a strategy yet to be developed.

The Ideal of Catholic Manhood

The issues discussed above sketch a picture of the type of masculinity considered dominant in the community. In an attempt to address men's behaviour and to overcome this type of popular masculinity, the church promotes moral values and alternative notions of manhood among men. Parishioners themselves also express religiously informed perceptions of masculinity. An ideal of Catholic manhood can be reconstructed by identifying the key notions. These are not so much well-defined concepts but rather the contours in which male identity and behaviour can be reshaped.

Responsibility

A key notion of the ideal of manhood is responsibility. When I asked men of different ages what it means to them to be a man, they often responded that it means being responsible. Of course, responsibility is a very broad concept. It is applied to almost all areas of life, such as the way a man deals with his sexuality, his roles in marriage and the family and his duties in the community. Growing up as a boy and becoming a man is understood in terms of a 'journey towards manhood', which leads a boy from childhood to the stage of 'responsible manhood'.[60] The sense of responsibility is thought to develop naturally in boys: 'As you grow older,

---

[58] Mpundu, *Men, Take Up the Challenge!*
[59] Interview with Fr Marc Nsanzurwimo, Lusaka, 28 July 2009.
[60] J. Kiura, *About Boys*, 4th reprint (Nairobi, 2007), 12.

you [will] feel an increasing need to lead, to take responsibility.'[61] Apparently, responsibility is considered to be a natural and essential characteristic of manhood. This is often explained with a reference to Genesis 1:28, suggesting that male responsibility is considered a God-given role from creation.[62]

What, then, is men's responsibility all about? This depends on one's age and stage of life. Young unmarried men understand their responsibility in terms of financial independence and self-reliance. As one of them explained: 'Nobody will come and take care of me when I am not responsible. I have to look for a job myself. I am a man; I just have to be responsible.'[63] This responsibility is perceived as quite tough, as it is difficult to find a job and to make an income. However, young men also realise that their ability to manage their own life is a way to prove that they are able to take care of a wife and a family.

For married men the notion of responsibility primarily focuses on a man's duty to take care of his wife and children. First of all this is about material issues: the common idea is that a man has to provide for the needs of the family, such as food, clothing, housing, and school fees. For example, one interviewee explained:

> I have to provide the resources. My wife, when she gives me children, that is enough for her. The economic failure of the family depends on the man. So if I am not able to send the children to school, I have failed in this lifetime. So it is my responsibility to take care of this.[64]

Men often emphasised that providing for the family is quite a difficult task. They may even feel 'burdened with an exceptionally heavy Cross'.[65] Yet when they are successful as providers, it adds to their status as a man. Male responsibility for the family, however, is not just material; it also concerns the emotional and spiritual aspects of men's role in the home (see below).

A man's responsibility concerns not just his direct family but stretches out to the wider circle of relatives – the extended family. In the words of one interviewee: 'If my in-laws have a problem I need to come in and to assist. Those are the responsibilities: you need to come in financially, materially, and to give advice.'[66] Concrete examples are the support of relatives who are less well off or the care of orphaned cousins. Several men noted that the demands on them have increased due to the HIV epidemic. As many relatives fall sick and die, 'the burden is growing

---

[61] Nganda, *Boys Growing Up*, 16.

[62] According to Genesis 1:28, humankind in general, male and female, received the command of God to rule over the earth. In the booklet this verse is applied to men specifically: they are said to have a particular 'need to lead and take responsibility' (ibid., 16).

[63] Interview with Justin Gondwe, Lusaka, 31 October 2008.

[64] Interview with Bensson Mbuzi, Lusaka, 11 November 2008.

[65] Mayblin, *Gender, Catholicism, and Morality in Brazil*, 114.

[66] Interview with Danny and Christine Mulikita, Lusaka, 25 July 2009.

for us who remain; our responsibilities are growing while our income is going down.'[67] Though challenging, the responsibility of a man for the extended family is felt as a moral duty. To ignore it, a respondent said, is against 'the African way of life' and is even a 'blasphemy in the Christian sense'.[68]

Last but not least, male responsibility is also applied to the area of sexuality. According to the booklet *About Boys*, 'as a young man you should realize that you also have responsibility for your sexual energies, and that you need to master them so that you don't create problems either for yourself or for a girl'.[69] In line with this, a youth leader expressed his concern that young men often engage in sexual relationships while they are not yet able to bear the responsibility for the possible consequences: 'They have not yet reached a level where they can be responsible parents. They can't take care of the wife and the child, both mentally and physically they are not ready.'[70]

Explaining why responsibility is so important for manhood, people often came up with cultural and religious arguments. They explained, for example, that 'African culture' and the Bible consider a man to be the head of his family, meaning that he bears responsibility for the economic and spiritual well-being of his wife and children. Likewise, the interviewee quoted above suggested that a man's responsibility for relatives in the extended family follows from both the African way of life and Christian teaching. Apparently, it is believed that African culture and Christianity correspond with regard to responsibility as a key aspect of manhood.[71]

Family Man

Apart from material aspects, the notion of male responsibility in marriage and family life also includes spiritual and emotional aspects of men's role in the family. These latter aspects are encapsulated in the picture of the family man. Asked to describe the ideal Catholic man, Nsanzurwimo responded: 'He is a family man, ... at home he lives by example and he prays with his family.'[72] Precisely these aspects of being involved in and praying with the family are also represented by St Joachim. Referring to his example, at a meeting of the St Joachim men's organisation it was stated that being a family man is a 'vocation'. This term often is used with regard to priesthood. Thus, the suggestion is that just as a priest is

---

[67] Interview with Raymond Malambo, Lusaka, 27 July 2009.
[68] Interview with Bensson Mbuzi, Lusaka, 11 November 2008.
[69] Kiura, *About Boys*, 29.
[70] Interview with Raymond Malambo, Lusaka, 27 July 2009.
[71] More generally, notions of Catholic manhood are articulated in the parish not so much in contrast to but rather in line with cultural notions. For the parishioners, to be a Christian and to be an African are integrated aspects of their identities as men.
[72] Interview with Fr Marc Nsanzurwimo, 4 November 2008.

called by God to serve the church, which is the Family of God, so laymen are called to serve their own families, the so-called domestic church.

Concretely, to be a family man is understood in terms of spending time with the family, showing interest in the children, sharing meals together as a family, saying prayers together, creating an atmosphere of communication and dialogue, and coming to church together as a couple. This is expressed, for example, in the testimony of a young man, who states: 'I pray to be a very good family man. That is that I truly love my wife and truly love my children and have time for them. That has been my priority.'[73] Organisations such as Marriage Encounter and St Joachim try to foster such attitudes among men. Members of these groups are likely to tell how they have come to appreciate family life. According to a Joachim member:

> You will find that in certain families where there is no prayer, in such families you will find that a man is on his own and the wife and the children are on their own as well. But in our families we are together. We eat together. And in that way you bring your family together.[74]

It is often suggested that a high level of family involvement is uncommon in traditional and present-day Zambian society. According to a female parishioner, men usually have their meals together as men, separated from the women and children, but 'in a Christian marriage they are expected to eat together as a family'.[75] Likewise, a couple of Marriage Encounter described how men generally do not look after their children and leave the task of upbringing to the mother, while 'we [in Marriage Encounter] teach them about the roles and responsibilities which they have as a parental couple together'.[76] Male family involvement is considered so important because it helps to build the stable marriages and families that, according to the church, can face the many challenges of today.

Closely related to the idea of being a family man is the notion of fatherhood, which specifically points to a man's relationship with his children. To beget offspring is considered a must for a man. Only then is he considered to have entered another stage of life, ready to receive the associated respect from the community. A young man explained that once you have fathered a child people will say: 'Now you are a grown man.'[77] Fatherhood is understood in terms of responsibility: first and foremost in the material sphere, but increasingly also in the emotional sphere. As a young woman commented, 'men mostly think that bringing up a child means going for work and buying what the child wants ... [but] I force my husband by saying "Can you hold the baby? Play with the baby, I am tired. It is not *my* child,

---

[73] Interview with Jack Mwale, Lusaka, 6 July 2009.
[74] Interview with Marc Bwali, Lusaka, 9 November 2008.
[75] Interview with Rosalyn Banda, Lusaka, 28 October 2008.
[76] Interview with John and Anne Machechali, Lusaka, 3 November 2008.
[77] Interview with Chaba Soko, Lusaka, 30 June 2009.

it is *our* child. She needs your affection as well".'[78] Clearly, a more active and caring form of fatherhood is advocated here – something that apparently is not that common. Inspiration for such a type of fatherhood may come from the belief in God as a heavenly Father who cares for his children. As one parishioner told me, he strives to be a 'godlike father', meaning that he follows the example of God's patience and love.[79]

Headship

The idea of male headship is often mentioned in discussions about manhood in Regiment parish. When talking about the position and roles of a man in the marriage and family setting, many parishioners point out that a man is supposed to be the head of the home. For them this means that he is responsible for the well-being of the family, materially as well as morally and spiritually. Headship is associated with roles such as being the breadwinner and providing for the material needs of the family, showing leadership and providing guidance to the family, and leading the family in prayer. The concept of male headship is not understood to mean that women cannot or do not play a role in these areas – it is often acknowledged that they do so, and this is appreciated. However, the general opinion is that in the end 'only one can be on top'.[80] One parishioner, a married man, stated: 'Of course the man is the head of the house. ... Though the woman also plays a very important role. ... But as a man you have to control things all the time.'[81]

People generally explained the idea of male headship with reference to Zambian or African culture and to Christian teaching. Culture and Christianity seem to be two authoritative canons that both support the idea of a man as the head of the home. However, a critical difference between both traditions is also indicated. The Christian concept of headship is thought to be less authoritarian than the cultural one. As one respondent, a married woman, explained:

> The headship is both cultural and biblical, but in the Bible it is a two-ways thing. The husband should first love the wife and then the wife should be submissive. But our tradition here in Africa just tells the wife to be submissive; it does not talk about love. You just should submit. Whether he beats you, he abuses you, the only thing is: you should be submissive.[82]

---

[78] Christine Mulikita, in the interview with Danny and Christine Mulikita, Lusaka, 25 July 2009.
[79] Interview with Raymond Malambo, Lusaka, 27 July 2009.
[80] Interview with John Kabonde, Lusaka, 24 July 2009.
[81] Interview with Haggai Mwansa, Lusaka, 6 July 2009.
[82] Christine Mulikita, in the interview with Danny and Christine Mulikita, Lusaka, 25 July 2009.

This account echoes the Pauline teaching on male headship in marriage. Here, husbands are not only called to be the head of their wives as Christ is the head of the church, but also to love their wives as Christ loves the church and gave himself up for it (Ephesians 5:23–27). This also seems to be the understanding of Nsanzurwimo, in whose perception male headship is not to be understood as a tool for domination but as 'a ministry, a way of service to the family and the community.'[83]

Many parishioners point out that there are different ways for men to practise headship. They distinguish between good and bad male family heads: the good ones understand headship in terms of taking up the responsibilities related to it, while the bad ones understand it in terms of power and ignore their responsibilities. Even though this distinction is made, in a discussion with a women's group it was emphasised that women should *always* respect their husbands as the head.

> Even when it is a bad man, you should respect him and follow good things and do things to him. That's why today many women have lost their marriage, because they show no respect. ... A woman is a woman. She always should be down, a man is the head.[84]

The members of this women's group not only support the idea of male headship but also explicitly relate it to a notion of female submission. They consider women's disrespect and lack of submission to their husbands as key factors in marital problems, separation and divorce.

The concept of headship in marriage defines the marital relationship in a hierarchical way. Precisely for this reason it is rejected, or at least criticised, by some parishioners involved in Marriage Encounter. Though they are a minority in the parish, they have an influential position as organisers of the (pre)marital courses. Several Marriage Encounter trainers explained that their teaching differs at one fundamental point from the traditional understanding of marriage in Zambia: on the point of male headship and the related notion of female submission. The distinction, as one member couple put it, is that 'Marriage Encounter emphasises partnership in marriage', through the promotion of communication, joint decision-making, sharing the finances, mutual sexual satisfaction, and co-responsibility for the upbringing of the children.[85] Some members of Marriage Encounter demonstrated a critical hermeneutical approach to biblical texts, which enables them to reject the notion of male headship even though it is found in the Bible. Referring to the Pauline epistles in the New Testament, a woman said: 'Those letters were written in that time, where the Jewish had their own problems. But

---

[83] Interview with Fr Marc Nsanzurwimo, Lusaka, 28 July 2009.

[84] Interview with members of the Nazareth group in Regiment Parish, Lusaka, 27 October 2008.

[85] Interview with John and Anne Machechali, Lusaka, 3 November 2008.

looking at our problems now, we should not take it as if he is the head of the house. We are partners and we complement each other.'[86]

The parish priest, Nsanzurwimo, showed sympathy for the progressive stance of Marriage Encounter and appreciation for their egalitarian approach.[87] However, he also suggested that this approach may be too radical for many people and might frighten them away from the organisation. For him, male headship is not so much an idea that should be either categorically rejected or actively supported; it simply exists and needs some revision so that it can function constructively. This pragmatic stance may be characteristic of the broader CC-Z. Male headship is not discussed, either positively or negatively, in the bishops' pastoral letters or in church publications; only men's misconduct, for example in the oppression of women, is addressed critically. A consequence is that male headship, even though it is not so much part of an officially promoted ideal of Catholic manhood, for many Catholics continues to define their culturally and religiously informed understanding of manhood.

Self-control

Another defining aspect of manhood is self-control or self-discipline. This notion is emphasised in view of all the temptations boys and men are faced with. Though certain feelings and attractions are considered natural, they need to be controlled in order for boys to become mature men. The booklet *Boys Growing Up*, for instance, presents the process of becoming a man as a growth in maturity. Referring to all the impulses and desires young men have, the booklet assures readers that these 'are good and should not be silenced'.[88] However, at the same time it underscores the need to control these impulses:

> In the beginning, you may not believe that it is possible to master all your impulses and desires. But as you grow older, you will be surprised at how self-controlled you can be. And then through experience, (which they say is not cheap at any price!), you will be able to agree that: Happy indeed is the person who has fully learnt to control his impulses and desires.[89]

The importance of self-control is highlighted in order to increase resistance to peer pressure among young men. Giving in to peer-pressure is considered unmanly: 'If you always keep following others, you are not a man. You are a sheep.'[90] In line with this, another booklet challenges young men to develop 'will power' in

---

[86] Linda Nyirenda, in the interview with Henry and Linda Nyirenda, Lusaka, 7 July 2009.
[87] Interview with Fr Marc Nsanzurwimo, Lusaka, 28 July 2009.
[88] Nganda, *Boys Growing Up*, 22.
[89] Ibid., 24.
[90] Ibid., 28.

order to say no to the pressures from their peers as well as to the internal impulses, emotions and 'sexual energies'.[91]

Self-control is considered particularly important in the area of sexuality. It is presented as a crucial means of preventing sexually transmittable diseases such as HIV. The well-known ABC-prevention message of Abstain, Be faithful or Condomise is re-defined as Always Be Chaste, with the clarification that 'chastity simply means sexual self-control'.[92] At the same time, condoms are rejected because these are considered a licence to have sex. One of the recommendations to young men in the booklet *About Boys* states: 'Avoid contraceptives at all costs, for they will lead you as a young man to seek pleasure devoid of self-control and responsibility, hence destroying your character.'[93]

The importance of self-control is not only underscored in booklets, but also confirmed by male parishioners. Recounting how they follow the moral teaching of the church, they talk of developing 'a certain mindset', making a 'resolution with the self', or 'disciplining their desires'. One of them even stated: 'I have put myself in the lifestyle of a monk', meaning that he avoids places of temptations and consciously isolates himself from peers with a different lifestyle.[94] It seems that the sense of urgency to discipline the self is reinforced by the HIV epidemic. Referring to fellow youths dying from the disease, one respondent said: 'I have found out that at this age the most important thing is discipline. ... Discipline is important to live long.'[95]

Of course, the emphasis on self-control is not surprising as religion – especially Christianity – is so often concerned with disciplining the body and has developed, in the words of Foucault, various technologies to regulate the bodily self.[96] Interestingly, however, in this social context of HIV and AIDS and contested forms of masculinity, bodily discipline appears to be a gendered practice in which the ability to control the *male* self becomes a way to perform manhood. Several young men suggested that the control over their sexuality reveals true male strength. 'I am strong enough to abstain', one of them stated firmly while speaking with a certain disdain about his peers who think they can prove their manhood through

---

[91] Kiura, *About Boys*, 24–25.
[92] M. Ochieng, *About True Love Waits*, 4th reprint (Nairobi, 2006), 9.
[93] Kiura, *About Boys*, 30.
[94] Interview with William Kunda, Lusaka, 11 November 2008.
[95] Interview with Titus Mundia, Lusaka, 26 October 2008.
[96] For Foucault, technologies of the self are the (often religious) practices 'which permit individuals to effect by their own means, or with the help of others, a certain number of operations on their own bodies and souls, thoughts, conduct, and way of being, so as to transform themselves in order to attain a certain state of happiness, purity, wisdom, perfection of immortality'. See M. Foucault, 'Technologies of the Self', in P. Rabinow (ed.), *Ethics: Subjectivity and Truth. Essential Works of Foucault, 1954–1984*, vol. 1 (London, 2000), 225.

sexual activity.[97] Talking about peer pressure, sexuality and the relationship with his girlfriend, another interviewee said:

> Her friends and my friends encourage us to do certain things, to cross the lines. So my friends say: "She is an attractive girl; why don't you do what you are supposed to do as a man?" And I say: "It's better for me not to be a man than to cross that line." Because when I cross that line I know: I won't be the man. For me, sticking to my rules makes me a man.[98]

So, in this perception 'sticking to the rules' is what makes one a man. This is not to say that there are no temptations or weaknesses – these are admitted by almost all interviewees – but restricting and controlling them is considered an indication of true manhood. This not only applies to youths. One interviewee, a man in his 60s, told me that some time ago he had come to a point where he has stopped drinking alcohol and having sexual affairs completely. He said that people often ask him how he changed. 'I do not tell them that it is God's power. Me, I just decided: this is the end. You have a strong free will; it is your mind.'[99]

Spirituality

'As a young man, you need to look after your soul.'[100] This is one of the pieces of advice given to boys as a way to build their character into that of a mature man. Apart from physical, emotional, social and material aspects of the 'journey towards manhood', the area of spirituality is also mentioned. Boys are challenged to strengthen their spiritual life. Apparently, spirituality is considered a crucial aspect of being a Catholic man. This is also evident from the St Joachim men's organisation, whose patron saint is considered a role model for Catholic men, among other things because of his prayerful life. The group aims to foster spiritual growth among its members.[101] The emphasis on men's spiritual life has to be understood from the above-outlined concern about lack of involvement in the church and the Catholic faith among men. However, there are two additional reasons.

First, it is believed that a rich spiritual life, consisting of daily prayer, Bible reading, regular taking of Communion and participating in the parish and SCC, will have a positive impact upon men's moral lifestyles. For example, the booklet *About Boys* says: 'Good reading, prayer and the Word of God will help the mind to be well disposed and oriented to ideas of value and good conduct.'[102] In other words,

---

[97] Interview with Titus Mundia, Lusaka, 26 October 2008.
[98] Interview with Chaba Soko, Lusaka, 25 June 2009.
[99] Interview with Kedrick Mbuzi, Lusaka, 14 July 2009.
[100] Kiura, *About Boys*, 27.
[101] *Constitution of St Joachim Catholic Men's Organization*, 8.
[102] Kiura, *About Boys*, 20.

it is hoped that spirituality will help one to 'become the man that God intends you to be'.[103] Furthermore, some particular spiritual means are recommended as ways of dealing with and overcoming temptation. The constitution of St Joachim men's organisation refers to prayer as 'a weapon of resistance to temptations'.[104] Indeed, a Joachim member described how when he is faced with sexual temptations he makes the sign of the cross and says, 'Get off from me, Satan.'[105] To call upon boys and men to look after their souls, as in the above quoted booklet, is not just a general call to develop a spiritual life. The idea of looking after the soul points to a particular understanding of spirituality. In Foucauldian terms it exemplifies the 'hermeneutic of the self', which is developed particularly in Christianity as here every believer 'has the duty to explore who he is, what is happening within himself, the faults he may have committed, [and] the temptations to which he is exposed'.[106] According to Foucault, Christianity is a confessional religion in which believers not only embrace a process of introspection but also confess to others the truth they discover about the self. In line with this, the St Joachim group can be considered a confessional community: a fellowship where men disclose to one another and discuss together their vulnerabilities and temptations and share their spiritual struggles. This hermeneutical and confessional practice re-creates the self. Thus, St Joachim is key to the spiritual formation of new Catholic male selves.[107]

Second, the need for men to develop their spiritual life is emphasised because men are supposed to be the spiritual leaders of their homes. This spiritual leadership is considered the key to building strong families. Men's spiritual life is not only a matter of individual devotion: as heads of their homes they are supposed to lead their families in prayer, or, as the Archbishop of Lusaka put it, 'to bring their families to the Lord'.[108] Nsanzurwimo considers the task of praying with the family as a crucial part of Catholic manhood.[109] The responsibility of leading the family spiritually is underlined in the St Joachim organisation time and time again. Members are recommended to pray the rosary because 'the rosary is a family prayer' and 'it would unite you as a family'.[110] Among the members, a deep awareness of their spiritual leadership can be found. Again, St Joachim is considered exemplary here, as his prayer according to tradition resulted in the

---

[103] Ibid., 30.

[104] *Constitution of St Joachim Catholic Men's Organization*, 1.

[105] Interview with Marc Bwali, Lusaka, 9 November 2008.

[106] M. Foucault, 'Sexuality and Solitude', in P. Rabinow (ed.), *Ethics: Subjectivity and Truth. Essential Works of Foucault, 1954–1984*, vol. 1 (London, 2000), 178.

[107] For a discussion on confessional practice and the formation of male subjectivity, see B. Krondorfer, *Male Confessions: Intimate Revelations and the Religious Imagination* (Stanford, 2010).

[108] Mpundu, *Men, Take Up the Challenge!*

[109] Interview with Fr Marc Nsanzurwimo, Lusaka, 4 November 2008.

[110] Diocesan meeting of St Joachim men's organization, Lusaka, 8 November 2008.

birth of Mary. Therefore he is considered a model figure, challenging all Catholic men to establish praying families.

Re-constructing a Theological Framework

A more systematic analysis of the notions of Catholic manhood identified above shows that they are informed by and embedded in the tradition of Catholic theology. The formation of masculinity takes place in a theological framework. A reconstruction of this frame makes clear that Regiment parish is part of a global church with a well-developed theological tradition.

Gender Ideology and a Creation-based Theological Anthropology

The understanding of masculinity, as generally expressed in interviews and publications, is informed by a gender ideology that takes as its starting point a theological anthropology of creation. This is demonstrated by the many references made to the Genesis creation stories. The creation-based anthropology gives rise to two notions that are key to the understanding of gender and, consequently, of masculinity: the equality of man and woman and the fundamental difference between man and woman.

Equal Human Dignity   In the parish, the idea of equality of the sexes is generally supported. In the pre-marital course provided by Marriage Encounter, values such as respect and partnership are taught, based on the notion of equality of husband and wife. As mentioned above, this teaching is considered a major difference with respect to traditional understandings of marriage. One respondent captured this difference by saying: 'In our traditional concept the man is a sort of the alpha and omega of the family, but the Bible tries to emphasise equality.'[111] Also in booklets and in the official letters of the Zambian bishops, the equality of male and female is frequently emphasised. Perceptions of women's inferiority and men's oppressive attitudes towards women are opposed.[112] Often, if not almost always, when the equality of the sexes it underlined, the reference is to Genesis 1:27, which reads, 'God created mankind in his own image, in the image of God he created them; male and female he created them' (NIV). The general interpretation of this verse is that humankind in general (thus women as much as men) is created in the image of God. This functions as the foundational theological argument for male–female equality. For instance, the booklet *About Boys* states: 'It is wrong for a boy to look

---

[111]   Interview with Jack Mwale, Lusaka, 6 July 2009.

[112]   The stance of the bishops on this issue may be influenced by the influential Jesuit Centre for Theological Reflection (JCTR) in Lusaka. This centre seeks to promote justice in society, including justice in gender relations. See the JCTR publication, *What does the Church Social Teaching Say about Gender Equality?* (Lusaka, 2008).

down upon a girl just because he is a boy and considers himself stronger. Boys should respect girls and not manipulate them just because they are female. God decided to create us differently, yet in his image and likeness.'[113] Likewise, the Zambian bishops say that the oppression of women is a denial of the 'fundamental Christian belief in the basic equality of human beings, a belief founded in the biblical revelation that all persons are created in the image and likeness of God.'[114] The strong emphasis upon 'the basic equality' of women and men may be inspired by the late Pope John Paul II who, in his apostolic exhortation *Ecclesia in Africa*, in the section on the family, stated:

> The dignity of man and woman derives from the fact that when God created man, "in the image of God he created him, male and female he created them" (Gen 1:27). Both man and woman are created "in the image of God", that is, endowed with intelligence and will and therefore with freedom. ... Having both been created in the image of God, man and woman, although different, are essentially equal from the point of view of their humanity. ... In creating the human race "male and female", God gives man and woman an equal personal dignity, endowing them with inalienable rights and responsibilities proper to the human person.[115]

This quotation shows that the 'essential equality' of women and men is understood in terms of an 'equal personal dignity'. It is about an anthropological essence of every human being, something that precedes or transcends the difference between male and female. Apparently John Paul II was concerned that women's human dignity is threatened. Therefore he called on the church in Africa to safeguard and foster women's dignity. The Zambian bishops have heard this call and quote with approval the Pope's statement on the dignity of women.[116] They continue to express a concern about the abuses of women and to emphasise women's dignity in more recent letters.[117] This also influences the discourse at grassroots level, such as in Regiment parish, where a similar concern about women's dignity can be found. At this level, respect for the dignity of women even becomes a characteristic of Catholic manhood as it is represented by saints such as Joachim and Joseph. Both saints are praised, among other things, because they respected their wives, even in difficult circumstances.

---

[113] Kiura, *About Boys*, 9.

[114] Catholic Bishops of Zambia, *You Shall be My Witnesses*, 254.

[115] John Paul II, *Post-Synodal Apostolic Exhortation Ecclesia in Africa of the Holy Father John Paul II to the Bishops, Priests and Deacons, Men and Women Religious and all the Lay Faithful to the Church in Africa and its Evangelizing Mission Towards the Year 2000* (Yaoundé 1995), no. 82.

[116] Cf. Catholic Bishops of Zambia, *Choose Life*, 378–9.

[117] See Catholic Bishops of Zambia, *That They May Have Abundant Life: A Pastoral Statement* (Lusaka, 2012), no. 16.

Because of his concern with the dignity of women, it has been suggested that John Paul II might be called a feminist thinker.[118] I have no intention to dispute this idea – this book, after all, is neither about John Paul II nor about feminism. However, the case study shows that the concern about women's dignity often comes with a limited understanding of the equality of men and women – something most feminists would perceive critically. For instance, Nsanzurwimo commented that equality should not be understood as a 'mathematical equality', which in his opinion easily ends up in dualism and competition between women and men.[119] For him equality means that men and women have to respect each other's human dignity, but this respect can also be given in a marital relationship characterised by male headship. In line with this, in an interview with a couple, the husband stated that while both man and woman are equal in the eyes of God, 'you can't say there is equality; they [women] will never get where the men are, because of the way God has made them.'[120] His wife supported his view, saying that 'it should not be like: "I should reach the level where my husband is." Then competition comes in. ... Equality does not mean to be at the same level.'[121] Thus, there is a sense of gender equality, but this is not interpreted in a radical way but, rather, is nuanced and toned down. This is not specific to Regiment parish but is informed more broadly by the complex relationship between the notion of equality and the conception of sexual difference that is at the heart of the Catholic understanding of gender.[122]

Sexual Difference The restricted understanding of gender equality is related to the notion of sexual difference, also derived from Genesis 1:27. This verse reads that humankind is not only created in the image of God but also created as male and

---

[118] T. Beattie, 'Carnal Love and Spiritual Imagination: Can Luce Irigaray and John Paul II Come Together?', in J. Davies and G. Loughlin (eds), *Sex these Days: Essays on Theology, Sexuality and Society* (Sheffield, 1997), 160.

[119] Interview with Fr Marc Nsanzurwimo, 29 July 2009.

[120] Danny Mulikita, in the interview with Danny and Christine Mulikita, Lusaka, 25 July 2009.

[121] Christine Mulikita, in the interview with Danny and Christine Mulikita, Lusaka, 25 July 2009.

[122] Illustrative is Catholic theologian Laurenti Magesa from Tanzania. He criticises African women theologians for a too radical ('western feminist') understanding of gender equality, which, in his perception, 'involves the tendency to reject the feminine in woman, turning woman into merely a mirror image of man, a very oppressive and non-liberating tendency indeed'. Magesa admits that woman and man have an equal human dignity but emphasises that this does not mean that man and woman are equivalents. In his perception, both are endowed by God with 'innate sexual qualities', leading to an 'essential complementarity' of the sexes rather than a radical equality. See L. Magesa, 'The Challenge of African Woman Defined Theology for the 21st Century', in N.W. Ndung'u and P.N. Mwaura (eds), *Challenges and Prospects of the Church in Africa: Theological Reflections of the 21st Century* (Nairobi, 2005), 100.

female. This notion gives rise to a binary and dichotomous understanding of gender. Actually, there is no gender, just sex: masculinity and femininity are not understood as social and variable constructs but are the distinctive essential characteristics of men and women respectively, related to the fundamental difference between male and female at the point of creation.[123] Such an understanding is expressed, for example, in the following quotation from the booklet *About Boys*: 'You are a boy or a man and when God created human beings, he distinctly created them male and female. By this definition, as a boy you will behave completely differently from a girl, because you are living your masculinity.'[124] The quotation does not make clear how this essential masculinity is understood, but clearly it is the opposite of femininity. Being a man is considered something completely different from being a woman. Therefore, marriage is essential in this theological line of thought, because it is in marriage that both sexes complement each other and become 'one body'.[125] In Catholic doctrine this complementarity of the sexes is understood not only biologically or psychologically but also ontologically. As John Paul II explained in his *Letter to Women*: 'It is only through the duality of the "masculine" and the "feminine" that the "human" finds full realization.'[126]

While the idea of complementarity ideally creates a balance between man and woman, 'the masculine' and 'the feminine', it tends towards a gender hierarchy. In the subtlety of official church documents, this is a hierarchy 'not so much in the sense that one party submits to the other but rather that the designated role for the female gender is one that is inherently more repressive'.[127] However, I found men in Regiment parish to be less subtle. They often referred to the Genesis 2 creation story, which tells that God first created man and then made woman from a rib of man. For them, the chronological order in this narrative is a principal order that constitutes a hierarchy of male and female. They say, for example, that because man was created first, in the sexual act 'always the man should be on top'.[128] For the same reason in marriage the husband is supposed to be the

---

[123] John Paul II, who has greatly developed Catholic doctrine on sexual difference, understands the bodily creation of humankind as male and female in terms of an ontological duality of masculinity and femininity (see John Paul II, *Man and Woman He Created them: A Theology of the Body* (Boston, 2006), 161). According to his theology, 'masculinity, femininity – namely, sex – is the original sign of a creative donation and at the same time the sign of a gift that man, male–female, becomes aware of as a gift lived so to speak in an original way' (ibid., 183).

[124] Kiura, *About Boys*, 8.

[125] B.C. Chilufya, 'Christian Marriage: What is it?', *The Parish Newsletter*, 114 (19 November 2006).

[126] John Paul II, Letter to Women (Rome, 1995), no. 7.

[127] A.H. Kalbian, *Sexing the Church: Gender, Power, and Ethics in Contemporary Catholicism* (Bloomington, 2005), 97–8.

[128] Interview with John Kabonde, Lusaka, 14 July 2009.

head while the wife is the helper.[129] Perceptions like these may be informed by booklets which, referring to Genesis 2, suggest that for boys the inclination 'to lead, to take responsibility, and even to be the boss' is completely natural.[130] Thus, in spite of an emphasis on equality, this gender ideology still allows for men to be 'on top', to be 'the boss' or 'the head' because this is considered part of masculinity as distinct from femininity. Only some parishioners, in particular those involved in Marriage Encounter, are critical of such views. They may even reject the concept of male headship because it contradicts the idea of equality of men and women. Generally, a hierarchical ordering of gender relations as such is not considered a problem in the parish. It is only emphasised that men should not misuse their position to oppress women. Putting it more positively, men are challenged to respect the equal human dignity of their female partners. Clearly, the theological anthropology derived from the Genesis accounts of creation results in an ambiguous gender ideology. It is in this ambiguous ideological space that masculinities are (re)defined and gender relations are (re)shaped in the parish.

Men, the Community and the Church as Family of God

As mentioned above, critical issues concerning men and masculinities are not very explicitly addressed in Regiment parish, and neither is an ideal of masculinity actively promoted. Moreover, documents from the Zambian bishops indicate a concern with *women's* issues but these are hardly analysed as *gender* issues and do not lead to an explicit concern about men and masculinities. Asked for an explanation, Nsanzurwimo pointed out that gender too often is understood in terms of the individual, as the equality of man and woman. He criticises this as a Western approach that easily leads to competition of women with men, in which women seek to become like men. According to Nsanzurwimo, the church opts for a different approach, which does not take the individual as a starting point but the family and the community. Describing this approach he says:

> [I]f we could really find a way to make everybody participate in the life of the family and the church and the community, that would be the ideal for me. So it is about participation in the community, and about the community allowing or promoting, making possible, for each individual, men and women, to give their best.[131]

---

[129] Cf. interview with Chaba Soko, Lusaka, 30 June 2009.
[130] Nganda, *Boys Growing Up*, 16.
[131] Interview with Fr Marc Nsanzurwimo (parish priest), Lusaka, 28 July 2009.

This communitarian approach to gender, which corresponds for example to the work of the influential Catholic theologian Bénézet Bujo,[132] implies that the concern of the church is not primarily with equal rights and power of women and men but with the participation of women and men in the community. As a consequence, it is not men's power as such that is considered a problem but the possible abuse of that power. As Nsanzurwimo put it, men's position of authority and headship is not intended to be 'a tool for domination' but 'a ministry, a way of service to the family and the community'.[133] This service is understood in terms of responsibilities and duties, some of which have been outlined above, which are related to men's position of authority. Problems only arise 'when the man does not match up to what is expected from him. That is when he exaggerates his role, forgetting the other people in the community.'[134]

The community ideal is reflected theologically in the ecclesiology of the church as the Family of God. Following the 1994 African Synod, this ecclesiology has been adopted by the Catholic Church in Africa and has become popular in African Catholic theology.[135] The metaphor of the church as family takes the human family as an image for being church. Even more, in this ecclesiology the human family is understood to be the 'domestic church' or 'the first cell of the living ecclesial community'.[136] Joseph Gelfer's observation of an ambivalence towards the family in North American Catholic men's ministries, which he explains by the Catholic preference for the church as a spiritual community (with a celibate clergy) over the natural family, apparently does not apply to the African context.[137] Here, the ecclesiology of the family of God presents an integrated understanding of the natural and the spiritual family. Though the celibacy of priests has implications for Catholic masculinity (see below), it appears that the supremacy of the family, and of the man's role within the family, is only confirmed by the metaphor of the church as a family.

When the metaphor is turned around, not only is the human family an image of the church but also the church is an image of the human family. The Catholic Church, as is clear from its organisational structure, is quite a hierarchical and patriarchal institution. Obviously, it is headed by priests, bishops and finally the Pope – all of whom are 'fathers'. What does this mean for the human family

---

[132] See B. Bujo, *The Ethical Dimension of Community: The African Model and the Dialogue between North and South* (Nairobi, 1998), especially chapter 7 entitled 'Preliminary Remarks on a Feminist Theology in Africa'.

[133] Interview with Fr Marc Nsanzurwimo, Lusaka, 28 July 2009.

[134] Interview with Fr Marc Nsanzurwimo, Lusaka, 4 November 2008.

[135] Cf. A.E. Orobator, *The Church as Family: African Ecclesiology in its Social Context* (Nairobi, 2000).

[136] John Paul II, *Post-Synodal Apostolic Exhortation Ecclesia in Africa*, no. 80.

[137] J. Gelfer, *Numen, Old Men: Contemporary Masculine Spiritualities and the Problem of Patriarchy* (London, 2009), 88.

and for the position of the man in the family? It seems that just as priests and bishops represent Christ as the head of the church, men as husbands and fathers are perceived as representing Christ in the 'domestic churches', that is, in their marriages and families. This idea is considered a crucial resource for responsible, serving and loving manhood – a notion that challenges men rather than affirming their position of power. For example, with reference to Ephesians 5:22–8 – where the relationship of husband and wife is presented analogously as the relationship between Christ and the church – a parishioner commented that 'what Paul is teaching is far more challenging for men than for women'.[138] In his opinion, for a man to truly love his wife is far more difficult than for a woman to submit to her husband. It appears that for men in the family, as much as for priests in the church as family of God, headship and leadership is modelled on Christ and is defined in terms of love, service and sacrifice. If men would take this seriously and practise headship in this way, Nsanzurwimo believes, 'the feminists would not have anything against Scripture'.[139]

As Aline Kalbian points out in her book *Sexing the Church*, in official Catholic writings metaphors of the church are powerful and have implicit or explicit meanings related to gender and sexuality.[140] Whereas the metaphor of the church as the people of God, which became popular in the RCC after Vatican Council II, is a 'profoundly democratic and egalitarian' image,[141] the metaphor of the church as (an African) family may be democratic but is not fully egalitarian. Both metaphors have a communitarian connotation, but in the family metaphor hierarchical relationships between men and women are not necessarily considered problematic. Following this metaphor, the concern is more about the participation of women and men – in their respective roles – in the family, the community and the church than about inequalities in gender relations as such. Yet out of this concern for everybody's participation in, and contribution to, the wellbeing of the community, the theological imaginary of the church as the family of God implicitly challenges oppressive types of masculinity and redefines male power from domination into love, sacrifice and service.

Saints and Religious Figures: Representations of Male Virtues

One of the characteristics of Catholicism is the role of saint figures derived from the biblical and Christian tradition. Gelfer found the devotion to saints, in particular St Joseph, a common feature of Catholic men's ministries in North America.[142] However, he does not elaborate on the significance of saints for the way Catholic masculinities are constructed. Sociologically, saints can be considered as

---

[138] Mr Nyirenda, in the interview with Henry and Linda Nyirenda, Lusaka, 7 July 2009.
[139] Interview with Fr Marc Nsanzurwimo (parish priest), Lusaka, 4 November 2008.
[140] Kalbian, *Sexing the Church*, 108–20.
[141] Ibid., 112.
[142] Gelfer, *Numen, Old Men*, 92.

constructions, meaning that 'they are remodelled in the collective representation which is made of them'.[143] As such they function as icons of holiness, objects of veneration and models for imitation. The constructedness of saints also draws attention to their political role: the particular meanings of a saint reflect the concerns and priorities of those who remember and venerate that saint and/or of those who promote the cult of a certain saint.[144] Therefore it is crucial to investigate male saints and the specific meanings they represent, and their implications for the construction of Catholic masculinity. In Regiment parish, St Joachim in particular plays a central role, though St Joseph is also frequently mentioned.

As the patron of the men's organisation, St Joachim is explicitly presented as an icon of Catholic manhood.[145] Actually it is a major objective of the group to promote its patron as the role model for Catholic men. As the constitution reads:

> Joachim is the model of every Catholic husband and father. He was a model of love, faithfulness, obedience, devotion, diligence, goodness, openness of husband and wife to one another. He is still a model of Catholic men. Joachim is a symbol of Christian life to all men who persevere to live happy marriages despite the shortcomings and misguiding from the other partner.[146]

When saints are remodelled, this quotation can be considered as an example of the collective representation that is made of the historical figure of Joachim. It is interesting, then, to observe the virtues associated with Joachim that make him a model for Catholic men: love, faithfulness, obedience, devotion, diligence, goodness, and marital openness. Apparently, these virtues, which largely correspond with the notions of responsibility, spirituality and the family man outlined above, are considered crucial for Catholic men today.

Members of St Joachim men's organisation indicate that their patron indeed functions as a role model. For them, Joachim embodies the virtues they seek to possess. Two exemplary qualities of Joachim are mentioned in particular: his piety and his commitment to his wife and family. As someone said: 'For me he is a role model in prayer, as he is an example in building a praying family, and he was a very loving husband as he was committed to his wife and his family.'[147] It is often mentioned that Joachim remained faithful to his wife Anne, although their marriage was childless for many years. In a cultural context where childlessness

---

[143] P. Delooz, 'Towards a Sociological Study of Canonized Sainthood in the Catholic Church', in S. Wilson (ed.), *Saints and their Cults: Studies in Religious Sociology, Folklore and History* (Cambridge, 1985), 195.

[144] Cf. S. Ditchfield, 'Thinking with Saints: Sanctity and Society in the Early Modern World', in F. Meltzer and J. Elsner (eds), *Saints: Faith Without Border* (Chicago, 2011), 185–8.

[145] See Van Klinken, *St. Joachim as a Model of Catholic Manhood*.

[146] *Constitution of St Joachim Catholic Men's Organization*, 1.

[147] Interview with Robert Kalumbila, Lusaka, 12 November 2008.

is associated with many taboos and is often a reason for separation or divorce, this is considered an example to follow. St Joachim embodies the 'new spirituality of marriage' that according to Catholic theologian Bujo is needed in Africa, especially among men.[148] Interestingly, the aspect of faithfulness is also applied to the context of HIV. For Joachim members, their patron saint demonstrates that HIV prevention through faithfulness is not only necessary but also possible.

As much as St Joachim is a representation of male virtues imitated by the members of the men's organisation, these members themselves appear as embodied representations of the same virtues associated with their patron. Though the Joachim members are small in number they are prominently present in the parish. They are particularly visible when wearing their blue uniforms, two Sundays a month, on Christian holidays including the Feast Day of St Joachim and St Anne (26 July) and at funerals. The meaning of the uniform colours is explained in the constitution: the main colour is light blue, the heavenly colour (which in Catholicism is also the colour of the Virgin Mary); the white blouse refers to faith, purity and goodness; the black belt symbolises the tying of sin, and the black shoes stand for the stamping down on sin.[149] The uniform symbolises the spiritual orientation in life of the members of St Joachim: they no longer set their hearts on earthly things but live up to different values. Clearly, when wearing the uniform with its symbolic meanings the Joachim members are performing the type of masculinity they are supposed to embody. Following the theoretical notion of the performativity of gender, wearing the uniform is an example of the 'stylized repetition of acts' through which gender identity is not just expressed but constituted.[150] To wear the heavenly blue uniform is not just an outward expression of an alternative religious masculinity but also a practice that re-constitutes the male self. The intention is that men come to embody internally the symbolic meanings associated with the uniform. In their uniforms, the Joachim members appear as living icons of holiness and in this way they also present an example to other men in the parish and community.

Besides St Joachim, St Joseph also functions as an icon of Catholic manhood. Several interviewees mentioned his name when asked for exemplary male figures. In particular, reference was made to the way Joseph responded to Mary after he found her pregnant:

---

[148] According to Bujo, the way African men influenced by cultural traditions and social expectations deal with childlessness in their marriage calls for 'a new spirituality of marriage' for Africa.' B. Bujo, *African Theology in its Social Context* (Nairobi, 1992), 111.

[149] *Constitution of St Joachim Catholic Men's Organization*, 6.

[150] J. Butler, *Gender Trouble: Feminism and the Subversion of Identity*, 2nd edn (London, 2006), 191. For a discussion on the performativity of masculinity, in particular the role of clothing, see T.W. Reeser, *Masculinities in Theory: An Introduction* (Malden, 2010), 81–90.

There was that social pressure when she got pregnant. Joseph had already decided to let Mary go, but silently. There was that consideration. And given the Jewish custom, the way they treated women, I think he did so because of that equality. I get inspiration from that. And then they go to Jerusalem as a family, even when Jesus was just born they went together, and they went to Egypt. You can see that commitment to his family.[151]

Likewise, Nsanzurwimo referred to 'the many rumours which husbands hear about their wives' and then mentions Joseph as a role model for Catholic men.[152] The virtues associated with St Joseph are patience, sacrifice, fidelity and commitment. These qualities, it is suggested, are the ones that enabled the Holy Family to come into being – and the Holy Family in turn is presented as the model for Catholic family life.[153]

Referring to the example of Joseph, in the quotation above the interviewee simply stated: 'I get inspiration from that!'[154] This illustrates how figures such as Joachim and Joseph function: They represent certain virtues and qualities which, through a devotional practice, come to inspire men who subsequently seek to model their lives on these heroes of faith. This devotion appears to be a gendered phenomenon: men tend to identify with male saints, and they understand the virtues represented by these saints as qualities of not only Christian life but also Catholic manhood.

Apart from saint figures, some interviewees also mentioned Jesus Christ as a role model. What exactly they gain from this model differs. Some refer to general virtues such as courage, sacrifice, patience and humility. Others refer more specifically to the way Jesus dealt with temptations (cf. Matthew 4:1–11). The very fact that Jesus was tempted provides a point of identification, and his ability to resist temptations is a point of inspiration and encouragement:

> When Jesus Christ got baptised he went through temptations. Jesus Christ is saying: I also went through temptations; I know where you are going through. So if he went through temptations, who am I? God is not protecting me from temptations; a lot of them are coming, so the question is how you face them.[155]

Clearly, for this man Jesus is a figure he can identify with and who gives him strength to face temptations and other challenges. The references to Jesus, Joseph

---

[151] Interview with Jack Mwale, Lusaka, 6 July 2009.
[152] Interview with Fr Marc Nsanzurwimo, Lusaka, 28 July 2009.
[153] According to Pope John Paull II, 'the Holy Family, which according to the Gospel lived for a time in Africa, is the prototype and example for all Christian families and the model and spiritual source for every Christian family'. Cf. John Paul II, *Post-Synodal Apostolic Exhortation Ecclesia in Africa*, no. 81.
[154] Interview with Jack Mwale, Lusaka, 6 July 2009.
[155] Interview with John Kabonde, Lusaka, 14 July 2009.

and Joachim illustrate the significance of the Catholic tradition of saints and other religious figures to the promotion of certain 'masculine virtues'. The examples of these figures set a high moral standard; because of their spiritual significance, they not only inspire men but also function as models of imitation.

Living Up to the Ideal

Having identified the ideal of masculinity and the related moral and spiritual virtues promoted among men in the parish, the question arises as to whether and how male parishioners live up to this ideal.

Popular Catholicism

The Archbishop of Lusaka was quoted above, saying that 'most Catholic men do not participate in a number of activities taking place in the parish'.[156] Apparently, popular Catholicism especially among men is not associated with a deep involvement in the church. Referring to the popularity of the rosary beads, a parishioner commented with some disdain that most people wearing a rosary are 'traditional Catholics' who actually never pray the rosary.[157] He referred to this as an illustration of the failure of the CC-Z to really impact on people's lives, both spiritually and morally. This corresponds with the statement of a parish marital counsellor, who said that the only difference the church makes is that Catholic men have girlfriends in secret while non-Christians do it openly.[158] It is also in line with the frequent reference to men as 'Sunday worshippers'. As one young man put it, 'our Christianity is most times like elastic. Only on Sunday we go to church and think about God, but during the rest of the week we are something else.'[159]

The widespread perception of Catholic men is that they drink and womanise, are hardly involved in the church and are not really committed to the Catholic faith. The suggestion is that Catholic manhood as the *lived practice* of the majority of men who identify as Catholic is characterised by a compromised loyalty to the church and a constant negotiation of its moral regulations. I do not argue here that this depiction is correct – that would require a different type of research. Most likely it is a generalised picture: levels of church involvement will vary, as will the ways in which men live up to the church's moral teachings. However, it is clear that the effect of the church's promotion of certain ideals and virtues among men should not be overestimated. The CC-Z is a mainstream church comprising a large part of the population. Most members became Catholic not by choice but by infant baptism. Combined with the inclusive ecclesiology in which the church is open to

---

[156] Mpundu, *Men, Take Up the Challenge!*
[157] Interview with Bensson Mbuzi, Lusaka, 11 November 2008.
[158] Interview with Rosalyn Banda, Lusaka, 28 October 2008.
[159] Interview with Gift Chilufya, Lusaka, 7 November 2008.

all people, this does not create a culture in which people en masse live up to the moral and spiritual standards of the church.

A Serious Devotion

Apart from Catholic masculinity as actually lived by a great number of Catholic men, it has become clear in this chapter that in the parish an alternative understanding of manhood is promoted. Though this ideal is not defined in a very explicit discourse, its characteristics have been identified above: responsibility, self-control, spirituality, and a deep commitment to the family and marriage. A number of men seek to live up to this ideal seriously. Several interviewees indicate a serious devotion and are dedicated to the moral and spiritual way of life promoted in the church. They say, for example:

> So it is very important for me to offer my life to God. That means: put God first; put God in your programmes. If you want to achieve a lot of things in your life, put God first, believe in God and ask God to lead you in your life. Pray to God through Jesus Christ and ask for the Holy Spirit. Whatever programme you do, it must be and should be the will of God because it is God who brought you in this world.[160]

> My role as a man is to try first of all to keep my baptismal vows. That is one role and from there everything flows. My involvement in Joachim is one way to live up to my baptismal vows. Also, being a man involved in church affairs, I do assist other men. Other men have noticed change in my life.[161]

Both men here express a serious commitment to what they consider a Christian life. The praxis of Christian life for these and other interviewees includes active church participation, having devotional time with prayer and Bible reading, personally and/or with the family, being faithful in their marriage, taking care of their family, and behaving in a responsible and morally proper way. Obviously, this reflects the virtues represented by exemplary saint figures such as Joachim and Joseph, and largely meets the ideal of manhood promoted in the parish.

Two interesting observations can be made on the basis of the accounts of these devout Catholic men – youths as well as adults. First, several interviewees indicate that in their serious devotion to the moral and spiritual ideal of the church, they differ from other men who engage in a more popular Catholicism. They distinguish themselves, claiming that they live up to different values and are more faithful husbands and more committed parishioners. The social consequence is that they sometimes feel isolated: 'Living up to the Christian values, sometimes it leaves

---

[160] Interview with John Kabonde, Lusaka, 14 July 2009.
[161] Interview with Marc Bwali, Lusaka, 9 November 2008.

you without friends.'[162] Another man told me: 'Normally what they do is they call me mad. Which means you are a lunatic, you are not normal, you are not indulging in what most of the people are doing.'[163] To provide men with an alternative 'safe' place for socialising, the parish has created social spaces, for example in the St Joachim fellowship and in the youth group. Here men meet, recreate and support each other to live up to the ideal. The church hopes to centre men's social lives on the church. In some cases the church seems to be successful, as is indicated by this statement of one young man: 'My life is just through our church. Even when I have a party, it is attached to church: a guy from church having a party at church.'[164]

A second observation is that several devout men indicated their church involvement is at least partly the result of the influence of their wives. For example, several members of St Joachim men's organisation recounted how they joined the group at their wives' insistence. As one of them told me:

> My madam was in St Anne and she encouraged me to join St Joachim. She felt guilty that I was not engaged that much in the church. I only went there on Sunday, but she wanted me to be involved in the small Christian community, too, and in a lay organisation. She thought this would help me to foster and to keep my faith. ... The lay group has kept me from immoral activities. I used to drink, but I stopped drinking when joining St Joachim. It also helped me to keep from womanising. Beer drinking easily makes one think about going after women, you know. Now I keep far from that.[165]

This personal account illustrates the statement in a Catholic youth magazine that women in marriage 'have the power to change a man'.[166] Women seem to be quite aware of this power. In a discussion about problems with men in marriages and families, and the way to overcome these, the women of the Nazareth group stated: 'When a man is married, the influence can come through us, from the wives to the husbands.'[167] Asked for an example of this influence, I was told that they often encourage their husbands to attend Mass and to participate in parish life, hoping that this will keep them away from the bars and will make them more faithful

---

[162] Interview with Raymond Malambo, Lusaka, 27 July 2009.
[163] Interview with Bensson Mbuzi, Lusaka, 11 November 2008.
[164] Interview with Chaba Soko, Lusaka, 25 June 2009.
[165] Interview with Robert Kalumbila, Lusaka, 12 November 2008.
[166] The youth magazine *Speak Out!* published an 'Open letter to my future wife' where the following statement was made: 'I know you have the power to change a man.' In the letter a young man encouraged his future wife to nurture him into the best husband and person he could be. See S. Kalunga, 'Open Letter to My Future Wife', *Speak Out!*, 26/3 (2009): 17.
[167] Interview with members of the Nazareth group in Regiment Parish, Lusaka, 27 October 2008.

husbands and fathers. It is an example of female agency in the transformation of masculinities. Success may be limited, but at least some men bear witness to their wives' efforts. Thanks to their wives, they have become more devoted and pious Catholic men.

Not too Strict ...

Interestingly, even those men who are seriously committed to the church and try to live up to its moral and spiritual ideals often indicate a flexible understanding of the church's moral regulations. To be sure, some interviewees show a radical commitment – one of them even said that he has put himself 'in the lifestyle of a monk',[168] but the more common attitude seems to be that moral restrictions are respected but are not taken and adhered to strictly. '[We are] not breaking the rule but bending it a bit', a young man stated when discussing how he and his girlfriend deal with intimacy.[169] Though he considers sexual intercourse before marriage unacceptable, he believes a certain level of intimacy is legitimate, even though he realises that it 'may lead us into something else'. Likewise, another young man stated that according to African culture and the Bible, 'the only thing you are not allowed to do before marriage is sex; the rest you can do', though he did admit that he has had sexual intercourse with his girlfriend several times.[170] He had to do so, he explained, in order to avoid the impression that he is not 'a good man'. Both interviewees seem to exercise their sexuality in a responsible way, but they clearly negotiate the strict regulations of the church. Their attitude may correspond with a more general understanding in the parish. Someone who has been working with parish youth for many years explained:

> I say to them: enjoy the days of your youth. When you are young, you can engage yourself in the activities for the youth, but time will come that you have to change. And if you are so involved in a wrong thing, it will be difficult to change. So you can do certain things while you are young, but remember: you have to stop this. With me, I am not too strict. And that is what they appreciate in me. I am correcting them, but not saying: don't do this. Just talking about things with them, giving them something to think about in a very friendly way.[171]

This relatively mild and flexible stance towards behavioural issues allows the youth some space to negotiate and to deviate from the moral regulations of the church. Hence, it also becomes understandable why an active parishioner told me that he has indeed enjoyed the years of his youth by having many girlfriends, adding that there is no need to regret this. Though stating that 'at a certain stage

---

[168] Interview with William Kunda, Lusaka, 11 November 2008.
[169] Interview with Chaba Soko, Lusaka, 25 June 2009.
[170] Interview with John Kabonde, Lusaka, 14 July 2009.
[171] Interview with Kedrick Mbuzi, Lusaka, 14 July 2009.

as a man you have to mature', for him it is equally true that 'of course when I was a bachelor I enjoyed myself'.[172] As mentioned above, the 'journey towards manhood' is viewed as a growth towards maturity.[173] How long the journey may take and what is allowed during the journey are not defined. However, the impression gained is that for youths (but possibly also for adults) it is considered acceptable, or at least understandable, that along this journey men will not always be able to fully control themselves.[174]

The Fear of AIDS and Divine Judgement

Though the moral regulations are not always interpreted and dealt with very strictly, men's motivation to follow these regulations appears to be reinforced by the reality of AIDS. Many interviewees indicate that they have been directly affected by the HIV epidemic, as they have lost relatives and friends and are faced with the challenge of taking care of cousins whose parents died from AIDS. Hence, several men acknowledged a realisation that 'AIDS is real'. Or, as a young man put it: 'Our elders are burying us, rather than we burying our elders.'[175] This realisation and the understanding that many people become infected because of risky sexual behaviour have both reinforced a commitment to the norms of sexual abstinence before marriage, or fidelity within marriage, and to the moral values promoted by the church in general. As one interviewee explained:

> I have lost several friends and relatives as a consequence of their lifestyle. They died because of HIV/AIDS, or because of an accident as a result of drinking. This reminded me that life can end easily, and that the question is where I will be then. I realised that I had to live with my Lord. The presence of HIV/AIDS in our community, and the suffering I have seen among friends, made me realise that faithfulness to your wife is crucial and life-protecting.[176]

Prevention messages sometimes explicitly allude to the fear of the reality of HIV and AIDS. For example, a booklet states: 'Unfaithfulness in married life opens

---

[172] Interview with Haggai Mwansa, Lusaka, 6 July 2009.

[173] Kiura, *About Boys*, 12.

[174] See, for instance, Nganda, *Boys Growing Up*, 22, which reads: 'You have not yet matured into a man. Being still in the maturing process, you have not yet succeeded in controlling your desires. Today you are eager to be helpful and kind. Tomorrow you are thinking of how you can avoid being bothered by anyone asking for help. At times you want to use the precious years of your youth to become a good and responsible person. But soon afterwards, you are filled with a strong desire to simply enjoy yourself with the girls, smoke, drink, and attend nightclubs.'

[175] Interview with Titus Mundia, Lusaka, 26 October 2008.

[176] Interview with Robert Kalumbila, Lusaka, 12 November 2008.

the door to the killer called AIDS.'[177] Likewise, in the men's organisation of St Joachim, it is underlined that 'AIDS comes about because of unfaithfulness' as a justification for the insistence upon marital fidelity among the members.[178]

The above quotation shows that there is more than just a fear of AIDS. The interviewee places his renewed commitment to marital fidelity in a religious discourse: he realised that he had to live with the Lord. This is not just informed by the confrontation with friends and relatives who are dying, but by the subsequent reminder that 'life can end easily' and the introspective question, 'where I will be then?' This reflects an awareness of personal judgement, and the related issue of salvation after death. Though this doctrine does not appear to be very prominent in the spirituality of parishioners nor in the church's teaching, it seems to be part of people's basic understanding of the Christian faith. Sometimes reference is made to the idea of judgment by God in order to underline the need to live up to the moral regulations of the church. For example, after *About Boys* has emphasised the need for boys to control their sexual energies, it reads: 'As a young man, you need to look after your soul. ... God will bring every deed into judgment, with every secret thing, whether good or evil.'[179] Ideas like this cultivate a sense of accountability to God for one's individual deeds. This seems to motivate at least some men to discipline themselves and live up to the moral norms related to Catholic manhood.

Conclusion

This chapter has provided what I called in Chapter 1 'a theological ethnography' of masculinity in a Catholic parish. The aim was to explore the contribution of Regiment parish to a transformation of masculinities in the context of the HIV epidemic. It can be concluded that the parish, though it has actively responded to issues of HIV and AIDS from an early stage, so far has not engaged in a proactive campaign to change men and transform masculinities. There is a concern in the parish and wider in the CC-Z about men and certain patterns of male behaviour, but critical issues are not so explicitly addressed, and when they are addressed it is in a relatively nuanced manner. The church makes some efforts to 'evangelise' men, trying to make them more familiar with the church's teaching and to increase their church involvement, but no well-defined alternative ideal of Catholic manhood is actively promoted. Rather than being preached and taught about, the moral and spiritual characteristics of manhood are symbolically presented by a saint figure such as Joachim, who is modelled as a pious and responsible family man.

From his comparative study of masculinities in Catholic and Evangelical men's movements in the United States of America, Joseph Gelfer makes two interesting

---

[177] O. Hirmer, *About the Killer Called AIDS* (Nairobi, 2001), 7.
[178] Interview with Marc Bwali, Lusaka, 9 November 2008.
[179] Kiura, *About Boys*, 27.

conclusions in light of the Regiment case study. First, he points out that Catholic men's ministries promote 'a broader spectrum of masculinity which is generally less patriarchal'.[180] Second, he argues that Catholic notions of masculinity are 'slightly queer', with queer not so much understood as gay orientation but – in line with queer theory – as 'a little strange', that which 'disturbs consistency'.[181] Though I will engage in a comparison of Regiment parish and the Pentecostal case study only in Chapter 5, here I want to briefly reflect on Gelfer's findings in relation to Regiment parish. First, though Regiment does not really *promote* various forms of masculinity, it is clear that because there is not one explicitly defined ideal of masculinity, the parish does allow for a broader spectrum of masculinities. Catholic men are left with space for different interpretations and perceptions and they can negotiate the moral norms of the church. The result is that different types of masculinity can be found in the parish and are considered more or less acceptable. For example, many men may consider themselves to be heads of their families, but some parishioners explicitly reject this notion. Drinking alcohol is considered acceptable by the church, but some parishioners take a radical stance and emphasise the need of self-control or abstinence in this area. With regard to the patriarchal character of Catholic masculinity, I have pointed to the ambiguous gender ideology underlying the understanding of masculinity and the organisation of gender relations in Regiment parish and wider Catholic circles: on the one hand, the equality or equal human dignity of men and women is emphasised, but on the other hand sexual difference tends to be ordered in a hierarchical way. Again, this leaves space for variation. The same can be said of the ways in which Catholic men are 'patriarchal'. Gelfer's second point, the queerness of Catholic masculinity, may be difficult to apply to a Zambian Catholic case study, as the concept of queer and its theoretical foundations are rather Western. However, queerness among others draws attention to the performativity of gender, which opens a new perspective on the St Joachim men's organisation. Here, men perform and come to embody an ideal of Catholic masculinity by wearing their uniforms, praying the rosary, showing devotion to Mary, etcetera. In their heavenly blue uniforms the Joachim members indeed are a little strange, both in relation to hegemonic forms of masculinity in society and to most of their fellow Catholic men. The blue colour, which clearly associates them with Mary (who is always dressed in blue), brings in a feminine element in their performance of masculinity, as does the red rose. If the Joachim members are an elite of Catholic men and St Joachim represents the ideal of Catholic manhood in the current Zambian context, Catholic masculinity – though obviously heterosexual – is indeed slightly queer. Queer or not, the members of St Joachim strive to be responsible husbands and fathers, taking their role in the church as the Family of God to begin in the 'domestic church' – that is, in their own families.

---

[180] Gelfer, *Numen, Old Men*, 94.
[181] Ibid., 95–6.

Chapter 4
Promoting 'Biblical Manhood': Masculinities in a Pentecostal Church

'The Bible tells that Adam was created first, and instructions were given to men, to the male. We men are the head, but you have to live up to it. We like to be the head, but we don't like to live up to the responsibility. That's our problem!'[1] If the politics of transforming masculinities can be captured in one quotation, it is this one, taken from Joshua Banda, bishop of Northmead Assembly of God, the second case study. The quote highlights the role of the Bible as the authoritative source and of Adam as an archetypal figure. It presents male headship as a central concept and shows how headship is associated with responsibility. This brief quote illustrates how the problem of men and masculinity is understood and gives an indication of the way this problem is addressed and how men are targeted for a change. The quote is from a sermon in a series on the theme *Fatherhood in the 21st Century*, preached by Banda. The preaching of such a series shows that fatherhood, and actually the broader topic of manhood, has become an explicit theme in the church, not at least as a response to issues raised by the HIV epidemic. This is what makes Northmead Assembly of God such an interesting case study.[2]

Northmead Assembly of God

Northmead Assembly of God (NAOG) is located in Northmead, one of the suburbs of Lusaka. Founded in 1971 as a Bible study group, the church has become one of the prominent Pentecostal churches in the city. Over the years it has grown into a congregation with a membership of over 2,000. The members of the church are relatively well educated and generally belong to the middle class. They come from all over the city and most of them live in the low-density areas of the suburbs. The majority of the people attending Sunday services are youths and young adults, including quite a number of students. Since 1995 NAOG has been under the leadership of Joshua H.K. Banda, who is the church's senior pastor and a bishop in the Pentecostal Assemblies of God in Zambia. The church's website portrays Banda as a high-profile leader with an international status:

---

[1] J. Banda, *Fatherhood in the 21st Century – Part 2* (Lusaka, 2008), DVD.

[2] This chapter is partly based on interviews. All names of interviewees mentioned in the footnotes are fictive except when referring to members of the church leadership (the bishop and pastors, who were interviewed in their professional role).

Now 45 years old and in his 26th year of Christian ministry, Bishop Banda has travelled widely in Africa and abroad. ... The Bishop has become a notable and influential voice on national issues in Zambia and is a highly sought after international conference speaker.[3]

In a recent study on Pentecostal Christianity in Zambia, Banda is indeed mentioned as one of the prominent Christian leaders in the country.[4] He can be found regularly in the media, commenting on national affairs. Banda is assisted by a team of eight pastors and by a number of elders and deacons. Each of them bears responsibility for a particular ministry, and together they form the church's governing body. Although the Pentecostal Assemblies of God in Zambia do ordain women, none of the pastors in NAOG is female. The bishop's wife does not have a formal position on the church board but she is actively involved in the church.

NAOG is associated with the Pentecostal Assemblies of God in Zambia. This fellowship of over 1,400 churches is a member of the ecumenically oriented Evangelical Fellowship of Zambia. The Assemblies of God stand historically in the tradition of North American classical Pentecostalism. NAOG shares the major theological characteristics of Pentecostal Christianity: the emphasis on personal salvation in Jesus Christ, the importance of the born-again experience, the transformation of one's life towards the holiness ideal, and openness to charismatic phenomena such as speaking in tongues, prophecy and healing.[5]

At the centre of the congregational life in NAOG are the church services. On Sunday morning two identical services are held in English, with the second being translated into a vernacular language. Each service consists of two main parts: worship and preaching. The church has various ministries that have their monthly meetings on Sunday afternoon: the men's ministry, the married couples' ministry, the singles' ministry and the women's ministry. There also is a youth ministry, which meets weekly on Saturday. All church members are expected to participate in a home cell group for weekly Bible study, prayer and fellowship. The vision of the church is 'to possess the land by reaching unreached peoples and nations'.[6] This indicates a strong missionary drive that is expressed through several evangelising

---

[3] 'Biographical Profile of Bishop Joshua H.K. Banda', website of Northmead Assembly of God, accessed 6 January 2009, http://northmeadassembly.org/index.php?option=com_content&task=view&id=13&Itemid=27.

[4] A.M. Cheyeka, 'Towards a History of the Charismatic Churches in Post-Colonial Zambia', in J.B. Gewald, M. Hinfelaar and G. Macola (eds), *One Zambia, Many Histories: Towards a History of Post-Colonial Zambia* (Leiden, 2008), 150.

[5] See J.K. Asamoah-Gyadu, 'Born of Water and the Spirit: Pentecostal/Charismatic Christianity in Africa', in O.U. Kalu (ed.), *African Christianity: An African Story* (Pretoria, 2005), 389.

[6] 'Missions', website of Northmead Assembly of God, accessed 23 February 2012, http://www.northmeadassembly.org/index.php?option=com_content&view=article&id=240&Itemid=29.

and church planting activities. However, propagating a holistic understanding of the Gospel, Banda emphasises that mission is not solely about winning souls but also about social issues. From this perspective, he considers the HIV epidemic a 'missionary opportunity':

> On the continent of Africa there is literally no family that is untouched. So if we give attention to the area of meeting needs related to HIV/AIDS, we will truly have an opportunity to meet human needs. And in a sense we will have an opportunity to do mission. We should not look at people just as candidates for heaven; they have a life to live here on earth.[7]

Out of this vision the church has established several 'outreach programmes'. Examples are the Circle of Hope Clinic for HIV testing and treatment, the Lazarus Project for street children, and Operation Paseli for the rehabilitation of sex workers. The church also has set up the radio programme *Choosing Hope* and the TV programme *The Liberating Truth*, based on the conviction that '[t]he church in the media can combat the depression, loss of focus, HIV/AIDS and many issues that our country and people are faced with'.[8] Realising that church members themselves are also at risk of contracting HIV, the church leadership has sought to create awareness in the congregation and encourages a preventive lifestyle. The basic notion of this lifestyle is that 'sexual purity guarantees you freedom from being infected'.[9] At the same time, Banda addresses popular and stigmatising perceptions such as that people with HIV have had an immoral past, that they bear the consequences of their own lust, that HIV is a curse and that it shows that God's judgement is still at work. Opposing these beliefs he states that every sickness including AIDS comes from 'the enemy' rather than from God.[10]

Where are Men and Masculinities Addressed?

In NAOG there is an explicit discourse in which men and issues related to masculinity are critically addressed and in which an alternative ideal of manhood is defined. Where this discourse is found precisely? In other words, what are the places where men are addressed and masculinities are reconstructed in the church?

---

[7] J. Banda, *HIV&AIDS and Stigma in the Church* (Lusaka, 2008), DVD.

[8] 'The Liberating Truth', website of Northmead Assembly of God, accessed 23 February 2012, http://www.northmeadassembly.org/index.php?option=com_content&view=article&id=246:the-liberating-truth&catid=51:liberating-truth&Itemid=43.

[9] 'Choosing Hope', website of Northmead Assembly of God, accessed 23 February 2012, http://www.northmeadassembly.org/index.php?option=com_content&view=article&id=263:about-choosing-hope&catid=57:choosing-hope&Itemid=53.

[10] Banda, *HIV&AIDS and Stigma in the Church*.

Sermons

Preaching is a crucial part of the Sunday services in NAOG. Sermons are usually delivered in series on specific themes. All kind of social and political issues are addressed that affect people's lives and society. Examples are alcoholism, HIV and AIDS, domestic violence, sexuality, the presidential elections, and the country's constitutional review process. According to Banda, the pulpit is a crucial place to address issues such as these in order to raise awareness among the people.[11] The sermons reach not only the congregation but the whole country, as they are broadcast in the church's TV programme *The Liberating Truth*. Frequently, men are specifically addressed in sermons. Whatever the topic, for example marital problems, sexuality, domestic violence, HIV, alcoholism, poverty or the moral decay of the country, particular reference is made to the role of men. Moreover, it is not just the role of men that is addressed, but also the popular types of masculinity in contemporary Zambia. Most explicitly this was done in a series of sermons delivered in 2008, entitled *Fatherhood in the 21st Century*. The series aimed to explore a vision of 'biblical manhood' in the light of a perceived 'distortion of manhood' in society.[12] Another interesting series in this respect is *Cultivating a Lifestyle of Truth*, preached in 2005. The sermons dealt with issues such as alcohol, sexuality, domestic violence and other topics concerning people's lifestyle, and time and time again men are addressed in particular. Banda frequently presents himself in his sermons as a role model, particularly as a model for how men should relate to their wives.

Youth Ministry

The church's youth ministry aims to nourish the faith of the youth and to raise them in what is considered a Christian, born-again lifestyle. There is a concern that youths are not really dedicated to this lifestyle, because they belong to a second generation of Pentecostals in Zambia, or because they are attracted by a 'modern' way of life. The teaching on lifestyle is applied specifically to the area of sexuality. Time and time again in youth meetings the need to abstain from sex, to protect virginity and to keep sexual purity is underscored. The ministry is coordinated by pastor Haggai Mweene, who understands his role as being 'a father for the youth'.[13] In his opinion, young people are faced with many pressures, and they hardly have any good father figures at home or in society to coach them.

---

[11] Interview with Bishop Joshua Banda, Lusaka, 6 November 2008.

[12] In this series Banda uses the concepts of 'fatherhood' and 'manhood' interchangeably. He frequently states that 'biblical fatherhood is rooted in biblical manhood'. I will use here the more general concept of manhood, except for those cases where I discuss fatherhood in particular.

[13] Interview with Pastor Haggai Mweene, Lusaka, 20 September 2008.

The weekly meetings are attended by 40 to 60 youths, aged between 16 and 25. Most meetings are like a service, with much time for worship, prayer and preaching, but there are also meetings that are more recreational. The youth ministry is a mixed group of young people, and the preaching is usually not gender-specific. However, the norms and lifestyle promoted in the ministry directly concern young males and impact on their understanding of themselves as young Christian men.

Singles' Ministry

For young adults not yet married there is a singles' ministry in the church, which also targets single parents and those who are widowed or who are single due to divorce or separation. In the monthly meetings and in other activities, singles share and discuss the particular challenges and opportunities of their single life. Because of the social norm of marriage, stigma is a major challenge. Another difficulty is the area of sexuality, which is considered a 'no-go area' for single people. The ministry aims to create a space where single persons can support each other and receive guidance through Bible study and discussion. Just like the youth ministry, the singles' ministry includes both men and women, and the preaching and discussions are mostly not gender-specific. Yet the discourse in this group directly affects the lives and behaviour of men participating in the ministry.

Men's Fellowship

The church has a men's fellowship called *Men of Truth*. This name was chosen 'to emphasise the need for men that are truthful and faithful to their marriage, their family and the community. Thus Men of Truth is designed to promote moral values among men.'[14] In order to have men live up to these standards, the fellowship has monthly meetings with Bible study and discussions on a wide range of topics, from marriage and sexuality to business and investment. Occasionally thematic conferences are organised. In 2005 and 2006, for example, two conferences addressed the theme 'The Quest for Sexual Purity and Integrity'. Furthermore, recreational outings are frequently organised to foster fellowship among men. Last but not least, the men's fellowship contributes financially and materially to the church and helps with renovating projects of the church building.

The meetings are generally attended by 30 to 50 men. The church leadership is concerned about the low participation of men in the ministry. The majority of men are said to lack the motivation to involve themselves actively.[15] However, according to the pastor in charge, the ministry itself is also to blame, because its activities are not attractive to most of the male church members.[16] Hence, in 2009 he presented a vision to transform the ministry into a more dynamic and

---

[14] Interview with Pastor Harold Gondwe, Lusaka, 12 November 2008.
[15] Interview with Bishop Joshua Banda, Lusaka, 5 November 2009.
[16] Interview with Pastor Boyd Banda, Lusaka, 15 July 2009.

attractive fellowship. The implementation will take time, but at least the plan shows that there is a creative search to make the ministry more effective in men's lives and more visible to the life of the church. Though numerically not that large, the ministry clearly is an important instrument for the church's work with men, addressing critical issues concerning masculinity, and promoting an alternative type of manhood.

The Marriage Ministry

Quite a large ministry in the church is occupied with issues related to marriage. Pre-marital counselling is provided to couples about to be married, and monthly meetings are organised for married couples. In cases of marital problems, pastoral counselling is provided.

The primary objective of the pre-marital counselling is 'to prepare couples for marriage in order for them to develop into an ideal husband and/or wife according to biblical standards'.[17] The topics covered vary from the spiritual life of the family to family-planning methods, and from the roles and duties of husband and wife in marriage to the question of how to deal with the extended family. Also the sexual aspect of marital life is discussed. Apart from the counselling as a couple, the husband-to-be and wife-to-be are supposed to be counselled separately by a member of the men's ministry and the women's ministry respectively (though the women's ministry seems to do better in carrying out this task than the men's ministry). Once married, a couple is supposed to attend the meetings of the marriage ministry. These aim 'to promote strong and healthy marriages in the church'.[18] According to one of the coordinators, 'strong marriages make strong churches and strong nations'.[19] In the meetings, a wide range of topics concerning married life are addressed, varying from joint investments and business as a couple, to tips for 'satisfying sex in a godly marriage'. This indicates that the church is concerned with all areas of marital life, from the financial and economic to the sexual aspects. The Marriage Ministry is an important instrument of the church to work with men as (future) husbands and fathers. Certain perceptions and practices concerning men's role and attitudes in marriage and the family are challenged here, and these are corrected by 'biblical teaching'.

---

[17] Premarital Counselling General Guide, Marriage Ministry, Northmead Assembly of God.

[18] 'Church Ministries', website of Northmead Assembly of God, accessed 18 March 2009, http://www.northmeadassembly.org.zm/ministry.html.

[19] Interview with Ragies Chipoya, Lusaka, 7 October 2008.

Addressing the 'Distortion of Manhood'

In the sermon series *Fatherhood in the 21st Century*, Banda frequently states that there is a 'distortion of manhood' in society. In the sermons, as well as in the other above-mentioned places in the church, several issues illustrating this 'distortion' are explicitly discussed.

Sexuality

In NAOG, issues of sexuality are often addressed. The concern with sexuality seems to be reinforced by the HIV epidemic. To emphasise the moral values concerning sexuality is, in Banda's words, a 'prevention strategy'.[20] However, the teaching on sexuality aims to safeguard people not just from the risk of contracting HIV but first and foremost from 'sexual sin' and to promote 'sexual purity'. Therefore the church principally teaches that God intended sexuality to be enjoyed only in the context of a marital relationship. This principle is taught in a typical Pentecostal discourse, where cultural criticism is mixed with biblical references (in this case to 1 Cor. 6:15):

> Sexuality before marriage is immoral. The body is not meant for sexual immorality. That is the way people are living, as if the body was meant for sexual immorality. Do you not know that your bodies are members of Christ himself? Let not Hollywood make you think that tasting sex outside marriage is exciting. Engaging in sex without a true union with God and without a true union in marriage, you are fracturing your life.[21]

Failure to live up to moral standards is considered immoral and sinful. According to Banda, this failure is so common nowadays that there is a 'culture of seduction' in society. Explaining this eschatologically, he says that the world is entering 'the final days' in which the devil uses the area of sexuality 'as a deadly moral trap' for people to depart from God.[22] The church's moral standard concerning sexuality prohibits not only sex before marriage but also masturbation and kissing. These strict guidelines are informed by a fear of the slippery slope. As one church member stated on the issue of kissing: 'As far as I know I think you have to wait. Because of the intention of kissing, it may lead to more than kissing.'[23] Because of this risk, people are called to build 'defence lines' and to observe strict boundaries.

Interestingly, when the topic of sexual behaviour is discussed, particularly men are addressed. The sermons on *Fatherhood in the 21st Century* denounce, time and

---

[20] Interview with Bishop Joshua Banda, Lusaka, 5 November 2008.
[21] J. Banda, *Making Relationships More Meaningful – Part 1* (Lusaka, publication date unknown), DVD.
[22] J. Banda, *Cultivating a Lifestyle of Truth – Part 5* (Lusaka, 2005), DVD.
[23] Interview with Clemens Kabunko, Lusaka, 3 November 2008.

again, popular perceptions in which manhood is understood as an 'an equivalent to the male sexual organ'.[24] According to this understanding, as one church member put it,

> If you are not producing, you are not a man. You have to make a woman pregnant. … Among youngsters there is the sense that sleeping with a girl makes you a man. There is a saying: This is a man. Culturally it is considered in this way.[25]

Opposing perceptions like these, Banda states that 'biblical manhood transcends and goes beyond human sexuality'[26] and that 'human manhood is not just defining yourself as a sex machine'.[27] Cultures and societies that do so are labelled by him as 'totally distorted'.[28] The definition of manhood in terms of sexual achievement is demythologised as being inferior and immature. It is said to be not only unchristian but also unmanly: a real man should be able to control his sexual desires.

While men's assumed preoccupation with sexual achievement is explained on the basis of socio-cultural definitions of manhood, Banda also points to a biological factor. In the series *Cultivating a Lifestyle of Truth* he presents a theory that men have a particular hormone that makes them look for women, arouses them and compels them to action:

> Men by their basic physiological and biological make up tend to have the initial attraction by the opposite side just by sex. … I did some reading and found out that men receive a chemical high as soon as they see some kind of a sexual image. As soon as they see a sexual image, something happens in the body of men. There is a hormone called epinephrine that is immediately released into the bloodstream as soon as men see a sexual image.[29]

This quotation indicates quite an essentialist understanding of manhood, in which it is considered natural for men to have problems controlling their sexual lusts. Men are compared with wild mustangs: both are 'roaming, running free and wild', meaning that they do not commit themselves to anybody.[30]

Whatever the reason for men's presumed preoccupation with sex and their difficulty in handling it, men are challenged to take control over the area of sexuality in their lives and to adopt an alternative understanding of manhood. The emphasis on moral boundaries concerning sexuality is accompanied by a radical

---

[24] See J. Banda, *Fatherhood in the 21st Century – Part 3* (Lusaka, 2008), DVD.
[25] Interview with Clemens Kabunko, Lusaka, 3 November 2008.
[26] Banda, *Fatherhood – Part 3*.
[27] Banda, *Fatherhood in the 21st Century – Part 4* (Lusaka, 2008), DVD.
[28] Ibid.
[29] Banda, *Cultivating a Lifestyle of Truth – Part 6* (Lusaka, 2005), DVD.
[30] Banda, *Making Relationships – Part 1*.

yet pastoral attitude towards men struggling in this area. They are not just called on to change their lifestyle, but are also encouraged to do so with the help of God:

> There are some men here who think that you cannot be free from bad thoughts, from extramarital affairs, from unfaithfulness and things like that. I want you to know that in this day and age you can live faithfully, you can be satisfied by one woman and be happy. It can be done in the name of Jesus.[31]

The possibility of conversion is emphasised, through which a man can overcome his problems in the area of sexuality and can re-commit himself to the promoted moral values.

The church encourages men not only to be faithful themselves, but also to prevent fellow men, such as colleagues and friends, from marital infidelity. Banda criticises the permissive attitude that, in his opinion, prevails in society and makes people shy away from addressing each other. He calls each man to be his brother's keeper: 'If you have that knowledge, God holds you responsible to reach that man and to say: Sir, what you are doing is wrong.'[32]

Homosexuality

Elaborating upon recent developments threatening 'the status and nature of fatherhood in the 21st century', Banda first of all points to issues related to homosexuality.[33] For example, he refers to the legalisation of same-sex marriages in some countries, to the debate on the ordination of homosexual priests and bishops in the Anglican Communion, and to some recent developments he has observed in Zambia that tend towards a growing acceptance of homosexuality. Discussing these issues, Banda emphasises that homosexuality is not original to Zambia, and he takes a political stance by stating that the legal ban on same-sex practices should remain intact because Zambia is a Christian nation. He clearly presents an example of popular African discourse where homosexuality is considered un-African, un-Christian and a Western invention.[34] However, this does not yet explain why the issue is addressed in a sermon series on fatherhood and manhood. A closer analysis shows that the topic is used in the discursive politics on masculinity.

As Banda understands homosexuality, it represents two of his main concerns about men: their preoccupation with sexuality, and their indifference towards the

---

[31] Banda, *Fatherhood in the 21st Century – Part 1* (Lusaka, 2008), DVD.
[32] Banda, *Cultivating – Part 5*.
[33] Banda, *Fatherhood – Part 2*.
[34] Cf. P. Jenkins, *The Next Christendom: The Coming of Global Christianity*, rev. edn (Oxford, 2007), 234–40; K. Ward, 'Same-Sex Relations in Africa and the Debate on Homosexuality in East African Anglicism', *Anglican Theological Review*, 84/1 (2002), 81–111.

male role they are to play. First, he develops a unique argument about same-sex sexuality, saying that

> the only reason why a man and a man come together in same sex relations is that because of their sexual preference they claim they are only attracted to men. It is a distortion, a serious distortion! The definition here is purely by sexual means, but God's order of marriage is not defined purely by sex.[35]

Thus, because homosexuals enter into relationships out of their specific sexual preference, according to Banda, same-sex relations are only defined by sex and homosexuals are only interested in each other sexually. He contrasts this with how God has defined marriage: not just in terms of sex but first and foremost in terms of companionship, commitment and love. The crux of the argument is that Banda, having stereotyped homosexuals as sex maniacs, calls upon the (assumed heterosexual) men in the church, insisting that they should not jump into relationships just because of sex.

The second argument starts from the principle of gender complementarity. According to Banda's line of thought, man and woman are put in different places and are assigned distinctive roles, and hence they can complement each other. Because homosexual relationships do not allow for this complementarity, they are considered contrary to the order of creation. For example, it is said that 'biblical manhood is rooted in creation. And in creation God made them male and female. It is Adam and Eve and not Adam and Steve. In creation we see a man and a woman in their respective roles.'[36] Referring to Genesis 2:24, Banda explains that, according to the divine order, a man is to leave his parents in order to be united with a woman in marriage. While arguing that homosexuals are opposing this order, men in the church are called to 'find joy and gladness and fulfilment in maintaining God's order' and to accept the role and position God has intended for them.[37] Clearly, in the sermons the homosexual is presented as a counter-example of biblical manhood, and used as an example to challenge men to live sexually straight and morally upright lives and to fulfil their God-given role.[38]

The Consumption of Alcohol

The drinking of alcohol is also addressed as a critical aspect of prevalent masculinities. The church's stance is quite clear: drinking alcohol is incompatible with being born again. 'If you know Jesus as the Saviour, there is no way alcohol

---

[35] Banda, *Fatherhood – Part 2*.
[36] Banda, *Fatherhood – Part 4*.
[37] Banda, *Fatherhood in the 21st Century – Part 6* (Lusaka, 2008), DVD.
[38] For a more elaborate discussion, see A.S. van Klinken, 'The Homosexual as the Antithesis of "Biblical Manhood"? Heteronormativity and Masculinity Politics in Zambian Pentecostal Sermons', *Journal of Gender and Religion in Africa*, 17/2 (2011), 126–42.

intake can become your lifestyle.'[39] Several motivations are given for this stance. There is a theological argument suggesting that alcohol is a direct threat to one's spiritual life. Both are considered to be mutually exclusive: either one is filled with alcohol, or with the Holy Spirit.[40] There is also a concern about the social effects of alcohol. For example, the impact of alcoholism on families is mentioned, with reference to economic impoverishment and to children being neglected by their parents. Also the effect of alcohol on sexual behaviour and the consequence this can have in the context of HIV are highlighted. Referring to the HIV prevalence rates in Zambia and to the reality of people dying because of AIDS, Banda rhetorically raises the question: 'How, then, can we make beer so fashionable to our people?'[41] The church's rejection of alcohol fits in the broader Pentecostal programme of a moral reordering of society. The prohibition turns the ordinary daily life of many urbanites, with common practices such as visiting beer halls and bars and drinking in public places, into an area of immorality. It further enables control of people's leisure time, and the redirection towards church activities of time saved from 'idleness'.[42]

Although it is acknowledged that alcoholism can also be a problem for women, particularly men are addressed. Elaborating on the impoverishment of families due to alcoholism, Banda says that 'the majority of our men spend their time on the bottle' while they leave the responsibility of providing for their families to 'the hard-working African woman' – a statement that can hardly apply to the middle-class men in the church, but seems to refer to men in Zambia generally.[43] In the same sermon he points out how alcohol causes men to intimidate women sexually and contributes to the spread of HIV. Exploring these issues Banda makes a strong appeal to men to change their attitude:

> Men of Africa, listen to me. As we continue in this way we will pay heavy prices before God almighty. Wake up! We pay a very heavy price and the days of drunkenness must be behind us in the name of Jesus. As we are to live as men of truth it must be behind us, and we must restore dignity to the African home.[44]

---

[39] Banda, *Cultivating a Lifestyle of Truth – Part 3* (Lusaka, 2005), DVD.

[40] Cf. J. Banda, '*Knowing God – Part 12*', website of Northmead Assembly of God, accessed 28 September 2009, http://www.northmeadassembly.org/index.php?option=com_content&view=article&id=269%3Atheme-knowing-god-part-12&catid=37%3Abible-study&showall=1.

[41] J. Banda, 'When the Grass Withers and the Flowers Fall', website of Northmead Assembly of God, accessed 23 March 2009, http://www.northmeadassembly.org.zm/ddata/news/viewnews.cgi?category=3&id=1037458688.

[42] Cf. R. van Dijk, 'Modernity's Limits: Pentecostalism and the Moral Rejection of Alcohol in Malawi', in D.F. Bryceson (ed.), *Alcohol in Africa: Mixing Business, Pleasure, and Politics* (Portsmouth, 2002), 260–61.

[43] Banda, *Cultivating – Part 3*.

[44] Ibid.

This quotation indicates that the opposition to alcohol is informed by a concern with the dignity of the family. In order to restore the family, men have to take their responsibility in their homes as husbands and fathers. They are challenged to reject everything that is a threat to the ideal of being 'men of truth'. In line with this, advertisements that present drinking alcohol as a sign of manhood are strongly denounced. Referring to the slogan of a beer brand – 'As powerful as the men who drink it' – Banda points to something that he believes to be far more powerful, and through which men can overcome their difficulty in the area of alcohol: the grace of God. 'This grace is powerful enough to keep you joyful and to keep you on a spiritual high that does not require you to get high on alcohol.'[45]

Domestic and Sexual Violence

Another issue related to masculinity that is addressed is domestic and sexual violence. In one church service, a sketch was performed to announce a marriage weekend organised by the marriage ministry. In this sketch, a woman was swathed in bandages, indicating that she had been battered. She tries to convince her husband to attend the marriage weekend together, but he responds: 'Then they will even teach us how to stop battering!' The sketch generated laughter – a laughter of recognition? – from the congregation.[46]

Although it is acknowledged that women can be involved in spouse battering, mostly men are addressed in this area. Referring to statistics of the Zambian police, Banda says that not only is domestic violence a serious problem in society, but also that it is largely perpetrated by men. He links this with the economic dependence in many marital relationships, saying that men often misuse their economic strength over the wives, who are dependent on their husbands for their income.[47] In the series *Fatherhood in the 21st Century*, the prevalence of violence against women is mentioned as an illustration of the impairment of 'true manhood' in Zambia.[48] Referring to pastoral experiences from the church's marriage counsellors, it is stated that domestic violence occurs not only outside the church but among church members as well. Thus men are challenged to mend their ways:

> There could be wife battering husbands here today! You are living between two worlds; your conscience is seared. God wants to set you free. There is hope for you, if you will recognise that a woman has as much a right to life as you do, even if you are the breadwinner, even if you're the one that brings food into the home. ... We have husbands who lift up their hands and sing "Glory hallelujah"!

---

[45] Ibid.
[46] Church service in Northmead Assembly of God, 19 October 2008.
[47] Banda, *Fatherhood – Part 1*.
[48] Banda, *Fatherhood – Part 1*.

But if you've been using your hands to batter your wife, God considers that an indecent violent and pervasive act and calls you to repentance here today.[49]

The use of violence in the home is considered inappropriate for a Christian man. Banda even calls it 'an insult to God's divine order' that will be judged by God.[50] His argument is that man and woman are created equally in the image of God, and that the divine image in women is defiled when they are violated or abused. He also states that according to 'the biblical order', men are supposed to protect women rather than beat them.[51]

Apart from violence of husbands against their spouses, sexual violence against siblings (incest) and against women in general is also addressed. In a sermon on 2 Samuel 13, which narrates the rape of Tamar by her half-brother Amnon, Banda draws a parallel between this story and what he observes taking place in society. In his observation, contemporary men, like the ancient Amnon, often approach vulnerable women in manipulative ways, violate them, and afterwards treat them viciously and do not show any remorse. Referring to God's judgement of Amnon, he calls upon men to repent of these things.[52]

Male Domination of Women

Apart from violence against women there is a more general concern about men's domination and feelings of superiority over women. In a sermon dealing with the relationship between man and woman, Banda emphasises the 'biblical principle' of male headship in marriage, but he underlines that headship should not be understood in terms of domination. Referring to both the context of marriage and the broader context of society, he strongly denounces the way men tend to exercise their authority and power: 'What we have seen most times is male domination. And it stinks in the nostrils of God. It is a distortion of God's order. Because male domination implies that the woman is less than the man, but that's not biblical.'[53] This observation is supported by a female church member involved in marriage counselling. In her opinion the majority of marital problems arise out of men's misunderstanding of male headship. For example, men hardly consult their wives when decisions have to be made. According to this marital counsellor, 'without us as a church giving guidance, almost by default men will

---

[49] J. Banda, 'Between Two Worlds – Part II', website of Northmead Assembly of God, accessed 24 March 2009, http://www.northmeadassembly.org.zm/ddata/news/view news.cgi?category=3&id=1041935291.

[50] Banda, *Fatherhood – Part 6*.

[51] Banda, *Fatherhood – Part 3*.

[52] Banda, *Between Two Worlds – Part II*.

[53] Banda, *Fatherhood – Part 6*.

appear to be very dictatorial in their approach towards issues. And I am talking about Christian men.'[54]

The tendency of men to dominate women and to exercise power in an oppressive way is often explained as being part of 'African culture'. As one of the pastors bluntly put it, 'from a cultural point of view a man is a tyrant'.[55] Where it is felt that traditional culture looks down upon women as inferior beings, it is believed that Christianity teaches the equality of men and women. Hence Banda labels male domination over women in marriage and in society as a violation of God's order. It is part of 'the past' born-again men have to break with.[56] Thus men are challenged to change their attitudes towards women: they are to respect women's dignity and to mobilise their capacities rather than to dominate.

Overall Irresponsibility

Another more general concern is that men often neglect their responsibilities and do not fulfil the roles they have as men. This irresponsibility is addressed in several areas of life.

First, there is the irresponsibility of men as fathers. Referring to men who make a woman pregnant without taking responsibility for the child, Banda calls upon his male audience, saying: '[Y]ou cannot continue to act irresponsibly: if you have fathered a child out of wedlock you are responsible for that child. ... You are being irresponsible and God calls you to repentance in Jesus' name.'[57] It is emphasised that a man should only engage in sex when he is ready for the responsibility of taking care of a child, in other words: when he has entered marriage. However, also in the context of marriage and the family, the way men exercise the father role is evaluated negatively. Men are challenged to take their role as a father in the home more seriously, and to pay attention to their children. Yet as a female church member commented: 'Very few men are responsible, because they leave everything to women. Very few men are concerned with the way their children are growing. They leave it to the woman to do the house thing, to teach the girls and the boys.'[58]

Second, there is the irresponsibility of men as husbands and as heads of their families. This is addressed, for instance, in relation to the role of men as providers. Illustrating the 'immature masculinity' he observes in society, Banda says: 'It is a shame to see a man sitting at home and the woman going out and bringing money back home.'[59] Similar statements are made with regard to men's role as protector

---

[54] Interview with Rosy Mbuzi, Lusaka, 29 October 2008

[55] Interview with Pastor Raymond Nyirenda, Lusaka, 22 October 2008.

[56] Cf. J.E. Soothill, *Gender, Social Change and Spiritual Power: Charismatic Christianity in Ghana* (Leiden, 2007), 189.

[57] Banda, *Between Two Worlds – Part II*.

[58] Interview with Isabel Lupiya, Lusaka, 8 July 2009.

[59] Banda, *Fatherhood – Part 3*.

in the home, when the issue of domestic violence is raised. Moreover, men are addressed for not practising their role as leader in the home in a responsible way: they either do not take this role seriously, or they practise it in a dominating way. Referring to the various responsibilities men have as heads of their families, Banda concludes: 'We men are the head, but you have to live up to it. We like to be the head but we don't like to live up to the responsibility. That's our problem.'[60]

Third, there is the irresponsibility of men as leaders in society. Referring to statistics indicating that men are in the majority of leadership positions in Africa and all over the world, and to the political oppression and the social problems that Africa and the world are faced with, Banda states: 'We seem to like authority but not the responsibility for the mess in which we are.' Hence he concludes that 'we men are doing a bad job'.[61] One of the major problems with men addressed in *Fatherhood in the 21st Century* is the 'abdication of leadership', and the series aims to challenge men to recapture their position and the related responsibilities.

The presumed irresponsibility of men in all these areas of life is a major concern for Banda, one that he shares with the congregation. It is this concern that led him to preach the series on manhood:

> The aim in the series was to handle this from the spiritual side, because I was feeling that these men have to be addressed by a higher power. Maybe when they understand that this responsibility is given to them by God, they begin to see that when they lay back they are actually sinning against God. So that they get to see: look, we have been given a divine role, let me get up and do it.[62]

Thus, the irresponsibility is understood to be a sin against God. Men are called to rise up and fulfil their 'divine role'. That is how the programme of born-again conversion brings about a transformation of masculinity, as will be explored below.

The Ideal of 'Biblical Manhood'

In NAOG, not only are problematic aspects of dominant forms of masculinity explicitly addressed and challenged, but also an alternative type of masculinity is actively promoted. This ideal is called 'biblical manhood', a term occurring in the sermons on *Fatherhood in the 21st Century* more than 20 times. What is 'biblical manhood' according to these sermons and the broader discourse in the church?

---

[60] Banda, *Fatherhood – Part 2*.
[61] Banda, *Fatherhood – Part 2*.
[62] Interview with Bishop Joshua Banda, Lusaka, 5 November 2008.

Responsibility

The concept of responsibility is one of the most central notions of manhood in the church. It is mentioned time and time again, not only in sermons and church meetings but also in interviews with church members. Responsibility is also the fundamental concept in the definition of biblical manhood presented and explored by Banda in the series *Fatherhood in the 21st Century*. He derives this definition from a publication by the American Baptist pastor and prolific writer, John Piper, who is associated with the American Council on Biblical Manhood and Womanhood.[63] According to Piper's definition, 'At the heart of mature masculinity is a sense of benevolent responsibility to lead, provide for, and protect women in ways appropriate to a man's differing relationships.'[64] Banda adopts this definition and unpacks it in a number of sermons. The notion of 'benevolent responsibility' means that men are (or should be) concerned with, and focused on the well-being of others. As stated in one sermon: men are 'to serve rather than to dictate'.[65] While Piper's definition defines men's benevolent responsibility only in relation to women, Banda applies it in a broader way to the areas of marriage, the family, sexuality, the community and society.

Of course, according to the church, women must also be responsible, as every human being is believed to be endowed with responsibility towards God, others and the self. Yet responsibility is a key notion defining manhood specifically. Following Piper, Banda emphasises that men, compared to women, have a *primary* responsibility.[66] He preaches that the man bears the primary responsibility to head the marital relationship, to provide for the material needs of the family, and to provide leadership. This idea is informed theologically by an interpretation of the Genesis 2 creation story. According to Banda, this account presents 'a vision of true biblical manhood' where Adam as the perfect man is 'placed at a location where he had to be responsible'.[67] Male church members reflect a similar understanding, as appears from the following quotation:

> [I]f you are a man, God expects a lot from you. When God made Adam, the Bible says: God made a garden and put the man in it. Adam did not find a mansion; he did not find a processing plant for juice. He found nothing, just a bush. He

---

[63] Piper is listed as a member of the governing body of this organisation. See 'Council Members', website of the Council on Biblical Manhood and Womanhood, accessed 7 May 2012, http://www.cbmw.org/Council-Members.

[64] J. Piper, 'A Vision of Biblical Complementarity: Manhood and Womanhood Defined According to the Bible', in J. Piper and W. Grudem (eds), *Recovering Biblical Manhood and Womanhood: A Response to Evangelical Feminism* (Wheaton, 1991), 36. This definition was quoted and explored by Banda in Parts 3, 4 and 5 of *Fatherhood*.

[65] Banda, *Fatherhood – Part 3*.

[66] Cf. Piper, *A Vision of Biblical Complementarity*, 37.

[67] Banda, *Fatherhood – Part 3*.

had to cultivate, he had to work it, to take care of it. He had to start using his engineering mind, innovation. For me that tells a lot about what God expects. God did not just tell: here Adam, everything is finished, here you are. So that is what a man should do: start from nothing, and do something. That is what every single man should do.[68]

According to this understanding, high expectations are put on men. This is not only because Adam was created first and received the responsibility of cultivating the garden. Reference is also made to God calling Adam to account after the Fall. Genesis 2 narrates how God calls Adam, saying, 'Adam, where are you?' Banda considers this to be 'question number one' to men in 'God's economy'.[69] Apparently, men's responsibility is based on their particular accountability to God. As part of his 'aesthetics of persuasion',[70] the bishop presents himself as someone who has answered God's question to men, preaching: 'Where are you? That is the simple question. Today I can answer the Lord: "I am where I am supposed to be." I am in the same house as where I brought a wonderful lady. I am in my marriage, but some of you have dislocated from their marriage.'[71] Note how he distinguishes himself from men in the church and presents himself as an example.

Apart from the figure of Adam, reference is also made to Jesus Christ to argue that responsibility is a defining notion of biblical manhood. Jesus Christ, according to Banda, is exemplary for men because he took up his God-given responsibility and hence fulfilled the divine role a man has to perform:

> Jesus Christ, when it was time to take his responsibility, he took responsibility. Then he said to his parents: I have a task. That is a picture of taking responsibility. And that is the role that a man should be able to fulfil. He had a commitment to humanity and a commitment to the restoration of people's life. And biblical manhood calls for men to rule and feed in these roles to making it better, making a better society. That role is given to men. Being a man is about taking up your responsibility, and that is what Christ did.[72]

Clearly, Jesus Christ is presented here not as a model for humankind in general but as a model of manhood. He is considered exemplary to men because of the responsibility he took. The above quotation illustrates how wide the notion of responsibility is perceived: it is concerned with the well-being of humanity and of society at large. Male responsibility, it seems, takes on messianic proportions.

---

[68] Interview with Philip Chime, Lusaka, 15 July 2009.
[69] Banda, *Fatherhood – Part 2*.
[70] B. Meyer, 'Aesthetics of Persuasion: Global Christianity and Pentecostalism's Sensational Forms', *The South Atlantic Quarterly*, 109/4 (2010), 754–8.
[71] Banda, *Fatherhood – Part 1*.
[72] Interview with Bishop Joshua Banda, Lusaka, 28 July 2009.

Jesus Christ, the man who took responsibility for others, presents a model of messianic masculinity that is to be followed by Christian men.

Where Banda presents responsibility as a fundamental notion of biblical manhood, church members indicate that it is also central to traditional understandings of manhood. As a young man recounted, his sense of responsibility developed when he grew up in a town and attended the meetings of the *Insaka*: 'This is the place where people of different ages meet. The elderly men are telling the younger about being a man. ... What they have told me is that being a man has a sense of responsibility. That sense considers you to be a man.'[73] Recounting the socialisation into gender roles during his upbringing in a rural set-up, another interviewee narrated how the boys were taught to be independent and to be responsible over others, which was 'different from what the women-folk was taught'.[74] Although the notion of male responsibility is not specifically biblical, as Banda suggests, but is also found in cultural traditions, various respondents indicated that Christianity makes a difference. The difference is that responsibility is considered a command of God to men. 'It becomes a responsibility from God. ... whereby if I don't do as I should do, then it becomes an issue in my spirituality.'[75] This suggests that the sense of male responsibility is reinforced by the church's teaching and becomes more imperative.

Various responsibilities   Responsibility is quite a general concept. In the church's teaching, it is applied to various areas of life: at the level of the individual, the level of marriage and the family, and the level of the community and society.

Though male responsibility is supposed to be benevolent to others, it is also concerned with the self. In concrete terms, it demands economic independence as well as moral maturity. As one young man explained: 'Graduating from a boy to a man is a stage where one is becoming responsible: looking for a job, for something to do; no longer depending on your parents but providing for yourself.'[76] Furthermore, it demands moral discipline over the self. Referring to the period in his life when he was smoking and drinking and had girlfriends, someone retrospectively said: 'I couldn't call myself a man because I wasn't responsible over my life.' However, after being born again, 'I became responsible. ... That is when I became a man because I started doing what God has purposed me to do.'[77] Apparently one is believed to become a man by taking responsibility over one's life, economically and/or behaviourally. Only when this maturity is reached, is one considered a real man who can establish a family.

With regard to marriage and the family, men's responsibility is understood in terms of provision and leadership. In the sermons on *Fatherhood in the 21st*

---

[73] Interview with Titus Kabunko, Lusaka, 3 November 2008.
[74] Interview with Jack Lungu, Lusaka, 7 November 2008.
[75] Interview with Henry Mwale, Lusaka, 15 November 2008.
[76] Interview with Gift Phiri, Lusaka, 21 October 2008.
[77] Interview with Danny Mulenga, Lusaka, 6 November 2008.

Century, it is frequently emphasised that a man has the *primary* responsibility to provide for the family – an emphasis that is informed by modern developments such as women's formal employment, as will be discussed later. The task to be the provider is quite demanding for men. A female interviewee explained that 'a man who is responsible will be very busy', as he has to make sure that all the needs of the family are provided for.[78] At the same time, she underlined that responsibility not only concerns the material needs: 'We [as women] have to remind them [men] to spend time with their children.'[79] Apart from the responsibility for their wives and children, various men told me that they look after siblings and support relatives in need. Interestingly, the church leadership does not pay much attention to a man's responsibility towards the extended family. Likewise, in the marriage ministry the high expectations on the part of the extended family are discussed as a burden to men and to married couples. The concern of the church clearly is with the nuclear family, which exemplifies Pentecostalism's modernising tendency.[80]

Lastly, male responsibility is applied at the level of the community and society. At a meeting of the men's ministry, men were challenged to 'commit their manhood to society'. The meaning of this was that men need to take responsibility not only in their family but in the wider society, too, 'in order to be the men God intends us to be'.[81] This responsibility in society is understood primarily in terms of leadership. Responsibility in the community is understood in terms of supporting people in the neighbourhood either materially or spiritually. It also includes providing moral guidance. This is apparent, for example, from Banda's call upon each man to be his 'brother's keeper', meaning that they have to speak to fellow men in the community when these engage in morally illegitimate behaviour.[82]

Headship

A second key notion defining the church's ideal of biblical manhood is headship. This concept particularly concerns men's position and roles in marriage and in the family. At every wedding ceremony in NAOG, the New Testament reading is from Ephesians 5, which reads: 'Wives, submit to your husbands as to the Lord. For the husband is the head of the wife as Christ is the head of the church, his body, of which he is the Saviour. Now as the church submits to Christ, so also wives should submit to their husbands in everything' (Ephesians 5:22–4, NIV). Referring to this Scripture, pastor Nyirenda, who is in charge of the marriage ministry, concludes that the headship of man in marriage is central to God's instructions for marriage:

---

[78] Interview with Isabel Lupiya, Lusaka, 8 July 2009.
[79] Ibid.
[80] See B. Martin, 'The Pentecostal Gender Paradox: A Cautionary Tale for the Sociology of Religion', in R.K. Fenn (ed.), *The Blackwell Companion to Sociology of Religion* (Oxford, 2001), 55.
[81] Meeting of Men of Truth, Northmead Assembly of God, 9 November 2008.
[82] Banda, *Cultivating – Part 5*.

These say: the man should be the head of that partnership. That is not negotiable. What is in the manual is not negotiable. We believe that marriage is instituted by God, and for us to live out this marriage we have to use God's manual for marriage, which is the Bible. The Bible says: the man is the head of marriage.[83]

In his sermons Banda also emphasises 'the principle of male headship' that should be part of God's order for creation.[84] Therefore he refers, again, to Genesis 2. The fact that Adam was created first and received the instructions for life, while Eve was given to him as a helper, is considered to illustrate the principle of male headship in marriage. Explaining the meaning of headship, Banda states that 'it is the man, not the woman [who] bears the primary responsibility to lead the partnership'.[85] According to the bishop, male headship does not apply to the public sphere. Here, women and men are equal. In Banda's opinion, a woman can be a church pastor, head of a company or even president of the nation, but at home she has to respect her husband as the head.[86] Headship is associated with several roles: the husband has to be the provider, the priest, the prophet and the protector of the family. Ultimately, it is about authority. Even when the wife brings in more income than the husband, because of the principle of male headship it should be the husband who has the final say in how the resources are used.[87]

Not surprisingly, male church members generally support the idea of male headship. Even when they are not yet married they make statements such as: 'Biblically a man is the head of the house. You can't compromise on that.'[88] However, women expressed similar opinions. Even a female interviewee who was rather critical of the actual behaviour of her husband still said: 'My husband is the head and whatever I do is in submission to his vision and what he is doing.'[89] The notion of male headship is accompanied here by the principle of submission on the part of the wife, as is common in Pentecostal discourse.[90] Indeed, this is part of the teaching of the church.[91] Conversations with women in the church indicate that they have generally internalised this perception of their role. Referring to the passage from Ephesians 5 quoted above, one of them stated that 'if you are not submissive to your husband, it means you are not submissive to Christ'.[92] What this concretely brings to bear on the daily relationship between

---

[83] Interview with Pastor Raymond Nyirenda, Lusaka, 22 October 2008.
[84] For instance, see Parts 2 and 6 of Banda, *Fatherhood*.
[85] Banda, *Fatherhood – Part 6*.
[86] Interview with Bishop Joshua Banda, Lusaka, 28 July 2009.
[87] Interview with Pastor Raymond Nyirenda, Lusaka, 17 July 2009.
[88] Interview with Gift Phiri, Lusaka, 3 November 2008.
[89] Interview with Rosy Mbuzi, Lusaka, 29 October 2008.
[90] R. Mate, 'Women as God's Laboratories: Pentecostal Discourses of Femininity in Zimbabwe', *Africa* 72:4 (2002), 556–7.
[91] Cf. *Premarital Counselling General Guide*.
[92] Interview with Febby Chibwika, Lusaka, 16 July 2009.

a husband and wife – whether indeed women are just submissive and men always are in charge – is of course a different question: the above-quoted woman, who was critical of her husband but yet said to submit to his vision, also told me she had opened her own bank account in order to be independent.

In the church there is anxiety about the fact that headship tends to be understood in terms of male superiority, which leads to men's domination over women. Marriage counsellors told me that they are faced with many marital problems arising from men's misunderstanding of headship as dictatorship and domination. Interestingly, this is often explained with reference to traditional Zambian cultures. Though male headship is considered both a cultural and a Christian principle, a major difference is emphasised. According to one church member, traditional headship results in 'a master–slave relationship' between the husband and his wife, whereas in a Christian marriage it should be expressed through mutual love and respect.[93] In line with this, Banda addresses the 'push for chauvinism' that he observes in 'African culture', with men as the heads looking down on their wives and treating them as inferior beings.[94] Thus, the critique of 'African culture', which is part of the break with the past that Pentecostalism wants to bring about, in NAOG particularly focuses on an assumed traditional, non-Christian pattern of male superiority and domination.[95] Therefore, in the church headship is redefined in a 'biblical' way.

In the process of redefinition, headship is dissociated from domination and re-interpreted in a more nuanced way, in terms of responsibility and leadership. Therefore, two theological notions are employed. First, headship is qualified christologically, in line with the text from Ephesians already quoted. Here, the relation of a husband to his wife is understood in analogy to the love of Christ for the church. Hence, Christ is presented as a model husband, showing men how to love, protect and take care of their wives.[96] Second, in order to prevent husbands from having feelings of superiority and dominating attitudes over their wives, Banda emphasises that men and women are created equal. This is derived from Genesis 1:26–7, which says that God created humankind in God's image, as male and female. Also, the narrative of Genesis 2, where woman is made from a rib of man and is accepted by man as 'bone of my bones, flesh of my flesh', is interpreted as an indication of equality.[97] Thus, where the creation stories first of all are used to found the primary responsibility and the headship of men, they are also used to argue for male–female equality. This notion of gender equality is understood in terms of an equal dignity of men and women and their equal status before God. According to the church leadership, this sense of equality is missing in African cultures but is characteristic of a Christian marriage: here, the husband is the head

---

[93] Interview with Moses Banda, Lusaka, 13 November 2008.
[94] Interview with Bishop Joshua Banda, Lusaka, 28 July 2009.
[95] Cf. Soothill, *Gender, Social Change and Spiritual Power*, 189.
[96] See Parts 4 and 6 of Banda, *Fatherhood*.
[97] Banda, *Fatherhood – Part 6*.

but there should be mutual respect and partnership in the relationship. This reflects a broader pattern in Pentecostal marriage, described by sociologist David Martin as 'patriarchalism in theory and consensuality in practice'.[98]

Where the church, on the one hand, opposes the assumed traditional understanding of headship as domination, on the other it rejects modern Western perceptions that do not accept the principle of headship. Banda strongly opposes 'extreme feminist views' that oppose God's order of creation, and he calls upon women not to fight but rather to accept male headship.[99] This call implicitly suggests that women do not always submit to their husbands as they should, according to the church. Indeed, there is a strong feeling that nowadays men's position as the head in marriage is threatened by women becoming more educated and being employed. Although the church is not against women pursuing a professional career, the concern is that they will start competing with their husbands at home.[100] Addressing this 'threat', pastor Nyirenda says:

> Even if the woman brings more money, that does not give her headship. But the sad thing about it is that there is so much hype about gender; that feminism thing that tries to zap God's order, it tries to zap the man's position. They are equal in the sense that none is more human than the other, but their roles are different. One has been given the role to provide leadership, and one has the role to support that leadership.[101]

Thus, apart from the notion of gender equality there is a notion of sexual difference that implies women are always to respect male headship in marriage. A gender ideology of heterosexual complementarity is indicated here, where a woman is supposed to complement the headship, leadership and primary responsibility of her husband.

Providing

One of the responsibilities a man has as head of the home is to be the provider. This appears to be a central aspect of 'biblical manhood', and it is discussed at length by Banda as well as by interviewees. The attention paid to the role of providing is informed by two concerns. The first is the observation of men's failure to fulfil this role. Banda critically addresses men who hang around in bars and leave the role of providing to their wives:

---

[98] D. Martin, *Pentecostalism: The World their Parish* (Malden, 2002), 98.

[99] Banda, *Fatherhood – Part 6*.

[100] A similar concern is found by Jane Soothill in charismatic churches in Ghana (Soothill, *Gender, Social Change and Spiritual Power*, 207).

[101] Interview with Pastor Raymond Nyirenda, Lusaka, 17 July 2009.

> The characteristic of many of our both rural and urban areas is that the majority of our men spend their time on the bottle. You find these men at 10 a.m. in the bar while in the meantime the precious lady is probably at the market ..., trying to make money.[102]

Hence, the call to men is to leave drunkenness behind and to take up their responsibility to provide. The second concern arises from the above-mentioned development of women increasingly being involved in formal employment, pursuing a professional career and bringing in an income that is sometimes even greater than the husband's. This is considered a threat to men's role of provider. The first concern seems rather rhetorical – after all, in a middle-class church like NAOG most men will not spend their time in bars while their wives are busy at the markets. Yet the second concern may be more relevant in view of the church membership. Out of these concerns, the church emphasises time and again that to provide income for the home is the primary and principal task of the man. This is considered part of African and biblical traditions and a fundamental principle in God's order. In the pre-marital counselling, reference is made to Ephesians 5:28–9, which calls on husbands to 'feed and care' for their wives just as Christ does for the church. Church members also consider providing a key role for men, but they predominantly relate it to cultural ideals. They say for instance: 'In African Zambian culture, in particular in Bemba culture, being a man means being able to provide, not only for your offspring but also for your family.'[103]

In spite of the cultural and biblical ideals, due to modern developments married men often find that their wives are employed and also bring money into the home. This sometimes creates tension in marriages. As mentioned above, a female interviewee told me she had opened a personal bank account where she deposits her income. She did so after some discussions with her husband about the household finances. The principle of the husband as provider is challenged by women's increasing participation in formal employment. It is interesting to see how the church deals with this, as it illustrates the negotiation with what is considered a biblical ideal. First, though Banda emphasises that 'man is the primary provider', at the same time he allows (and even seems to encourage) women to bring in a 'supplementary income'.[104] Thus women, too, can provide for the family, but it remains primarily a task of men. This view is reflected by interviewees who say, for instance: 'For me it's not an option whether to work or not to work ... [but] my wife has a choice.'[105] In other words, as a man you have to be able to provide for the needs of the family whether your wife contributes or not. A second strategy is to subtly broaden and redefine the meaning of providing. Then it is not just about the material needs of the family – which can also be

---

[102] Banda, *Cultivating – Part 4*.
[103] Interview with Gift Phiri, Lusaka, 21 October 2008.
[104] Banda, *Fatherhood – Part 5*.
[105] Interview with Henry Mwale, Lusaka, 15 November 2008.

provided for by the wife – but also about the emotional and spiritual needs that the head of the home has to provide. This shift is indicated by the association of 'providing' with 'protecting' in the sermons on *Fatherhood in the 21st Century*. In one of these sermons Banda also speaks about 'the responsibility to provide an enabling environment for initiatives', which reflects a much broader understanding of providing.[106] One church member commented that 'being the provider goes with leadership', meaning that even when a wife brings in more income than her husband, it is the latter who is supposed to plan and prioritise how the income is spent (though in consultation with his wife).[107] These shifting meanings indicate that the church seeks to allow for modern developments in the household economy, but at the same time wants to maintain 'the biblical order'.

Leadership

Central to 'biblical manhood' is also the notion of leadership. According to Piper's definition used by Banda, leadership is one of the characteristics of 'mature masculinity'. As previously mentioned, the headship of men in marriage includes, among other things, providing leadership to the family. However, male leadership has a wider scope than the context of family life. It also concerns the community, society and the nation. At all these levels, it is said, men's role is to lead. This role is emphasised because the church is extremely concerned about the 'abdication of leadership' among men in society. 'The sons of Africa and the sons of Zambia have failed to take the lead.'[108] Therefore Banda wants men to understand their role in the family and society: 'God has given them a role to lead, not to triumph but to lead, to facilitate the society to grow.'[109]

To ground the idea of male leadership, Banda draws from Genesis 3, which narrates the Fall of humankind in paradise. In contrast to traditional Christian interpretations of Genesis 3, which tend to blame woman for the Fall,[110] in Banda's reading man is blamed. Adam in Paradise neglected his leadership role. As he had received the instruction from God not to eat from the tree of knowledge of good and evil, Adam should have prevented Eve from taking a fruit from the tree.[111] That God after the Fall goes to Adam and calls him to account, rather than Eve, is

---

[106] Banda, *Fatherhood – Part 4*.

[107] Interview with Moses Banda, Lusaka, 13 November 2008.

[108] Banda, *Cultivating – Part 5*.

[109] Interview with Bishop Joshua Banda, Lusaka, 5 November 2008.

[110] See A.-M. Korte, 'Paradise Lost, Growth Gained: Eve's Story Revisited. Genesis 2–4 in a Feminist Theological Perspective', in B. Becking and S. Hennecke (eds), *Out of Paradise: Eve and Adam and their Interpreters* (Sheffield, 2010), 142–5.

[111] This interpretation is also found by Jane Soothill in charismatic churches in Ghana, and by Joseph Gelfer in the evangelical men's movement in the United States. Apparently, Banda's reading of the story is in line with broader strands of Pentecostal and Evangelical theology. Cf. J. Gelfer, *Numen, Old Men: Contemporary Masculine Spiritualities and the*

understood as an indication of the leadership that God has given to man. Because biblical manhood is rooted in creation, as Banda states frequently, the leadership and accountability of Adam applies to all men. Hence, the question from God to Adam is put to men in general, and is applied to the observed crisis of male leadership in global society:

> All over the world men are in the majority of leadership positions, but look at the level of oppression, so we are doing a bad job. It is a very serious problem. … God is seeking to correct that. He says to the man: "Where are you?" Today I ask you: men, where are you? Don't blame your wife for a relationship that is not working. Don't blame your son for things that you know you have the opportunity to protect. I know that they have a role, but however, in God's economy question number one is "Where are you?"[112]

Clearly, the so-called abdication of leadership by men is traced back to Adam's failure in the Fall. At the same time, the fact that God holds Adam accountable for the Fall is considered an indication of men's leadership role. Parallel to this, on the one hand men are addressed for 'the mess' in society, while on the other they are challenged to take responsibility and to turn things around.

The notion of male leadership is buttressed further by Christology. Jesus Christ is presented as the second Adam, being the one who has answered God's question to men, 'Where are you?' Hence, the way Jesus practised leadership is presented as a model for men, which reflects an ideal of messianic masculinity.[113] The primary aspect is that of leadership through service. Ephesians 5:25 is cited here, which reads: 'Husbands, love your wife as Christ loved the church and *gave himself up for her*' (NIV; emphasis added). From this verse it is said that 'loving is about giving' and that male leadership should be characterised by service and sacrifice.[114] The second aspect taken from Jesus' model is that leadership is not concerned with superiority but seeks to mobilise the strength of others. Hence, it is said that men as leaders have to create an atmosphere where the initiatives of all – including those of women – are encouraged, in order for the family and for society to grow.[115]

Among men there is a deep awareness of their leadership role. They understand this role in terms of providing guidance and direction to the wife and family, as controlling and influencing situations, and as the ability to realise things in society. In the family, male leadership means that a man has the responsibility 'to track a

---

Problem of Patriarchy (London, 2009), 58; Soothill, *Gender, Social Change and Spiritual Power*, 186.

[112] Banda, *Fatherhood – Part 2*.
[113] See Banda, *Fatherhood – Part 4*.
[114] Banda, *Fatherhood – Part 4*.
[115] Banda, *Fatherhood – Part 5*.

course for his family' and to 'influence things into the right direction',[116] but it is also related to managing the finances of the family. At the level of society, it is understood in terms of moral leadership, giving a good example and encouraging others to live morally upright, and 'making a difference' in people's lives, in the community and in the nation. The feeling is that leadership in all these areas is a crucial role that men have to play. As was stated at a meeting of the men's ministry: 'We have no option but to lead. When we withdraw, when we lie back, we create a vacuum.'[117] Clearly the notion of leadership is a gendered concept, as it characterises manhood in distinction to womanhood. In the words of one church member:

> I so much feel that God has put a higher premier, a higher demand on the man than on the woman. Saying: If you do not lead, she will not follow. So the demand for men is higher, to develop real character. To which the woman will come to complement. There has to be one leader, isn't it?[118]

The perception of a higher demand placed on men by God is often explained by reference to the leadership role that God has given to Adam. Although leadership is thought of as a male role, men frequently indicate that it should be practised in a democratic way that also gives space to women. For example, though the notion of leadership attaches decision-making to men, pastor Nyirenda, who is responsible for the marriage ministry, underlines that the husband should always consult his wife and seek for consensus. Only in case of an impasse should the man use 'his additional vote'.[119]

When it is about leadership at the level of society, especially young people are addressed. The youth is considered a new generation, which is to restore things that have gone wrong because of men's abdication of leadership. In one of his sermons, Banda extensively elaborates on the moral decay of Zambia, after which he challenges youth by saying: 'Let's change the face of Africa in the name of Jesus. It can be done. ... I want you to dream big; I want you to know that God can put into your hands the ability to turn things around.'[120] Although here both young men and women are addressed and are called to be leaders in society, the discourse on leadership is clearly masculine. Leaders are seen as social and spiritual *father* figures in society, and leadership is mentioned as a key characteristic of biblical manhood.

---

[116] Interview with Rosy Mbuzi, Lusaka, 29 October 2008.
[117] Meeting Men's Ministry, 9 November 2008.
[118] Interview with Charles Muleya, Lusaka, 13 July 2009.
[119] Interview with Pastor Raymond Nyirenda, Lusaka, 17 July 2009.
[120] Banda, *Cultivating – Part 5*.

Self-control

Yet another notion central to the church's ideal of manhood is self-control. Self-control is supposed to help men to live up to the ideal of biblical manhood. It should prevent them from behaving in ways considered immoral, especially in the area of sexuality. In his sermons Banda frequently denounces men's inability to control themselves. For example,

> Who says that this is the way men must behave, unable to control their sexual desire? ... So who told you that men can never keep themselves pure? Who says that men cannot be satisfied by one woman, that there always must be an extra one? ... You and I can change, today![121]

Hence, men are called to take control over their own lives and to master their desires. Contesting the popular opinion among men that they cannot control their urges, the church emphasises that men *have* strength and *can* take control. 'You have the capacity to control yourself.'[122] Thus the ability to control the self becomes a feature of male character.[123] Referring to Job 31:1, which reads: 'I made a covenant with my eyes not to look lustfully at a girl', Banda challenges men to reset their minds and to make a covenant with their eyes. In a Foucauldian frame this can be called a mental technique of the self, as the body is disciplined by mastering the mind.[124] Where Banda initially explains men's sexual weaknesses in relation to the hormone epinephrine, he then states that this hormone needs to be conquered through maintaining control over the eyes and desires.[125] It is underlined that men cannot blame the devil for their failure in this area. 'We want to demonise everything, to explain it away ... [but] it is just a man who is failing to have control over his lusts.'[126]

It is interesting to see how the general Christian practice of disciplining the body becomes a characteristic of born-again masculinity. Pointing out that for their peers sexuality is a major place to manifest manhood, male church members indicated that a real man should be able to control his sexual urges, as this expresses true male strength. Self-control is mentioned as a crucial difference between the periods before and after becoming born again. 'Before that time it was the opposite, the promiscuous ways and all the lack of control. But now there

---

[121] Banda, *Fatherhood – Part 1*.

[122] Banda, *Cultivating – Part 6*.

[123] A similar emphasis on character, especially that of the young male, is mentioned by D. Maxwell, *African Gifts of the Spirit: Pentecostalism & the Rise of a Zimbabwean Transnational Religious Movement* (Oxford, Harare and Athens, 2006), 201.

[124] See Chapter 3, note 96.

[125] Cf. Parts 6 and 7 of Banda, *Cultivating*.

[126] Banda, *Between Two Worlds*.

is control, and righteous living has become a joy.'[127] This is not to say that there are no more temptations when one has been born again. Feelings are normal, is the general opinion, but the challenge is to control them. In one youth meeting, the self-control that men are supposed to develop was captured in the metaphor of circumcision. The guest preacher delivered a talk on *Raising the Remnant for the Lord*, with 'the remnant' referring to what he called 'a new generation of men and women of morality'. He especially elaborated upon sexual morality, and then he began to address young men in particular: 'When we talk about raising the remnant, we seek for men that are circumcised. Circumcision is a painful process. You need to be a man of the Lord. You cannot just go on with your life!'[128] Here, male circumcision is used as a metaphor of how a young Christian man is supposed to be: capable of controlling his sexuality, saying 'no' to temptations and reserving sex for marriage. Self-control, it appears, is all about a moral discipline of the body through which men, metaphorically speaking, are circumcised.

Re-constructing a Theological Framework

Identifying the key notions of the ideal of biblical manhood as promoted in NAOG, already attention has been paid to some of the underlying theological thoughts. A more systematic analysis shows that 'biblical manhood' is a theological construct embedded in and related to some major lines of thought in Pentecostal theology.

Gender Ideology and a Creation-based Theological Anthropology

The many references to the biblical creation stories in sermons and interviews indicate that the ideal of manhood is inspired by an ideology of gender that takes its theological starting point from the account of creation. Another indication is that the figures of Adam and Eve in Genesis 2 and 3 are literally presented as the models of biblical manhood and womanhood respectively. The creation-based theological anthropology entails four notions that are crucial for the understanding of gender and thus also of masculinity: difference, complementarity, heterosexuality and equality.

There is a strong perception of men and women as fundamentally different from each other. This perception is based on Genesis 2, which, according to Banda, presents 'the first surgery of human history' through which man, who was created first, received woman as a helper.[129] According to Banda, this 'surgery' resulted in woman being made from the rib of man but as a 'differently abled version'.[130] This difference, which is applied to women in general, is not only physiological, but

---

[127] Interview with Charles Muleya, Lusaka, 13 July 2009.
[128] Youth meeting, 11 October 2008.
[129] Banda, *Fatherhood – Part 6*.
[130] Banda, *Fatherhood – Part 5*.

also psychological and emotional. In all these areas, women are said to be weaker than men. The difference between men and women is understood especially in terms of roles. As Nyirenda puts it: '[T]heir roles are different. One has been given the role to provide leadership, and one has the role to support that leadership.'[131] In the same way, Banda, following the definition of manhood and womanhood from Piper, defines manhood in terms of providing, leading and protecting women, and womanhood in terms of receiving and affirming the leadership, provision and protection by men. It appears that the notion of gender difference is used to legitimate the primacy of men in gender relations. That Adam, according to Genesis 2, was created first is understood as meaning that 'there is something higher and bigger given to men'.[132] Likewise, the fact that, in this creation story, it is man who names the new creature woman, is presented as an illustration of the principle of male headship.[133]

It is believed that man and woman, as fundamentally different beings assigned with different roles, are intended to complement each other. Marriage is considered the primary setting for this complementarity to take place, as here a man and a woman become 'one body'. However it appears to be especially the wife who is supposed to complement the husband. This is indicated not only in interviews, but also in the text of the marriage liturgy. While the groom is addressed as 'God's most elaborate creation – a man', the value and role of the bride is phrased only in terms of her contribution to the life and success of her husband: 'You can be able to lift him to the highest of God's plan for him.'[134] Complementarity in marriage turns out to be rather one-sided.

The rhetoric on gender complementarity in the church clearly is 'a language of presumptive heterosexuality'.[135] It is believed that only a man and a woman can complement each other and become one body in which each fulfils the respective roles. The more explicit politics of 'compulsory heterosexuality', as so often inspired in Christianity by the Genesis account of creation, are demonstrated in Banda's discussion of same-sex relationships. Here he states that 'in creation God made them male and female. It is Adam and Eve and not Adam and Steve.'[136] This quote shows that 'biblical manhood' is a heteronormative construction of masculinity. Homosexuality, according to Banda, is a violation of God's order of creation. Referring to Genesis 2:24, which says that a man will leave his parents to be united with a woman, he points out that marriage is not only a divine institution but also is unchangeably heterosexual.[137] Because the complementarity

---

[131] Interview with Pastor Raymond Nyirenda, Lusaka, 17 July 2009.
[132] Banda, *Fatherhood – Part 1*.
[133] Banda, *Fatherhood – Part 6*.
[134] Standard Liturgy for Wedding Service, Northmead Assembly of God.
[135] J. Butler, *Gender Trouble: Feminism and the Subversion of Identity*, 2nd edn (London, 2006), xxxii.
[136] Banda, *Fatherhood – Part 4*.
[137] Banda, *Fatherhood – Part 6*.

of the sexes is missing in same-sex relations, Banda argues that these relationships do not mirror God's image and therefore should be condemned categorically. This theological view directly influences his political opinions, expressed in his sermons, such as when he states that same-sex practices should continue to remain a crime in Zambia, or when he opposes a plan to do research on HIV transmission among men having sex with men.[138]

Apart from the notions of gender difference and complementarity, the church also derives a notion of gender equality from creation theology. This equality is based on Genesis 1:27, which says that God created humankind in God's image as male and female, and on Genesis 2:23, where Adam recognises Eve as 'bone of my bones and flesh of my flesh' (NIV). In the church's perception this equality does not break down the fundamental difference between man and woman. They are believed to be 'different yet equal'. The equality is that they both bear and represent the image of God, meaning that 'none is more human than the other'.[139] In this context Banda refers to George Orwell's *Animal Farm* where all animals are equal, but some are more equal than others. In Banda's argument, the world is *not* an animal farm because it is God's world, and therefore men and women are in principle equal.[140] It does not become clear, however, how the notion of gender equality is to be reconciled with the concept of male headship and leadership. Though the sense of equality is used to give space to the emancipation of women in society and to accept female pastors in the church, in the context of marriage male–female relations are understood in terms of male headship versus female submission. And even outside marriage, men in general are said to have a primary responsibility, as God has placed a higher demand on men. This suggests that actually, in the view of the church, God's world *is* an animal farm where men and women may be equal but with the former in fact being more equal than the latter. Clearly, there is a contradiction in the gender ideology of the church. But it is also obvious that men, in the ambiguous space between headship and equality, are prevented from misuse of their power at the expense of women and children.

Jesus Christ as the Second Adam

As mentioned above, in the church Adam is presented as the exemplary model for manhood. At the same time, he is blamed for the Fall of humankind because he neglected his leadership role. Following traditional Christian theology, the Fall has brought sin into the world. In the words of Banda, God's perfect order of creation has been violated and humankind now is in a fallen 'Adamic nature'. Interestingly, he applies the latter term specifically to men. Discussing the problems caused by men in society, in one sermon he states: 'What we are struggling with is the state

---

[138] The latter is particularly critical considering Banda's position as the chair of the National AIDS Council in Zambia.

[139] Interview with Pastor Raymond Nyirenda, Lusaka, 17 July 2009.

[140] Banda, *Fatherhood – Part 4*.

of men after the Fall into an Adamic nature.'[141] Evidently, the figure of Adam after the Fall has become problematic as a model for manhood.

In order for men to overcome their current sinful Adamic state, Banda develops a soteriology of male redemption, for which he creatively employs the Pauline theology of the first and the second Adam (cf. 1 Corinthians 15). Here, the first Adam refers to the figure of Adam in Genesis 2–3, and the second Adam refers to the person of Jesus Christ. In Banda's interpretation, Jesus Christ has come as the second Adam to restore the ideal of manhood that was impaired by the failure of the first. It is believed that Jesus is the one responding to God's question, 'Adam, where are you?', and therefore is the new archetype of manhood. As Banda puts it: 'God decided to keep a provision for the re-innovation of masculinity through the fact that the second Adam came, so he could deal with our Adamic nature. So there is a restoration there, where we can see what God desires in fatherhood truly restored.'[142] Although Jesus is presented as the embodiment of 'biblical manhood', he is not really masculinised. In contrast to some American Evangelical men's movements, Banda's sermons employ no warrior, military or heroic metaphors for Jesus Christ.[143] Rather, he is presented as someone who shows men how to take responsibility, practise leadership-through-service, and be wholeheartedly committed to the ones entrusted to them. Likewise, following Ephesians 5:25, the sacrificing love of Christ for the church is presented as the example for husbands in relation to their marriage and family. In all these aspects, Jesus Christ shows how God has intended manhood to be. What has been lost with the Fall of the first Adam is restored by the second.

Jesus Christ as the second Adam is believed not only to restore the ideal of biblical manhood, but also to liberate men from their Adamic nature and to nurture them into the ideal of manhood he embodies himself. The root problem of the Adamic nature, which causes men to sin, is believed to be solved with the resurrection of Jesus Christ. Men do not have to live 'under the mould of a default type of manhood' any longer but can be elevated to a higher level.[144] Referring to certain mindsets of men, to prevailing opinions in the media and society, to curses that may run through the lineage and to certain habits passed on from father to son, Banda points to the power of the second Adam, which can break down all the realities in which men can be entrapped:

> Today I call you, because I don't see how a man who has truly come to know Jesus can be of the kind of attitude and circumstances that we see around. Something is wrong. The second Adam does a special work. ... The second Adam can break the mindset and that curse that makes men think that they must act like animals out there, unable to control their sexual desires. We are better

---

[141] Banda, *Fatherhood – Part 3*.
[142] Cf. Banda, *Fatherhood – Part 4*.
[143] Gelfer, *Numen, Old Men*, 55.
[144] Interview with Bishop Joshua Banda, Lusaka, 28 July 2009.

than that, we are higher than that, and we are more elevated than that because God gave us a provision in the second Adam. I want men here today to agree in their hearts and to understand that this Jesus can set you free. Today and now.[145]

Jesus Christ as the second Adam is considered the one who can change men, if only they would open themselves to his transformative power. If there is a masculinisation of Jesus, it is in the sense that he is presented as a powerful male saviour of men.

With his application of the Pauline symbolism of the first and the second Adam, Banda stands in the tradition of Pentecostal theology, where the figures of the first and the second Adam, according to Ogbu Kalu, have 'enormous spiritual and political powers'.[146] However he further develops this tradition in an innovative way. The Adam symbolism is usually applied to the Fall and redemption of humankind in general, but Banda applies it to *man*kind as a gendered category. He employs the theme of the first and second Adam to develop a theological framework for the redemption and transformation of masculinity.[147] In this framework, Jesus Christ is presented both as the new archetype of manhood and as the one who liberates and elevates men into the 'true masculinity' that he embodies himself.

Being Born Again and the Ideal of Holiness

In NAOG, as in Pentecostal theology in general, 'born again' is a central theological concept, just as is the closely related notion of holiness. Time and time again, the importance of being born again and living a holy life is emphasised.

Born again Being born again is a prerequisite to becoming a member of the church.[148] Consequently, the whole membership can be expected to be born again, but actually this is often questioned in sermons. According to the church's theology, being born again should result in a different way of life. However, the church is aware of many critical issues in the behaviour of its members, especially of men. Therefore it is questioned whether people are really born again. Observe, for instance, the following quotation from a sermon in which men's 'macho-masculinity', expressed through sexual conquest and domestic violence, has just been addressed:

---

[145] Banda, *Fatherhood – Part 1*.

[146] O.U. Kalu, *African Pentecostalism: An Introduction* (Oxford, 2008), 221.

[147] Soothill (*Gender, Social Change and Spiritual Power*, 186) found that the figure of Adam also is used in Charismatic churches in Ghana in a discourse on men and masculinities. However, here reference is only made to the Genesis figure and not to Jesus Christ as the second Adam. Banda uses the Adam symbolism in a more elaborate and systematic way; for him, it is a theological framework not only to address men and issues of masculinity critically but also to transform masculinities constructively.

[148] *Church Constitution – Excerpt of Key Articles*, Northmead Assembly of God.

> There has to be a true encounter between you and Jesus. You can't claim to be a born again Christian man and do what I described earlier. Where it seems to be no difference for you: your language has not changed, you still beat your wife, you still act recklessly. Then something has not happened, you haven't met the true Christ.[149]

As this quotation indicates, being born again is understood in terms of a meeting, a 'true encounter', with Jesus Christ and is considered a unique, once-in-a-lifetime experience. Indeed, this experience is well remembered by church members and they are eager to narrate it. From these stories it appears that in the born-again experience, one accepts Christ as a personal Saviour and commits one's life to Christ. This event is mentioned as a moment of change. On the one hand, this is a change in one's mind and orientation in life, which indicates individual agency in becoming born again. On the other hand, this change is said to be initiated by God, as God has the power to release people from the 'bonds' in which they can be caught. As Banda preaches: 'There is a God in heaven who came in the person of the Lord Jesus Christ who, when allowed entrance into your life, is the deliverer, is the hope of glory; he can set you free from unhealthy passions and desires.'[150]

The change that takes place when becoming born again results in a second beginning of one's life. In the words of one church member: 'When being born again you start with an empty page. Justified in Christ, I am a secondary virgin.'[151] The image of a restored virginity is meaningful because it symbolically illustrates, first, the radical new start one can make after born-again conversion, and second, the enormous concern in Pentecostal circles with sex and sexual morality. It appears that the born-again experience is understood as a crucial marker of the beginning of Christian life. This event makes a distinction, both in a person's life (between the period before and after becoming born again) and between people (those who are and who are not born again). In other words, being born again functions as a symbol of Christian identity, at the level of both the individual and the group. Anthropologically, the born-again discourse is a discursive regime in which people break with the past, leave former friends behind, make a radical new start in life and build a social network of other born-again Christians who together follow Christ and experience the Holy Spirit.[152] This regime involves an aspect that anthropologist Ruth Marshall, following Foucault, calls *askêsis* or 'an active work of the self on the self'.[153] It is noteworthy that this work on the self is a gendered process that, in the case of men, brings about new born-again male selves. This is illustrated in the following born-again story of an interviewee:

---

[149] Banda, *Fatherhood – Part 1*.
[150] Banda, *Cultivating – Part 3*.
[151] Interview with Charles Muleya, Lusaka, 13 July 2009.
[152] For the notion of born-again as a discursive regime, see R. Marshall, *Political Spiritualities: The Pentecostal Revolution in Nigeria* (Chicago, 2009), 36.
[153] Ibid., 146.

> I used to drink, to smoke, to have girlfriends; I used to mess around. I couldn't call myself a man because I wasn't responsible over my life and the life of others, and the feelings of others. But when I changed I became responsible and started to say: when I do this, my family is not happy; when I smoke I may get sick; this is not good for me. That is when I became a man because I started doing what God has purposed me to do.[154]

The story shows how, in the born-again programme, not just a new moral subject is created but a new male gendered subject, inspired by an alternative understanding of masculinity.[155]

Holiness As a marker of the beginning of Christian life, the born-again concept is closely related to the notion of holiness that, according to the church, characterises Christian life. Holiness points to the process of sanctification by which one's life becomes pleasurable to God. Hence it especially concerns one's behaviour and lifestyle. Theologically, the importance of holiness is informed by two lines of thought. First, reference is made to the biblical commandment to believers to be holy because God is holy (cf. Leviticus 11:44 and 1 Peter 1:15–16). This verse is understood to mean that only when a person is holy he or she is able to be connected with God. Thus holiness is a pre-condition for the relationship with God. At the same time it is believed that in the human–divine relationship, God's holiness is reflected upon the believer. As Banda puts this dialectic: 'When we are close to God, God demands us to be holy and at the same time his holiness is reflected upon us. … It is something to strive for and something to receive. He gives us the capacity by our union with him.'[156] Ultimately, in Banda's line of thought, human holiness is rooted in our creation in the image of God. However, because of the Fall of humankind, this reflection is damaged. Only through becoming born again and living according to God's intentions can the reflection of God's holiness in one's life be restored, it is thought.

The second theological concept is the New Testament metaphor of the human body as a temple of the Holy Spirit and as part of the Body of Christ (cf. 1 Corinthians 6:15–20). This perception of the body reinforces the urgency to keep the body 'clean' and 'pure' by preventing it from being involved in sin. For example, it is said that sex before marriage desecrates the body as a temple of the living God.[157] Put positively, this perception also means that a person can

---

[154] Interview with Danny Mulenga, Lusaka, 6 November 2008.

[155] For a more elaborate discussion, see A.S. van Klinken, 'Men in the Remaking: Conversion Narratives and Born-Again Masculinity in Zambia', *Journal of Religion in Africa* 42/3 (2012): 215–239.

[156] Interview with Bishop Joshua Banda, Lusaka, 28 July 2009.

[157] Pastor Raymond Nyirenda in the meeting of the single's ministry, 28 September 2008.

'glorify God with the body' through living in a God-pleasurable way.[158] Church members often apply the notion of the body as a temple to the area of sexuality. They perceive sexual misconduct as a sin against not only God's will, but also their own bodies (cf. 1 Corinthians 6:18). Although it is believed that every sin can be forgiven by God, 'when you sin against your body it leaves a scar'.[159]

The metaphor of the body as a temple has a specific gender dimension, as men are not only called to sanctify their own bodies but also are given a responsibility towards women's bodies. Young men are called on not to explore the bodies of their fiancés before marriage.[160] In line with this, one male youth talking about his relationship explained: 'When I would insist on sex, I am not respecting her body.'[161] In order for men to keep their bodies clean and to protect the bodies of the women in their lives, they are called to develop self-control over their bodily desires. At the same time it is stated that God helps and gives strength to believers to sanctify the body. 'When the body is a temple of the Holy Spirit, the Spirit will help to protect that temple, to clean it and prevent it from certain things that you want to defile your temple with.'[162] It appears that holiness is an ongoing process of sanctification and transformation of one's life, which is initiated through the born-again event. Along this process, men are believed to grow towards the ideal of 'biblical manhood'.

Judgement of God

The notion of divine judgement is not very prominent in preaching, but is crucial in the accounts of church members. Banda only now and then refers to this thought, especially to underline the urgency of following the born-again lifestyle promoted. For example, when preaching about drinking alcohol, he says that according to the Bible, drunkards shall not enter into the kingdom of God.[163] Likewise, in the series *Fatherhood in the 21st Century*, he uses the notion of divine judgement to motivate men to take up their responsibilities:

> It is the man who has the primary responsibility to lead the partnership in a God-glorifying direction. Which means: gentlemen, we will be judged before God for how we lead in this partnership. And from the beginning, you know, we have not done too well in leading this partnership; we have not done very well as men. And we must remember that we will be judged in this area.[164]

---

[158] J. Banda, *Cultivating a Lifestyle of Truth – Part 8* (Lusaka, 2005).
[159] Interview with Moses Banda, Lusaka, 13 November 2008.
[160] Banda, *Cultivating – Part 8*.
[161] Interview with Danny Mulenga, Lusaka, 13 November 2008.
[162] Interview with Gift Phiri, Lusaka, 21 October 2008
[163] Banda, *Knowing God – Part 12*.
[164] Banda, *Fatherhood – Part 6*.

Although reference is made to judgement, this notion is hardly an articulated line of thought. It does not become clear how divine judgement is considered to take place. Talking about homosexuality, Banda refers to Sodom and Gomorrah as an illustration of God's punishment for sin. However he does not argue that today God is punishing people in such a direct way, and he explicitly rejects the understanding of HIV as a manifestation of God's judgement at work.[165] The reference above to drunkards not entering the kingdom of God indicates that Banda understands judgement in terms of individual eschatology: it is about a person entering the kingdom of God or not, about going to heaven or to hell. As stated in the church's constitution: 'We believe in the eternal conscious bliss of all true believers in Christ and also in the eternal conscious punishment in the lake of fire of all Christ rejecters.'[166]

Though the notion of divine judgement is not very prominent in preaching, among church members it is a reality they often refer to. They live in the awareness that they are answerable to God and will be judged by God for everything they do. Actually, the awareness of God's judgement over one's life is mentioned as a motivation for becoming a Christian. For example, recounting his born-again experience, one young man narrated: 'I realised that I should have gone to hell. So I thought: let's give up this bad behaviour, this bad life.'[167] Once born again, the realisation that God will judge one's actions reinforces the commitment to live up to God's instructions for life. Good moral conduct is not just an issue of outward appearance to others, but primarily of accountability to God. '[Even] when nobody knows you, you must remember that your primary responsibility is to God.'[168] The awareness of accountability to God and of divine judgement is a crucial part of the church's religious framework. It is within this frame that people are called to live up to the prescribed way of life and indeed are motivated to do so.

Living Up to the Ideal

The question arises as to how men live up to the ideal of manhood promoted in the church. Is 'biblical manhood' just an ideal or does it really change men and transform their male identities?

A Lack of Commitment?

Men's commitment to the ideal of biblical manhood is questioned critically by the church leadership, which is concerned about the low level of participation of men in the church. Indicators of this are the small number of men participating

---

[165] See Banda, *HIV&AIDS and Stigma in the Church*.
[166] Northmead Assembly of God, *Church Constitution – Excerpt of Key Articles*.
[167] Interview with Robert Cherwa, Lusaka, 27 July 2009.
[168] Interview with Henry Mwale, Lusaka, 15 November 2008.

in the men's ministry, especially when compared to the women's ministry, and the difficulty of involving men in church work. According to Banda, this is not a problem specific to his church, but a universal phenomenon. He aimed to address this 'recessive attitude' in the series *Fatherhood in the 21st Century*. As he says in one of the sermons:

> In church, when we ask for volunteers, there are more women than men. Make an altar call and there are more women than men. Today I am making an altar call for men only. Listen, this is about recapturing our position. The world needs us, gentlemen, to perform a better role that what we are performing.[169]

Note how in this quotation men's lack of church involvement is understood directly in terms of men not assuming their role in society. Apparently, in order for a man to 'recapture his position' he is supposed to be an actively participating church member.

The concern of the church leadership about men's church involvement is shared by various church members. They give different explanations. For example, men are said to be so busy that they 'use every minute to make money and don't want to spend time in the men's fellowship'.[170] It is also suggested that men prefer other ways of spending their leisure time, such as watching football or visiting friends or relatives. An interesting explanation is the materialism and career-making among men. See, for instance, how a woman recounts how her husband strayed from the church and lost his commitment to the Christian faith:

> But when he started ascending in his profession, when things became better, the need for God stopped. ... He was overtaken by the flow of material things, and in the process he was in wrong company. He started having friends at work who were not believers. That is what affected him. Not just that he chose to go away from church; it just started small and he thought to overcome it, but he didn't manage. Men don't know how to balance wealth and God. I have seen it. It happens to so many men.[171]

The suggestion here is that a process of secularisation takes place among men who are professionally and economically successful. The concern of the church is that for many men the church is not a top priority. As one of the pastors puts it: 'Men think that church is for Sunday, that it has nothing to do with their life.'[172] In other words, even when men are involved in the congregation and identify as Christians, they are not seriously committed in their daily life to Christian values and principles. Some church members are said to observe 'a life of pretence'

---

[169] Banda, *Fatherhood – Part 1*.
[170] Interview with Ezra Kambole, Lusaka, 21 October 2008.
[171] Interview with Febby Chibwika, Lusaka, 16 July 2009.
[172] Interview with Pastor Boyd Banda, Lusaka, 15 July 2009.

among fellow Christian men, suggesting that for men Christian life is often about keeping up appearances.[173] All this is addressed critically in the church, but it is realised that perhaps 'it is the willingness of men where[in lies] the problem.'[174]

Apparently it cannot be assumed automatically that male church members live up to the promoted ideal of 'biblical manhood'. There are gradations in the commitment to this ideal and in the involvement in the church. The problem might be, however, that the church leadership perceives both in a close relation: the commitment of men to the ideal of manhood is evaluated by their level of church involvement. In personal conversations some male church members complained about the high demands of church membership: they are expected to attend not only Sunday services but also the home cell groups, to participate in the men's ministry, in the marriage or singles ministry, and so on. Several men pointed out that they do not know how to meet all these expectations while at the same time fulfilling their responsibilities in their marriage, family and employment.

Serious Intentions

Though it cannot be taken for granted that male church members generally live up to the expectations of 'biblical manhood', in interviews many of them at least show a serious intention to do so. They demonstrate a willingness to take seriously the church's teaching on moral norms and behaviour, and they point out that this distinguishes them from fellow men in society. How serious their commitment is may be illustrated by the following quotation from an interviewee talking about the period before he entered into marriage: 'So in terms of relating to ladies and going beyond, I haven't had any intimate relationship; that was definitely out of order because I set my mind to pleasing God in that area; it was something I decided consciously to do.'[175] For this man, living up to the norm of sexual abstinence before marriage has been an issue of self-control. It is about taking a conscious decision, developing a certain mindset, out of a desire to please God by fulfilling what is considered God's commandment.

The commitment men have to what they perceive as a Christian lifestyle seems to be strongly affirmed by their born-again experience. In interviews men often distinguish between life before and after becoming born again, and the difference is often described in terms of moral behaviour. For example, in the words of a young man recounting his born-again story:

> Before that [becoming born again] I used to drink, I used to smoke, I was a bad boy, I was womanising, had a lot of girlfriends. After a certain incident in my life, I decided that the life I was leading was not a good life. ... I thought: let me just give up alcohol and drugs and this kind of life, and become a Christian.

---

[173] Interview with Gift Phiri, Lusaka, 21 October 2008.
[174] Interview with Isabel Lupiya, Lusaka, 8 July 2009.
[175] Interview with Moses Banda, Lusaka, 13 November 2008.

From my upbringing I was a Christian, my family are Catholics, but I wasn't serious with that. ... But then I had that incident, and I decided to change.[176]

Note the aspect of individual agency in this account: becoming born again is presented as a personal decision to change. The story also demonstrates that becoming born again is not so much about a change in beliefs or doctrines, but a change in lifestyle. The new commitment to Christian life is understood in terms of obeying the commandments of God, following Jesus Christ, becoming more serious, focused and careful in life. The time before becoming born again is often referred to as 'the former life', which not only illustrates the power of the born-again discourse to frame life stories but also shows that people seriously think that they have left behind 'the sins of the past'.[177] If born-again stories are biographical reconstructions, as Henri Gooren points out, the above story shows how, in this autobiography, the male self is reconstructed from 'a bad boy' into a serious Christian.[178]

Though interviewees generally indicate that they are committed to a born-again lifestyle, this does not mean that they uncritically follow the moral teaching of the church. One young adult man, when discussing this, emphasised that choices concerning behaviour and lifestyle are ultimately between the individual and God. This view reflects the classic Protestant idea of individual responsibility to God, which today reappears in Pentecostal circles and is an important theological factor in the much debated links of Pentecostalism to modernisation and individualism.[179] The sense of individual moral agency inculcated by Pentecostal religion may explain the success of the born-again project of conversion.[180]

Interestingly, elaborating upon the impact of Christianity on their life, some men put this in terms of a transformation of their perception of manhood. One interviewee stated that he has been 'remodelled' as a man, which he explained as follows:

I had to learn right and wrong because of God. I've had to learn to live the Christian culture, of what the expectation of the man should be. I am expected to be good standing in society. I am expected to be a model for young people.

---

[176] Interview with Robert Cherwa, Lusaka, 27 July 2009.

[177] Cf. B. Meyer, 'Make a Complete Break with the Past. Memory and Post-Colonial Modernity in Ghanaian Pentecostalist Discourse', *Journal of Religion in Africa*, 28:3 (1998), 316–49.

[178] H. Gooren, 'Conversion Narratives', in A. Anderson, M. Bergunder, A. Droogers and C. van der Laan (eds), *Studying Global Pentecostalism: Theories and Methods* (Berkeley, 2010), 93.

[179] See Chapter 10, 'Pentecostalism: A Major Narrative of Modernity', in D. Martin, *On Secularization: A Revised General Theory* (Aldershot, 2005), 141–55.

[180] Cf. Marshall, *Political Spiritualities*, 129.

I am expected to exemplify a godly character, trying to do everything that God wants me to do.[181]

Another respondent claimed that 'being a Christian has really helped to mould me into a better man'.[182] He pointed to his renewed sense of responsibility and the control over his sexual urges as proofs of his new, better type of manhood. It seems that Christian life, in the perceptions of these men, has resulted not just in a change of their behaviour but also of their type of manhood. They perceive themselves now as mature men, because of the responsibilities they fulfil and the self-control they practise. By observing Christian values they have discovered the 'true identity of being a man'.[183] It appears that the church-promoted type of manhood really is an alternative to which these men consciously try to live up to. It is realised that this is not a stage that is achieved automatically when becoming born again, but that it is a process: 'Being a man, for me, it has to take God. You have to accept Christ, and that is when God is going to make a man out of you. ... I can't say: I have arrived. I have my mistakes. I am still a man in the making.'[184] In the process of growth towards 'mature' or 'biblical' manhood one is not only a subject actively working on self-transformation, but also an object of God's transformative power.

The Weakness of the Flesh

Where male church members indicate their serious intentions to live a Christian way of life, they also point out that they do have their weaknesses when faced with temptations. They are engaged in an ongoing struggle, balancing between what is perceived as the Christian moral code of conduct and the fleshly desires. To live as a Christian man, an interviewee explained, feels like being Spiderman, because you have to look constantly for the delicate balance. He illustrated this with the issue of kissing:

> From the pulpit it is told: don't do it, because one thing leads to another. But we do it, the majority of the guys do it. And we end up feeling sorry about it. Because they say, "Don't do it". It's a constant struggle. Good and evil. You can't constantly regulate yourself. ... You want to do it, and the next day you don't want to do it. Indeed I do it, but that is as far as it goes.[185]

Striking in this quotation is not only the apparent fact that kissing is considered an issue of good or evil. The quotation most aptly shows how the church's

---

[181] Interview with Marc Mwila, Lusaka, 22 October 2008.
[182] Interview with Jack Lungu, Lusaka, 7 November 2008.
[183] Interview with Clemens Kabunko, Lusaka, 3 November 2008.
[184] Interview with Danny Mulenga, Lusaka, 6 November 2008. For a detailed analysis of the conversion narratives of born-again men, see Van Klinken, *Men in the Remaking*.
[185] Interview with Marc Mwila, Lusaka, 22 October 2008.

moral teaching results in men constantly struggling to live up to the ideal while negotiating their desires. They may give in to the desire of kissing, but 'that is as far as it goes', meaning that they continue to struggle with other issues.

Several interviewees indicate that they have developed strategies to cope with temptations and to control the self. For some, this is an issue of developing the appropriate mindset in order for feelings not to reach a critical level. Certain energies are channelled by concentrating on other things, for example through prayer. Personal prayer seems to be a central technique to discipline the self. Explaining how to deal with temptations, one interviewee told me: 'You handle it through prayer. ... You go out to meditate, just being with God and thinking about the things of God.'[186] Apart from this individual technique, some church members have involved other people to prevent themselves from committing sin. One adult man, who often travels for business, told me that he has established a network of friends all over the country. When visiting another town, he will meet with one of these friends rather than go to 'bad places'.[187] Another example is a young man who, realising that he is weak in the area of sexuality, has consciously opted for a girlfriend who supports the principle of abstinence before marriage: 'As for me, as a man it is dangerous to be close to a girl, unless you are with somebody who has principles. ... It comes to women to be strong in this area. I don't know for others, but I am weak in this area; I am not strong.'[188] Thus, the awareness of their weaknesses makes men develop strategies in order to stick to the moral principles they consider to be part of Christian life.

Although men often indicate that it is challenging to live a Christian way of life, they also show a certain optimism about the possibility of doing so. They find it difficult but not impossible. Bishop Banda is referred to by church members as an exemplary figure showing that it is possible to live up to the ideal. 'He is able to indicate that the pressure can be faced, and it is actually not impossible for you to actually overcome it', one male interviewee told me.[189] Likewise, a woman, referring to the bishop, pointed out that men in the church no longer have any excuse when they misunderstand their roles or mistreat their wives.[190] Banda himself is keen to foster this idea. As a true charismatic preacher, he presents himself as an example to the male folk in the church, saying: 'I have experienced this in my life; I have seen that he [Christ] has helped me to condition my mind as a man, to be a faithful husband. Beloved, it can be done today and now in the name of Jesus.'[191] Thus, as a kind of 'charismatic saint', the bishop is the living

---

[186] Interview with Bernard Kamanga, Lusaka, 30 June 2009.
[187] Interview with Henry Mwale, Lusaka, 15 November 2008.
[188] Interview with Robert Cherwa, Lusaka, 27 July 2009.
[189] Interview with Moses Banda, Lusaka, 13 November 2008.
[190] Interview with Febby Chibwika, Lusaka, 16 July 2009.
[191] Banda, *Fatherhood – Part 2*.

proof that it is indeed possible for men to resist temptations and to live a Christian life through Christ.[192]

The Sword of Damocles

Men's commitment to live up to the ideal of Christian life is motivated by different reasons. First and foremost there is a religious motivation. Men often express a desire to live a holy and responsible life, in accordance with God's commandments. Talking about this they frequently refer to certain male figures in the Bible who are inspiring models of manhood. For example, David because he admitted his mistake, asked God for forgiveness and improved his life; Joseph because he handled situations wisely and took responsibility; Jesus because he had a clear direction in life and stood up for what he believed in. On the contrary, the figure of their own father is mentioned by some interviewees as a bad example, functioning as a counter-role model that encourages them to engage in a different type of manhood.[193] For instance, referring to his father who left his family and separated from his wife, one interviewee said: 'It made me aware in my mind that I should always care for my wife ... and not do something that will split up the family and destroy the family.'[194]

It appears that men's motivation is reinforced by two realities that function as a kind of 'sword of Damocles'. These are HIV and the belief in divine judgement. The HIV epidemic has reinforced the commitment of men to live up to the teaching in the area of sexuality. Many of them have seen friends and relatives die because of AIDS. The confrontation with the harsh reality of the epidemic has a strong impact upon their lives. As one interviewee recounted: 'I used to be careless. I thought AIDS is just for those who are unfortunate. But when it was coming closer, to my family and to friends, I changed.'[195] Another told me that the presence of HIV has led him to realise that 'a few minutes of passion can mean death, can ruin your dreams'.[196] It seems that male church members, against the background of the HIV epidemic, have come to understand that the church's emphasis on sexual abstinence can make a difference between life and death and is therefore highly urgent. Clearly, personal health motives reinforce men's religious motivation to abstain from sex or to be faithful in marriage.

---

[192] The notion of 'charismatic saints' comes from anthropologist Simon Coleman, who emphasises that spiritual exemplification of Charismatic leaders is a profoundly relational process. It is not only the pastor who presents himself as a moral and spiritual model, but also the believers who affirm this and who indeed are inspired by and imitate the pastor. See S. Coleman, 'Transgressing the Self: Making Charismatic Saints', in F. Meltzer and J. Elsner (eds), *Saints: Faith Without Borders* (Chicago, 2011), 76.

[193] Cf. Soothill, *Gender, Social Change and* Spiritual *Power*, 186.

[194] Interview with Henry Mwale, Lusaka, 15 November 2008.

[195] Interview with Danny Mulenga, Lusaka, 13 November 2008.

[196] Interview with Marc Mwila, Lusaka, 22 October 2008.

Though HIV may be something to fear, interviewees indicated that the epidemic should not be the sole or primary reason to live up to the moral teaching of the church. They pointed to 'the fear of God' as the most paramount motivation to do so: '[B]eyond HIV/AIDS and beyond attracting these other STDs, there is somebody that I am actually answerable to.'[197] The sense of accountability to God, of course, concerns not only the area of sexuality but moral behaviour more broadly. All deeds that are considered to be immoral are thought of as sin, meaning that they critically impact upon one's relationship with God. There seems to be a constant awareness that 'for everything you do you are going to be judged'.[198] As pointed out above, the fear of divine judgement over one's life is a major stimulus for men to become born again and to live up to the church's ideal of 'biblical manhood'.

Conclusion

Through a detailed analysis of the case of Northmead Assembly of God, this chapter has explored a Pentecostal trajectory and theology through which masculinities are transformed in contemporary Zambia. An important conclusion is that the transformation of masculinities is an explicit project in which the church is actively engaged, as is most clearly demonstrated in the sermon series *Fatherhood in the 21st Century*. In these sermons, as in the broader church discourse, men are blamed for many social problems, such as violence against women, alcoholism, the spread of HIV, disrupted families, failing political leadership, etcetera. These issues are mentioned as illustrations of the 'distortion of manhood' in society, which is explained theologically from the 'Adamic nature' of mankind. An alternative ideal of 'biblical manhood' is defined and promoted, according to which men have to recapture their God-given position and to live up to the related responsibilities. Jesus Christ as the second Adam is presented not only as a model of 'biblical manhood' but also as one who possesses the spiritual powers to liberate men from their 'Adamic nature'. Through Christ, men can become born-again and their masculinity as intended by God is restored.

The discourse on men and masculinity in NAOG in many ways fits in a broader pattern of Pentecostal and Evangelical gender and masculinity politics. For example, there are many similarities between NAOG and the Ghanaian churches studied by Jane Soothill: a similar concern about male behaviour in relation to a perceived moral and social crisis in African families and societies; a similar association of 'African culture' with male domination and irresponsibility; a similar interpretation and use of the Genesis creation story about Adam and Eve; a similar redefinition of male headship and leadership from domination and authority into responsibility, service, sacrifice and self-giving love; a

---

[197] Interview with Moses Banda, Lusaka, 13 November 2008.
[198] Interview with Danny Mulenga, Lusaka, 13 November 2008.

similar shift in focus from the extended to the nuclear family as the centre of a man's responsibility and loyalty; and a similar focus on joint-decision making, partnership and love in marriage.[199] Banda's use of the writings of John Piper on 'biblical manhood' further shows that the discourse in NAOG is directly influenced by American conservative evangelicalism, which exemplifies the globalisation of gender discourses in global Christianity. At the same time it is important to observe that the political intention of Banda's teaching of 'biblical manhood' is different from Piper's. Where Piper and the Council on Biblical Manhood and Womanhood with which he is associated develop their vision of 'biblical manhood and womanhood' as a conservative response to 'evangelical feminism' (that is, gender egalitarian views in American evangelical circles),[200] Banda uses their idea of 'biblical manhood' in his constructive quest to overcome popular types of masculinity in Zambia and the related social problems. Where Piper is explicitly anti-modern, the type of discourse Banda presents is modernising in the Zambian and wider African context, as I will explain later in this book. Even though there is no direct link, the discourse on men and masculinity in NAOG also shows striking similarities with the Promise Keepers, an evangelical men's movement that in the 1990s was popular in the United States. According to John Bartkowski, the Promise Keepers are 'bargaining with patriarchy', meaning that some aspects of hegemonic masculinity are affirmed while others are undermined; traditional and progressive elements are mixed.[201] Because of this ambiguity, there has been much discussion among scholars about the interpretation of the Promise Keepers: 'Are they really moving towards egalitarian relationships between men and women, but still clinging to residual, traditional "headship" language, or are they seeking to undo the gains that women have made and to restore patriarchy in the home?'[202] Similar questions can be raised with regard to NAOG where the 'principle of male headship' is emphasised while at the same time male–female equality is underlined. How to understand the ambiguous discourse on masculinity in NAOG is a question that I will take up further in Chapter 6: can notions such as 'bargaining with patriarchy', 'soft-patriarchy' and 'neo-traditional', which all have been used for the Promise Keepers and similar American evangelical men's movements, also be applied to NAOG and broader African Pentecostal discourse? Here, I just conclude that the case of Northmead Assembly of God reflects the gender paradox observed by sociologist Bernice Martin in global Pentecostalism: 'An unresolved tension remains between the *de jure* system of patriarchal authority in

---

[199] See Soothill, *Gender, Social Change and Spiritual Power*, 181–218.

[200] See 'About us', website of the Council on Biblical Manhood and Womanhood, accessed 7 May 2012, http://www.cbmw.org/About-Us.

[201] J.P. Bartkowski, *The Promise Keepers: Servants, Soldiers, and Godly Men* (New Brunswick, 2004), 74–86.

[202] W.H. Lockhardt, '"We Are One Life", But Not of One Gender Ideology: Unity, Ambiguity, and the Promise Keepers', in R.H. Williams (ed.), *Promise Keepers and the New Masculinity: Private Lives and Public Morality* (Lanham, 2001), 73.

church and home and the *de facto* establishment of a way of life which decisively shifts the domestic and religious priorities in a direction that benefits women and children while morally restraining the traditional autonomy of the male and the selfish or irresponsible exercise of masculine power.'[203] The '*de jure* system of patriarchal authority' here refers to the notions of male headship and leadership that are theologically supported in NAOG. The *de facto* transformation Martin observes is clearly visible in the church, with men being transformed towards an ideal of responsible manhood. As with the Promise Keepers, the fact that this ideal is 'embedded in the familiar and culturally powerful narrative of Christianity' will increase its transformative power.[204]

---

[203] Martin, *The Pentecostal Gender Paradox*, 54.
[204] J.L. Newton, *From Panthers to Promise Keepers: Rethinking the Men's Movement* (Oxford, 2005), 231.

Chapter 5
Comparing the Trajectories and Theologies to Transform Masculinities

The different trajectories and theologies for transforming masculinities presented in the preceding chapters will in this chapter be subjected to a comparison. I will analyse the similarities and differences in the ways the churches and the theologians understand the problem of men and masculinities in times of HIV and AIDS and how they envision and work towards a transformation. This will be done in two steps. First, I will attend to the two case-study churches and, second, I will compare the case studies with the account of the African theologians on masculinities in the context of the HIV epidemic.

Comparing a Catholic and Pentecostal Trajectory

The case studies in Regiment parish and Northmead Assembly of God (NAOG) present a Catholic and a Pentecostal example of how local churches address men and issues related to masculinity, and how they promote Christian ideals of manhood as alternatives for popular forms of masculinity. What are the similarities and differences in the masculinity politics of the two churches? Exploring this question, I discuss the case studies in relation to broader characteristics of Catholicism and Pentecostalism in Africa. This helps to better understand the discourses found in the churches. It also shows that the case studies are part of broader Christian traditions and therefore have a significance that extends into a wider sphere.

A Shared Concern with Men's Moral Lifestyles

Both churches share a deep concern about some patterns of behaviour in men. They address similar issues, such as men's sexual lifestyles and the excessive consumption of alcohol; men's disrespect of, and violence towards, women; men's overall irresponsibility; and men's lack of involvement in the church and commitment to the faith. Apparently, the churches have quite a negative perception of 'the Zambian man' and the prevalent type of masculinity in Zambia. According to the representation of men in the church discourses, Zambian men generally tend to enjoy themselves in bars with alcohol and girls, spend money for amusement rather than using it for the family, dominate women in marriage, are largely absent from the family, often abuse their power and are out to prove their virility. Of course, this is a generalised account. Men's behaviour and the related hegemonic ideals of masculinity are not analysed in-depth in the churches. Some simple explanations are given, pointing to 'African culture' (especially in NAOG), to social factors such as poverty and unemployment (especially in Regiment parish), as well as to the media, modernisation and 'Western culture'. Both churches consider it to be their task to address men about their behaviour. To different extents, they both oppose and contest popular notions of masculinity by promoting Christian values. Clearly, the churches' concern with men is focused on men's private and public moral lifestyles. These are evaluated negatively because they are considered incompatible with Christian moral values (Regiment parish) or with the born-again ideal of holiness (NAOG).

Obviously, the critical perception of men in both case studies is reinforced by the HIV epidemic. Without HIV and AIDS, the churches would probably still address issues concerning sexual behaviour and teach certain moral norms, but the HIV epidemic has made it a priority. Though they do not present an elaborate gender analysis of the epidemic, both churches seem to perceive men's sexual lifestyles as more critical than women's. Consequently, this is a major item in the discourses about men and masculinity. Both church discourses seek to correct men's observed tendency to engage in indiscriminate sexual activity by teaching the norms of abstinence before and fidelity in marriage and by presenting self-control as an essential characteristic of manhood. The use of condoms is prohibited, as this would contradict the values promoted.

The discourse on sexuality and HIV that targets men is in both churches a *moral* discourse. Though the churches do not uphold the belief that HIV is a punishment from God for sexual immorality, they still address it as a consequence of sexual irresponsibility and, indeed, immorality. Of the several discourses on HIV and AIDS that can be distinguished, both churches primarily engage in the 'medico-moral discourse', which promotes HIV prevention 'through individual-centered behaviour change' but opposes the use of condoms as a public health prevention method.[1] This is remarkable, as the leadership in both churches also acknowledges structural factors such as poverty, unemployment and gender inequality. Out of this awareness, Regiment parish has established a community school and a youth training centre, and NAOG has established an HIV clinic and the Lazarus project. However, when HIV is addressed within the congregation, the churches primarily opt for a moral discourse. Individual behaviour is considered the level at which the church can influence its members. The fact that men in particular are addressed might be a result of the awareness of the gendered dimension of HIV. However, it seems to be mainly motivated by a concern about men's sexual lifestyles. In both churches this concern is informed by a particular, biological essentialist understanding of male sexuality: in Regiment, booklets presents men's 'carnal

---

[1] B. Schmid, 'AIDS Discourses in the Church: What we Say and what we do', *Journal of Theology for Southern Africa*, 125 (2006): 96–7.

desires' for sexual satisfaction as part of the natural 'masculine pattern',[2] while in NAOG Bishop Banda points to a particular hormone that makes men to act like 'sex machines'.[3] This biological factor is not presented as an excuse for men, however. Rather, it is emphasised that men have the ability, of course with the help of God, to control their desires through the mind.

The concern about men and male behaviour in both churches is reinforced by the epidemic. However, it is informed by a broader awareness of social problems facing Zambia, such as alcoholism, broken marriages, the impoverishment of families, and disease. Both the sermons in NAOG and the letters of the Zambian Catholic bishops clearly demonstrate a general concern with the poor state of Zambian society. More or less explicitly, this situation is explained in relation to men, male behaviour and dominant versions of masculinity. With the notion of responsibility as key to the ideal of manhood, the churches somehow blame men and their irresponsible behaviour for Zambia's deprived conditions.

An Overlapping Alternative Vision of Masculinity

In addition to their corresponding criticism of men and male behaviour, the churches also show concurrence regarding the ideals of masculinity they promote. Central to the definition of Pentecostal masculinity in NAOG as well as of Catholic masculinity in Regiment parish are notions such as responsibility, headship and self-control. With these notions, the churches seek to promote an ideal of masculinity among men that is opposite to the popular types of masculinity in Zambia. They develop a male ethics of responsibility – responsibility for oneself, one's marriage and family, and the community. Through several church programmes this ethic is promoted among men.

In both churches, there are men who take the church's teaching seriously and try to apply it in their lives. In so doing, they come to embody a type of masculinity that is different from the hegemonic ideals of masculinity in society. What sociologist Bernice Martin notices with regard to men in Pentecostal churches, in my observation not only applies to born-again men in NOAG but also to the practising Catholic men in Regiment parish:

> Pentecostal men must put themselves under novel restraint. Much of what the church expects of them would stigmatize them as unmanly among their unconverted peers: giving up alcohol, drugs, gambling, sexual adventures, and the opportunity to sire children in many households, putting the family and fellow believers before themselves, and so on.[4]

---

[2] C.N. Nganda, *Boys Growing Up*, 5th reprint (Nairobi, 2007), 57.

[3] J. Banda, *Cultivating a Lifestyle of Truth* – Part 6 (Lusaka, 2005), DVD.

[4] B. Martin, 'The Pentecostal Gender Paradox: A Cautionary Tale for the Sociology of Religion', in R.K. Fenn (ed.), *The Blackwell Companion to the Sociology of Religion* (Malden, 2001), 55.

It appears from the case studies that men put themselves under this restraint because it gives them a new identity and dignity, not just as Christians but also as men. In both churches several men expressed the feeling that since living up to the ideal of Christian masculinity they are more appreciated by their wives, are respected in the community, are assigned tasks in the church, and will be blessed by God. This seems to compensate for the possible loss of 'manly status' among peers. In Regiment parish, the new dignity given to men is clearly expressed by the members of the men's group of St Joachim: in their blue uniforms they embody the ideal of Catholic manhood and are highly esteemed in the community.

In the churches the ethical notion of responsibility is related to the concepts of male headship and leadership, which are informed by biblical and cultural traditions. The combination of concepts such as headship and leadership with an ethic of responsibility that involves men in marriage and family life bears resemblance to the process of the 'domestication of men' observed by sociologist Bradford Wilcox in evangelical Protestantism in the United States, and to the 'reformation of machismo' examined by anthropologist Elizabeth Brusco in evangelical Christianity in Colombia.[5] Though completely different contexts, the general pattern is that a certain authority is ascribed to men, which is linked to an ethic of male familial involvement and of more peaceful and constructive male behaviour. Apparently, this is a more commonly used strategy in religious communities and movements to transform hegemonic forms of masculinity. Most often in the literature, this strategy is associated with Protestant-evangelical and Pentecostal Christianity, but the case study in Regiment parish shows that a similar approach can be found in Catholic circles.[6]

It is noteworthy that the case-study churches in their definition of a Christian ideal of manhood depart from what they consider to be 'tradition' or 'culture' on exactly the same issue: male–female relationships. The churches correspond in their criticism that traditional cultures in Zambia do allow dominating attitudes of men towards women, in marriage and in the broader social sphere. The cultural notion of male headship, according to this criticism, entails male superiority and domination of women, and easily gives rise to violence against women. This

---

[5] W.B. Wilcox, 'Religion and the Domestication of Men', *Contexts*, 5/4 (2006): 40–44; W.B. Wilcox, *Soft Patriarchs, New Men: How Christianity Shapes Fathers and Husbands* (Chicago, 2004); E.E. Brusco, *The Reformation of Machismo: Evangelical Conversion and Gender in Colombia* (Austin, 1995).

[6] For a similar observation with regard to the Catholic Church in Peru and El Salvador, see A.L. Peterson, M.A. Vasquez and P.J. Williams, 'The Global and the Local', in A.L. Peterson, M.A. Vasquez and P.J. Williams (eds), *Christianity, Social Change, and Globalization in the Americas* (Piscataway, 2001), 216. Refining Brusco's argument on the reformation of machismo in evangelical churches, these authors point out that 'in both progressive and relatively conservative parishes, Catholic pastoral programs can have many of the same consequences that Brusco and others have described for Evangelical Protestants, such as domesticating men and generating more peaceful patterns of behaviour'.

is contrasted with a Christian version of headship, which is said to be about responsibility, protection and servant leadership. In line with this, both churches describe gender relations, for example in marriage, in terms of equality, mutuality and companionship, and they contrast this with traditional customs. It is believed that Christianity, compared with the traditional set-up, supports more equal relations between a husband and wife and between men and women generally. Much can be said about whether or not the churches' idea of gender inequality in Zambia's traditional cultures is correct. The discourse on 'African culture' in Christian churches should always be viewed critically. However, my point here is a different one. The case-study churches, by promoting a nuanced version of male headship and supporting a sense of gender equality, engage in a pattern of Christian masculinities described by some scholars as 'soft patriarchy'.[7] The concept of soft patriarchy indicates that the churches do not support a brutal form of patriarchy that confers indefinite power to men and legitimates male supremacy. Rather, they present a nuanced patriarchal ideology, in which notions such as male headship and leadership are used to remind men of their 'God-given' responsibilities. Men are challenged to respect women and to contribute constructively to their marriages, families and communities. This soft patriarchal ideology allows the churches to respect what they consider to be the biblical order of gender relations, on the one hand, and to oppose and correct the dominating and destructive male behaviour they observe in society, on the other.

A Shared Understanding of Gender from Creation

In terms of theological anthropology, the ideal of masculinity promoted in the churches is informed by a gender ideology based on the account of creation, with Genesis 2 as a foundational text. According to this understanding, God has created humankind as male and female and has designed both with different but complementary characteristics. This gives rise to a dualist perception of gender and to normative and essentialist perceptions of masculinity and femininity. Actually, according to the theology of these churches there is no such thing as 'gender' (as a socially and culturally variable construct): there is only 'sex' (as a biological given that distinguishes men and women as differently created human beings). Of course the churches are aware that empirically there are different understandings and practices of being a man and being a woman. However, in their perception there is an essential type of 'manhood' and 'womanhood' designed by the creator God. An illustration of this perception is Banda's talk about 'restoring manhood': socially prevailing types of masculinity are considered deviations from the original

---

[7] Joseph Gelfer observes an ideology of soft patriarchy in both the Evangelical and the Catholic men's movement in the United States. See J. Gelfer, *Numen, Old Men: Contemporary Masculine Spiritualities and the Problem of Patriarchy* (London, 2009), 57–8, 87. See also Wilcox, *Soft Patriarchs, New Men*, who observes the emergence of a soft patriarchy in American evangelical Protestantism.

version intended by God, which is to be restored.[8] Although in Regiment parish the discourse is less developed, the perception of masculinity is informed by a similar understanding of sexual difference as rooted in God's creation of humankind as male and female. Remember, for example, how one of the booklets, with a reference to creation, says that 'as a boy you will behave completely differently from a girl, because you are living your masculinity'.[9]

Because of the essentialised and binary understanding of sex/gender, in both churches being a man is considered something fundamentally different from being a woman. Feminist understandings of gender equality are criticised for ignoring the differences between men and women. Indeed, both churches support a notion of male–female equality, based on the idea of humankind being created in the image of God (Genesis 1:27), but this equality is understood in a restricted way. It is about an equal human dignity (Regiment) or equality in personhood (NAOG), which respects the 'fundamental difference' between man and woman. This difference, however, is understood more or less hierarchically in both churches, which is informed by the same account of creation. The creation narrative in Genesis 2 saying that Adam was created first and that Eve was created from Adam's rib is interpreted as a divinely ordained natural order that is to be maintained. This results in an anthropological scheme of male primacy, understood in terms of responsibility, headship and leadership, which has to be accepted and respected by women. Clearly, both churches represent what feminist theologian Rosemary Radford Ruether has called the 'ambiguous structure of Christian anthropology'.[10] The ambiguity is that while the equality of the sexes is recognised, at the same time sexual difference is ordered hierarchically.

As gender theorist Judith Butler points out, the construction of gender as a binary system is informed by an 'epistemic regime of presumptive heterosexuality'.[11] In the case-study churches, this regime is founded upon the creation narrative of Genesis 2 and its notion of male–female complementarity. The idea is that man and woman, because they are created differently, are to complement each other in order to be fully human together. Marriage is considered the institution where this

---

[8] Cf. J. Banda, *Fatherhood in the 21st Century* – Part 4 (Lusaka, 2008).

[9] J. Kiura, *About Boys*, 4th reprint (Nairobi, 2007), 8. Kiura further underscores her essentialist understanding of gender when she says: 'This sexual nature is yours from the moment of conception until death. You may undergo changes as you mature but your sexuality does not change. You remain male.'

[10] R.R. Ruether, *Sexism and God-talk: Towards a Feminist Theology* (Boston, 1983), 93. Ruether describes this ambiguity as follows: 'On the one hand, deeply rooted in Christian thought is an affirmation of the equivalence of maleness and femaleness in the image of God. This has never been denied, but it has tended to become obscured by a second tendency to correlate femaleness with the lower part of human nature in a hierarchical scheme of mind over body, reason over passions.'

[11] J. Butler, *Gender Trouble: Feminism and the Subversion of Identity*, 2nd edn (London, 2006).

complementation is to take place. In Regiment parish, compulsory heterosexuality is clearly at work in the discourse on marriage and family life, and in the promotion of a heterosexually married saint as the model of Catholic manhood. The idea of sexual complementarity is central in Catholic anthropology and is often used in Catholic circles to argue against same-sex relationships.[12] However, different from NAOG, in the parish homosexuality is hardly discussed. In NAOG there is an explicit discourse on homosexuality in which it is argued that same-sex relationships are a violation of God's order of creation. Clearly reinforcing the norm of heterosexuality and more or less actively opposing homosexuality, the case-study churches are no exception in African Christianity. Biblical scholar Masiiwa Ragies Gunda, for example, found that in the public debate on homosexuality in Zimbabwe there is an 'overwhelming use of the creation stories to justify the normativity of heterosexual sexual practices'.[13] Gunda's study and the case studies presented in this book reveal the continuing power of the creation stories to reinforce 'a compulsory and naturalized heterosexuality'.[14] Obviously, the above outlined epistemic regime has direct implications for the politics of masculinity. Not only is masculinity differentiated from, and put in a hierarchical order with, femininity, but also it is defined as a normatively heterosexual category that leads to the silencing of same-sex desire and the discrimination against men involved in same-sex relationships. On this critical issue, the case-study churches reinforce rather than transform hegemonic masculinity.

Different Discourses and Ecclesiologies

Apart from the similarities identified above, there are also some obvious differences in the way the case-study churches deal with men and engage in a transformation of masculinities. For example, though they largely correspond in their negative depiction of men, the churches differ in the way they address men and contest the type of masculinity considered problematic. In NAOG there is a far more explicit discourse in which issues concerning men and masculinity are addressed critically,

---

[12] For example, Tanzanian Catholic theologian Laurenti Magesa refers to an 'essential complementarity' of man and woman because of the 'innate sexual qualities which God has endowed each sex'; hence, he argues that 'this is perhaps where homosexuality falls short: not only on the biological level, but more essentially on the psychological and spiritual levels. If homosexuality means the total rejection of either woman or man, [...] either the feminine or masculine, then one must say that it is theologically and spiritually seriously flawed.' See L. Magesa, 'The Challenge of African Woman Defined Theology for the 21st Century', in N.W. Ndung'u and P.N. Mwaura (eds), *Challenges and Prospects of the Church in Africa: Theological Reflections of the 21st Century* (Nairobi, 2005), 100.

[13] M.R. Gunda, *The Bible and Homosexuality in Zimbabwe: A Socio-historical Analysis of the Political, Cultural and Christian Arguments in the Homosexual Public Debate with Special Reference to the use of the Bible* (Bamberg, 2010), 205.

[14] Butler, *Gender Trouble*, 31.

and in which men are challenged to change their lifestyles. At times, this discourse employs dramatic language, with terms such as distortion, deception, abdication, and violation being used in reference to socially prevalent types of manhood. The case of NAOG, then, confirms the finding of Jane Soothill from research in Ghana that charismatic or Pentecostal discourses particularly address 'the role played by irresponsible males in what is perceived by the churches as the social and moral crisis in African family life'.[15] In NAOG, the social and moral crisis is considered in an even broader way: it is not just a crisis in the family but in society at large. In contrast to this is Regiment parish, where a dramatic discourse on men and masculinities is absent. Compared with NAOG, the discourse that addresses men and masculinity issues is less developed and not prominently present. Furthermore, this discourse is more nuanced on several issues, for example when it comes to the consumption of alcohol.

The difference between an explicit, somewhat dramatic discourse and a more implicit, nuanced discourse can be explained on the basis of the different ecclesiologies of both churches and the related fundamental difference in church types. Regiment parish is part of the Catholic Church, which is a mainstream church in Zambia comprising a substantial part of the population. Furthermore, the Catholic Church has an inclusive ecclesiology, understanding itself not as separated from but as closely connected to the community. A sociological result of this is that numerous men who identify as Catholics actually embody, in various degrees, the type of masculinity prevalent in society. Though the church may be fairly critical of popular masculinity, it will not radically oppose it but rather seek to 'evangelise' it gradually, because the church understands itself not in contrast to but as part of society. As Ghanaian Catholic theologian Peter Addai-Mensah puts it in his book on the church's mission among male youths: '[T]he church is not a haven of saints. Rather, it is a place where people come in to encounter the Lord Jesus Christ in order to be formed so that they can be transformed into the image and likeness of God.'[16] Pentecostal churches such as NAOG have a completely different ecclesiology. In line with the theology of holiness, they consider the church as a holy place in the midst of a sinful world.[17] All church members are supposed to live holy lives. One has to be born again, that is, to have left the former life behind, before joining the church. Hence, there is a strong tendency to demarcate the lines between the church and 'the world'. In NAOG this results in a discourse that strongly contests the popular, 'worldly' versions of masculinity and promotes a radically different, Christian ideal that is typically called 'biblical manhood'.

---

[15] J.E. Soothill, *Gender, Social Change and Spiritual Power: Charismatic Christianity in Ghana* (Leiden, 2007), 186.

[16] P. Addai-Mensah, *Mission, Communion and Relationship: A Roman Catholic Response to the Crisis of Male Youths in Africa* (New York, 2009), 172.

[17] Cf. V.M. Kärkkäinen, *An Introduction to Ecclesiology: Ecumenical, Historical and Global Perspectives* (Downers Grove, 2002), 90.

The observed difference between Regiment parish and NAOG transcends both case studies and points to a fundamental difference between Catholicism and Pentecostalism in general. Comparing both strands of Christianity globally, sociologist David Martin points out that where Catholicism is characterised by territoriality, birthright membership and continuity, Pentecostalism presents a church model based on individual choice, strict group boundaries, conversion and discontinuity. 'This means', says Martin with regard to Catholicism, 'that it places a sacred canopy over the average and the religiously relaxed, and lacks a defined and incisive edge.'[18] These broad characterisations of Pentecostalism and Catholicism respectively help to understand the different starting positions and strategies of Pentecostal and Catholic churches to function as moral communities and to bring about change in the behaviour and lifestyle of their members. The case studies show how this impacts on the ways men are critically addressed and the degree to which popular masculinities are challenged in churches.

A Strict Ideal versus a Broad Direction

When it comes to the alternative to hegemonic masculinity promoted in both churches, the difference between an explicit, quite radical and a more implicit, nuanced discourse appears again. In NAOG a Pentecostal ideal of masculinity is presented in terms of 'biblical manhood', claiming that it is derived from the Bible (and suggesting that it is opposed to 'African culture'). This ideal is defined in sermons and is promoted in the various ministries of the church, such as the youth ministry, the men's ministry and the marriage ministry. In Regiment parish, on the other hand, there is no precise definition of an ideal of masculinity. If there is such a thing as 'Catholic manhood' – and I have tried to reconstruct its meaning – it is a diverse outcome of men's commitment to the tradition of faith and the moral values of the church rather than a clearly articulated ideal. Rather than being preached about, it is symbolically represented by ancient figures such as St Joachim and St Joseph, who embody the moral and spiritual virtues considered important for Catholic men. The difference in discourse leaves men in Regiment parish, compared to men in NAOG, with more space to navigate and negotiate the ways they understand and perform masculinity within a range that is more or less acceptable to their church. Compared with the well-defined and actively promoted ideal of masculinity in NAOG, Regiment parish allows for relatively diverse masculinities.

Not specifically writing on masculinities, Robert Garner has observed that Pentecostal churches are more successful than mainline churches in HIV prevention. He explains this in terms of four key factors: indoctrination, religious experience, exclusion and socialisation. He considers the first factor, indoctrination (which is to be understood 'without pejorative undertones' as 'the methods and depth

---

[18] D. Martin, *Pentecostalism: The World their Parish* (Malden, 2002), 18.

of the group's educational programme'), the most powerful.[19] This underscores the importance of the explicit discourse and well-defined ideal of masculinity that is found in NAOG.[20] The indoctrination in teaching on manhood is further strengthened by the above-mentioned exclusivity of the church in relation to society at large, the social spaces in the church where men are encouraged to live up to the ideal of Christian manhood, and by the fact that this ideal is defined in relation to the religious experience of becoming born again and the subsequent process of sanctification that is characteristic of Pentecostal spirituality. In other words, NAOG's engagement with masculinities and their transformation largely meets the four factors for successful HIV prevention mentioned by Garner. This is in line with Ezra Chitando, who – though quite critical of Pentecostal masculinity, as will be explored later – praises the engagement of Pentecostal churches like NAOG for inculcating 'progressive masculinities'. From research in Zimbabwe, Chitando observes that the 'Pentecostal engagement with masculinities offers a lot of promise in the struggle against the HIV epidemic'.[21]

Does this mean that Regiment parish, or the Catholic Church in general, compared with NOAG and other Pentecostal churches, is less effective in realising change among men, because it does not promote a well-defined ideal of masculinity and does not engage in a proactive campaign to transform masculinities? I have already noted that the ideal of masculinity promoted in Regiment parish largely corresponds with the one promoted in NAOG. The parish also provides social spaces for men to be educated in this ideal and to encourage each other to live up to it. However, the level of what Garner calls indoctrination is obviously lower than in NAOG because of the absence of an explicit discourse on issues related to masculinity. Additionally, in contrast to NAOG, Regiment parish does not seem to impose strict social and/or spiritual sanctions on those who violate the norms set by the church. On the one hand, this may imply that the parish is less prepared to effectively transform masculinities in the face of the HIV epidemic and other social challenges. On the other, however, Regiment parish, precisely because of its inclusive ecclesiology and rather broad ideal, may be well positioned to reach

---

[19] R.C. Garner, 'Safe Sects? Dynamic Religion and AIDS in South Africa', *The Journal of Modern African Studies*, 38/1 (2000): 48.

[20] Though the promotion of a clear ideal of manhood is likely to add to the effectiveness of a transformation of masculinities, there is also a risk that the ideal is too high and becomes unrealistic. In that case, living up to the high moral standards might become no more than an issue of keeping up appearances (cf. J. Sadgrove, '"Keeping Up Appearances": Sex and Religion Amongst University Students in Uganda', *Journal of Religion in Africa*, 37/1 (2007): 116–44).

[21] E. Chitando, 'A New Man for a New Era? Zimbabwean Pentecostalism, Masculinities and the HIV Epidemic', *Missionalia*, 35/3 (2007): 121. By 'progressive masculinities' Chitando means the Pentecostal effort to socialise boys and men to be 'counter-cultural in terms of their values', especially their values concerning matters of sexuality, violence and gender relations (ibid., 117).

men in the community and to gradually effect change – particularly among those men who are frightened away by the radical approach of Pentecostal churches such as NAOG.

An Individual versus a Communitarian Approach

Another significant difference between the case-study churches is the use of either a more individual or a more communitarian approach to issues of gender, men and masculinities. An indication of this difference is the reluctance demonstrated by the parish priest in Regiment parish to target men as a specific group to be addressed. Explaining this, he says that in Catholic thought 'the starting point is the family' rather than issues of gender or men and women as individuals.[22] This is a meaningful comment, especially in contrast to the explicit discourse on masculinities in NAOG and the direct ways Banda calls upon men as individuals.

In Regiment parish, the starting point is the family rather than the individual. As outlined in Chapter 3, the concept of the family is rather broad, as it points to all levels of the church as the family of God: from the nuclear and extended family to the community and society. The individual is principally thought of as a member of the human community. As a result, the ideal of masculinity is the model of the family man, with family being understood in this broad way. Masculinities are defined and evaluated in terms of men's contribution to the community. This approach can be understood from the way African cultures traditionally understand the relation between the individual and the community. Referring to the traditional philosophical principle that 'I am because we are, and since we are therefore I am', Addai-Mensah underscores the need for the Catholic church 'to point out to male youths that individualism is not according to their nature' and that young men need to understand their existence in relation to, and as contributing to, the existence of others.[23] In NAOG, the approach is precisely the other way around. The starting point is the individual who has to make a break with the past to become born again and to live a holy life. Certainly, the ideal of masculinity in the church emphasises the role of men in the family, the community and society. However, fulfilling these roles is considered the responsibility of the individual, while in Regiment parish there is an idea of an organic community where men and women play their respective roles.

The observed difference between the two churches can be understood in relation to a fundamental divergence between Pentecostalism and Catholicism observed in scholarly literature. Scholars of Pentecostalism have often argued that this religious movement somehow advocates 'modernity' in Africa and in other parts of the world, among other things through the promotion of individualism. In the words of David Martin, Pentecostalism reflects the 'major narrative of modernity' as it represents individual self-consciousness and agency, and underscores a new

---

[22] Interview with Fr Marc Nsanzurwimo, Lusaka, 29 July 2009.
[23] Addai-Mensah, *Mission, Communion and Relationship*, 103.

religious identity that implies a break with social bonds.[24] He contrasts this with Catholicism, which embodies 'the realities of organic community, located in territory and uniting religious with social identity'.[25] Where African Pentecostalism is concerned with 'rebuilding the individual',[26] Catholicism in Africa embraces the idea that '[i]n African culture and tradition the role of the family is everywhere held to be fundamental'[27] and hence insists upon the 'promotion of the family and protection of the sacredness of family life'.[28]

The broad association of Pentecostalism with 'modernity' and of Catholicism with 'tradition' is also reflected in the case-study churches. A case in point is the different perception of the family. NAOG tends to focus on the nuclear family, while Regiment parish tends to have a broader scope. In both churches there is reference to the demands made by relatives in the extended family, and church members indicate they consider these a serious responsibility. However, in NAOG, both in the formal discourse and in the accounts of church members, the duties to the extended family tend to be considered problematic. There is a sense that a man as head of his family first and foremost should concentrate on his marriage and small family, rather than sharing his resources with relatives (yet he is supposed to contribute substantially to the church, which might suggest that the church replaces the extended family[29]). In Regiment, on the other hand, these demands are considered as inherent to a man's position in the community and cannot, therefore, be neglected. Even though people realise that due to economic hardship it is often difficult to respond to these demands, they still consider them a responsibility that cannot simply be ignored.

---

[24] D. Martin, *On Secularization: Towards a Revised General Theory* (Aldershot, 2005), 141. See also Martin, *Pentecostalism*, 17ff.

[25] Martin, *On Secularization*, 144.

[26] O.U. Kalu, *African Pentecostalism: An Introduction* (Oxford, 2008), 213–15. This is not to say that Pentecostalism is not concerned with a rebuilding of society or the nation. As appears in the chapter on NAOG, clearly there is such a concern. However, the starting point is the individual, and a rebuilding of the nation is thought to be realised through a spiritual and moral renewal of individuals.

[27] John Paul II, *Post-Synodal Apostolic Exhortation Ecclesia in Africa of the Holy Father John Paul II to the Bishops, Priests and Deacons, Men and Women Religious and all the Lay Faithful to the Church in Africa and its Evangelizing Mission Towards the Year 2000* (Yaoundé, 1995), no. 43.

[28] Catholic Bishops of Zambia, 'You Shall be My Witnesses: Pastoral Letter of the Catholic Bishops of Zambia to Mark 100 Years of Catholic Faith in Zambia (9th July 1991)', in J. Komakoma (ed.), *The Social Teaching of the Catholic Bishops and Other Christian Leaders in Zambia. Major Pastoral Letters and Statements 1953–2001* (Ndola, 2003), 253.

[29] Indeed, David Maxwell, in his study on the Zimbabwean Pentecostal Assemblies of God, observes that among urban Pentecostals, 'the church becomes the believer's extended family while ties with kin diminish as energies are refocused on the nuclear family'. See D. Maxwell, *African Gifts of the Spirit: Pentecostalism & the Rise of a Zimbabwean Transnational Religious Movement* (Oxford, Harare and Athens, 2006), 201.

The Relation between Christianity, Tradition and Modernity

As mentioned above, the difference between an individual-centred and community-centred approach and between a focus on the nuclear and the extended family can be understood in relation to the broad orientation of Pentecostalism towards 'modernity' and of Catholicism towards 'tradition'. As anthropologist Birgit Meyer points out, the different appreciation of what is perceived as African tradition and culture distinguishes Pentecostalism from Catholicism and mainline Protestant Christianity in Africa:

> While other groups in society, among them leaders of the Catholic and Protestant mission churches, try to come to terms with local traditions and to reconcile new and old ideas in order to develop a genuinely African synthesis, Pentecostalists oppose this revaluation of tradition and culture. They emphasize the "global" character of this variant of Christianity and the necessity to break away from local traditions.[30]

It appears from the case studies that the observed different appreciation of culture directly affects how the relation between 'African' and 'Christian' manhood is considered in local church communities.

In NAOG, the ideal of biblical manhood tends to be defined, especially by the church leadership, in contrast to 'traditional' Zambian or African types of masculinity. While the latter are associated with extramarital sex, domination over and violence towards women, laziness, irresponsibility and so on, a Christian man is supposed to be born again and to live a totally different type of life. This corresponds with Soothill's observation that Pentecostal churches hold African culture, specifically the traditional perceptions of the superior status of men, responsible for the moral and social crisis they perceive in African societies and families nowadays.[31] The churches demand a definite departure from tradition, and this is considered as having particular implications for male converts. For them, 'a break with the past is conceptualised in terms of their attitudes towards women and the rejection of role models established by their fathers'.[32] The departure from local traditions and the orientation towards global Christian discourses is further illustrated in Banda's definition of 'biblical manhood', developed in several sermons, which he borrowed from the North American evangelical author John Piper.[33]

---

[30] B. Meyer, '"Make a Complete Break with the Past": Memory and Post-colonial Modernity in Ghanaian Pentecostalist Discourse', *Journal of Religion in Africa*, 28/3 (1998): 317.

[31] Soothill, *Gender, Social Change and Spiritual Power*, 189.

[32] Ibid.

[33] This is in itself an example of the globalisation of gender ideologies within contemporary world Christianity. Such a globalisation also takes place in a transnational

In Regiment parish the continuity in, rather than the distinction between, Christianity and African culture is highlighted. This is in line with the Catholic idea of inculturation, which presumes a basic positive attitude towards local cultural traditions and their compatibility with Christianity. Drawing from the concept of inculturation, Addai-Mensah argues that for the Catholic Church in Africa, in the light of 'the crisis of male youth', there is a missionary responsibility to employ the religious-cultural traditions in the formation of identity among young men:

> [I]f the church is to respond effectively to the plight of male youth in Africa, it must attend to the cultural dynamics of Africa [*sic*] Religious Tradition (ATR) mindful of the fact that having been born into the religio-cultural reality of ATR, young men are not well-served by denying this reality or relegating it to the background of their lives. In the past, ATR contributed to the formation of their ancestors[;] in the present its philosophical insights and traditional religious wisdom must be recognized as a critical component of their identity formation from birth to adolescence and from adulthood to the grave.[34]

Though this proposal for a Catholic evangelisation of male youths by means of African religious and cultural resources is not formally implemented in Regiment parish, the positive attitude to, and the constructive use of, indigenous traditions is also found in the parish. However, even though traditional cultures and religions are perceived positively, the project of inculturation is intended to be a *critical* correlation between 'gospel' and 'culture'. In the process, some elements in African cultures are accepted but others are rejected or changed, thus bringing about a Christian transformation of culture.[35] In Regiment parish this is also applied to the type of masculinity that is considered traditional: on the one hand, its assumed notions of responsibility and provision are embraced, while on the other hand its assumed notions of male supremacy and domination are criticised because they do not recognise the equal dignity of men and women. Some parishioners go as far as to reject the notion of male headship for this reason (in particular the parishioners involved in Marriage Encounter – a movement considered to be more middle class, modern and Western).

One may conclude that Regiment parish promotes a Christianised version of traditional masculinity, while NAOG promotes a modern Christian masculinity. However, it is too simple to say that Pentecostalism advocates 'modernity'. First, such a statement assumes a singular (Western) notion of modernity, while in

---

institution such as the Roman Catholic Church. Discourses on gender in Regiment parish clearly reflect wider Catholic thought. However, in Catholic circles in Africa there is a tendency to mediate the church's teaching in relation to local cultures and traditions (inculturation), which is more or less missing in Pentecostalism.

[34] See Addai-Mensah, *Mission, Communion and Relationship*, 176.

[35] Cf. L. Magesa, *Anatomy of Inculturation: Transforming the Church in Africa* (Maryknoll, 2004), 144.

contemporary Africa there are multiple ways of being modern, as is acknowledged in the plural notion of 'African modernities'.[36] Second, anthropological research shows that the relation of Pentecostalism to what is often considered 'modern' is rather complex and ambiguous. As Rijk van Dijk puts it, 'Pentecostalism in modern African societies is both a debate within modernity as well as a discourse on modernity'.[37] The complex relation between Pentecostalism and modernity is illustrated, for example, in the way Bishop Banda of NAOG deals with the modern notion of gender equality. In one and the same sermon he can emphasise the fundamental 'equality of male and female' and criticise feminist movements for fighting God's order of male headship.[38] Banda's attempt to 'reconcile' the notion of male–female equality with the notion of male headship is not so much an example of an African Pentecostal pastor being stuck halfway toward modernity. Rather, it exemplifies the construction of alternative modernities in African Pentecostal circles. This process is a negotiation between modern socio-economic developments, new opinions brought about by Western (but globalising) discourses, and traditional values and beliefs. An example of such a negotiation is the understanding of men's role as providers for the family. More so than in Regiment parish, where this notion is simply confirmed, in NAOG it is subject of discussion. One explanation may be that a middle-class church like NAOG is affected to a greater degree by recent developments in Zambia such as the increasing level of education among women, the consequent increased involvement of women in formal employment, and women's pursuit of a professional career. These socio-economic changes are brought about by modernity and urban life, and they impact on gender relations in marriage. As outlined in Chapter 4, NAOG responds to these changes in an ambiguous way. On the one hand, the church allows, and even encourages, women to be educated, employed and to pursue careers. On the other, the church wants to maintain the male role of providing. This is not primarily because it is thought to be 'African' but because it is regarded as 'biblical'.[39] Thus, the church ends up allowing women to contribute a substantial or even the major part of the household income, while at the same time insisting that they respect their husbands as heads and primary providers in the home.[40] In

---

[36] J.G. Deutch, P. Probst and H. Schmidt (eds), *African Modernities: Entangled Meanings in Current Debate* (Oxford, 2002).

[37] R. van Dijk, 'Time and Transcultural Technologies of the Self in the Ghanaian Pentecostal Diaspora', in A. Corten and R. Marshall-Fratani (eds), *Between Babel and Pentecost: Transnational Pentecostalism in Africa and Latin America* (Bloomington, 2001), 218.

[38] J. Banda, *Fatherhood in the 21st Century* – Part 6 (Lusaka, 2008).

[39] Cf. J. Banda, *Fatherhood in the 21st Century* – Part 3 (Lusaka, 2008), DVD: 'The principal income is for the man. That's the biblical order. He is provider and protector of the homestead.'

[40] Like NAOG, charismatic churches in Ghana are found by Soothill to be 'critical of married women who try to "boss" their husbands because their income matches or even

order to make the latter reasonable, the male role of providing is redefined: the emphasis subtly moves from providing for the economic needs of the family to the need for spiritual and moral leadership. This process of negotiation over, and changing meanings of, traditional gender roles illustrates the need to move beyond the question of whether Pentecostalism is modern or not, and to focus on the ways in which Pentecostalism brings about new forms of modernity.[41]

As much as NAOG and Pentecostalism in general do not merely advocate but negotiate and recreate modernity, Regiment parish and the Catholic Church in Africa more generally do not simply embrace 'tradition' and oppose 'modernity'. The project of inculturation can be considered a particularly Catholic way of negotiating Christianity, African cultural traditions and modern values and developments.[42] As a result, parallel processes of creating African modernities can be found in African Catholic and Pentecostal circles. The Catholic navigation of modernity may be more positive towards African cultural traditions, but this positive stance is only insofar as the beliefs and practices in these cultures do not conflict with Catholic thought (which itself originates from the West but has a complex relationship to Western modernity). As the case studies have shown, both in Regiment parish and NAOG a Christian ideal of masculinity is defined that moves between the local and the global, between tradition and modernity, but with somewhat different outcomes.

Religious Leaders as Role Models of Manhood

A final but important difference between the two case studies concerns the role played by the leaders of the churches in the promotion of the ideal of manhood. In NAOG, a prominent role is played by Banda. That men and issues of masculinity are addressed so explicitly and that the church actively promotes an alternative ideal of masculinity have largely arisen from his concerns and vision. As the senior pastor of the church, which *is* his personal ministry, he is in the position to put his vision into practice, for example by delivering a series of sermons on 'biblical

---

exceeds that of their spouse' (Soothill, *Gender, Social Change and Spiritual Power*, 207). Soothill explains this from the situation of economic decline, where traditional masculinities are threatened because men are not able to be the breadwinners as tradition expects of them, while at the same time women engage in the informal sector and may bring in the greater part of the income. Though similar cases are referred to in NAOG, the concern in this church with the male role of providing is not informed primarily by the situation of economic hardship but rather by women's increased involvement in *formal* employment in modern urban Zambia.

[41] Cf. J. Robbins, 'Anthropology of Religion', in A. Anderson, M. Bergunder, A. Droogers and C. van der Laan (eds), *Studying Global Pentecostalism: Theories and Methods* (Berkeley, 2010), 168–73.

[42] Cf. A.J. Paolini, *Navigating Modernity: Postcolonialism, Identity, and International Relations* (London, 1999), 173–5.

manhood'. Furthermore, as the prominent charismatic and high-profile leader of the church, he functions as a role model for church members in general and particularly for men. Banda not only preaches about biblical manhood; according to both men and women in the church, he also embodies this ideal himself. Male church members take him as an example to follow, and female church members refer to him when correcting their husbands. Indeed, in sermons Banda frequently presents himself as an example, particularly in the area of marriage and family life. He can possibly be considered an example of what anthropologist Simon Coleman has called 'charismatic saints' – Charismatic preachers who exemplify the principles of holiness and whose lives and words are mirrored in the lives of their followers.[43]

Different from Banda is Nsanzurwimo, the priest in charge of Regiment parish. As a parish priest in a worldwide, hierarchically organised and liturgically centred church, his position is far less prominent and his power is limited. His role is first and foremost to celebrate the sacraments. He may function as a spiritual role model to his parishioners, but because of his celibate lifestyle it is difficult for male parishioners to take him as an example in the critical areas of sexuality, marriage and family life. In contrast to Banda, Nsanzurwimo does not seem to function as a role model of manhood. Male parishioners may identify with him as Catholics, but probably not specifically as Catholic *men*. It might be that among Catholic men, the bishop rather than the parish priest is a primary figure with authority and a role model function.[44] This is indicated, for example, by the eagerness of members of St Joachim to provide assistance in diocese-related gatherings where the archbishop of Lusaka is acting. However, like the parish priest, the archbishop will also be a spiritual role model rather than a model of masculinity. Compared with the charismatic pastors in a Pentecostal church such as NAOG, the celibate clerics in a Catholic church such as Regiment parish seem to be less appealing to male believers as models they can identify with as men. However the Catholic Church has its saint figures that function as role models representing certain male virtues. Though originating from ancient times, their traditions are revitalised in the light of today's challenges, as the case of St Joachim clearly shows.[45] Compared to the charismatic Pentecostal church leaders, the advantage of these saint figures is, of course, that they will never fall from their pedestals.

---

[43] S. Coleman, 'Transgressing the Self: Making Charismatic Saints', in F. Meltzer and J. Elsner (eds), *Saints: Faith Without Borders* (Chicago, 2011), 73–96.

[44] This is suggested by Joseph Gelfer with regard to the Catholic men's movement in the USA. See J. Gelfer, 'Identifying the Catholic Men's Movement', *Journal of Men's Studies*, 16/1 (2008): 52.

[45] Cf. A.S. van Klinken, 'St. Joachim as a Model of Catholic Manhood in Times of AIDS: A Case Study on Masculinity in an African Christian Context', *CrossCurrents*, 61/4 (2011): 467–79.

Comparing the Case Studies to the African Theologians

Chapter 2 has shown that the African theologians working on issues of gender and masculinities are, on the one hand, critical of churches for reinforcing patriarchal masculinities, while are, on the other, positive about the potential role churches could play in the transformation of masculinities. This calls for a closer analysis of the ways the theologians and the case-study churches understand and seek to overcome the 'crisis of masculinity' as revealed by the HIV epidemic. How do the case-study churches actually relate to the trajectory and theology of transformative masculinities presented by the theologians? What are the convergences and divergences in the way the churches and the theologians address men and masculinities?

A Shared Concern about Men and Masculinities

Among the African theologians, Ezra Chitando has most explicitly expressed the view that the HIV epidemic challenges African churches to rethink their mission towards men. He considers it crucial for 'AIDS-competent churches' to challenge hegemonic masculinities and to engage in an 'evangelisation of men' and a transformation of masculinities.[46] The case studies show that some local churches have indeed been challenged to engage in a mission towards men. This is most obvious in NAOG, where the transformation of men and masculinities is an explicit project in which the church is engaged, though to a lesser extent it is also true for Regiment parish. Both churches, as concluded above, show a critical awareness of the role played by men in various problems facing society, and they try to change men and to promote alternative forms of masculinity. As far as this criterion is concerned, Regiment parish and NAOG can be considered as examples of the AIDS-competent churches Chitando is looking for.

With regard to specific critical aspects of masculinities, African theologians point to issues such as men's engagement in violence against women, their domination of women, and male sexual behaviour. Precisely these issues are also addressed in the case-study churches. South African theologian Beverley Haddad calls on churches to break the silence on violence against women and to challenge men to take responsibility for their sexual behaviour.[47] Both case-study churches meet this call, as has become clear in the former chapters: they address men's perpetration of domestic and sexual violence, they challenge men to behave sexually in a responsible way and they promote men's control of their sexual desires. Where Ezra Chitando, Sophie Chirongoma and Fulata Moyo employ the

---

[46] E. Chitando, *Acting in Hope: African Churches and HIV/AIDS 2* (Geneva, 2007), 40–54.

[47] B. Haddad, 'Choosing to Remain Silent: Links between Gender Violence, HIV/AIDS and the South African Church', in I.A. Phiri, B. Haddad and M. Masenya (eds), *African Women, HIV/AIDS and Faith Communities* (Pietermaritzburg, 2003), 155.

concept of machismo to capture the hegemonic masculinity that in their opinion is destructive in the context of HIV and AIDS,[48] expressions of this machismo among men are critically addressed in the churches. It can be concluded, then, that the churches and the theologians largely correspond in their perception of the critical role of men and of the problematic aspects of popular masculinities in relation to the HIV epidemic and other challenges in society.

A Shared Quest for Alternative Masculinities

Apart from addressing men and contesting hegemonic forms of masculinity, the case-study churches as well as the theologians want men to embrace an alternative masculinity. With regard to the churches, this is most obviously the case in NAOG, where there is an explicit discourse on what is called 'biblical manhood' and where male church members in several ways are actively challenged to engage in this ideal. But it is clear that Regiment parish also upholds certain ideals that differ from popular versions of masculinity. So when Chitando argues that 'churches need to engage with men in order to transform dangerous ideas about manhood in Africa', both churches meet this need, though in different ways and to different extents.[49]

As mentioned above, with regard to Pentecostal churches Chitando indeed acknowledges their engagement with the transformation of masculinities. He evaluates this positively in view of the impact in contexts of HIV:

> Pentecostals seek to empower men to realise that abstinence and faithfulness are realistic options in the HIV era. The Pentecostal teaching on mutuality and communication in marriage is also critical in the HIV era. ... The Pentecostal engagement with masculinities offers a lot of promise in the struggle against the HIV epidemic in Zimbabwe.[50]

Chitando speaks about the Pentecostal movement in Zimbabwe, and does not refer to churches from other Christian traditions. However, he seems to suggest that in their engagement with masculinities, Pentecostal churches distinguish themselves from other churches. This suggestion is supported by the case studies: more so than Regiment parish, NAOG is explicitly engaged in a transformation of masculinities as a response to the HIV epidemic and other social challenges. However both churches foster values such as abstinence and fidelity among men, and teach

---

[48] Cf. E. Chitando and S. Chirongoma, 'Challenging Masculinities: Religious Studies, Men and HIV in Africa', *Journal of Constructive Theology*, 14/1 (2008): 58; F.L. Moyo, 'Sex, Gender, Power and HIV/AIDS in Malawi: Threats and Challenges to Women Being Church', in I.A. Phiri and S. Nadar (eds), *On Being Church: African Women's Voices and Visions* (Geneva, 2005), 131.

[49] Chitando, *Acting in Hope*, 46.

[50] Chitando, *A New Man for a New Era?*, 121.

notions like partnership, mutual respect and communication in marriage. Where Chitando concludes that Pentecostal churches play 'a major role in challenging men to adopt masculinities that do not threaten the well-being of women, children and men',[51] this study shows that a Catholic church such as Regiment parish also plays a significant role, albeit in a way that is different from a Pentecostal church such as NAOG. As both case-study churches engage constructively in a mission towards men and seek to realise change among men, it can be concluded that they somehow meet the basic demand of the theologians that churches should challenge hegemonic masculinities and promote alternative types.

An Individualist versus a Structuralist Analysis

Though Chitando acknowledges the major role played by Pentecostal churches in a transformation of masculinities, his overall judgement of the engagement of these churches with masculinities in the context of HIV is rather critical. His criticism is interesting as it clearly illustrates some of the most fundamental divergences between the theologians and the case-study churches in their analyses of and visions for masculinities.

One of the critical issues mentioned by Chitando concerns the difference between an approach that analyses men primarily as individual moral subjects, and a structural approach of men as gendered subjects involved in powered gender relations. As mentioned above, the case-study churches correspond in their concern about men's moral lifestyles and they both seek to change the moral behaviour of men. In that sense, they both address and transform masculinities at the level of the individual. Interestingly, Chitando in his criticism of Pentecostal efforts to transform masculinity praises this focus on the individual but at the same time evaluates it as insufficient:

> One of the most persuasive aspects of African Pentecostal rhetoric on masculinities in the context of HIV is its focus on the individual. He is encouraged to undertake a commitment to become "a new man". However, this might downplay the reality that numerous factors can constrain a man's capacity to act differently. Thus, there is a clear need for Pentecostalism to address structural factors, while encouraging individuals to become new creations. Socio-cultural definitions of masculinity and femininity need to be deconstructed.[52]

According to Chitando, and other theological scholars such as Tinyiko Maluleke and, recently, Jairos Hlatywayo, there is an urgency for churches to adopt a structural approach to men and masculinities that takes into account the problematic

---

[51] Ibid., 124.
[52] Ibid., 123.

male behaviour deeply rooted in structures of gender and power in society.[53] This approach is in line with the tradition of African women theologians, who have always addressed gender inequality as embedded in social, economic and political structures and in cultural and religious ideologies. Hence the theologians now engage in a thorough and critical analysis of masculinities. Their focus is not just on the critical behaviour of individual men, but more broadly on the social structures in which this behaviour is embedded. The case-study churches hardly do so: while they are concerned with the way men engage in gender relations, they are not concerned with structures of gender and power as such. While they do address the abuse of power by men, such as through violence or domination, rather than analysing this critically in terms of structural and powered gender inequalities, they seek to correct it by focusing upon men's responsibilities.

The observed difference between the churches' individualist and the theologians' structuralist analyses of men and masculinities corresponds with their different understandings of the HIV epidemic. Though the churches demonstrate some awareness of structural issues underlying the epidemic, they tend to deal with HIV primarily at the level of people's moral attitudes towards sexuality. Thus, they critically address individual behaviour, teach certain Christian moral values and insist on responsibility and self-control. In so doing, they specifically target men, as men's sexual lifestyle is considered so problematic. The theologians on the other hand, as explored in Chapter 2, have developed an HIV and AIDS liberation theology that explains the epidemic primarily from unequal social and economic structures. In the tradition of liberation theologies, these structures are interpreted theologically in terms of 'social injustice' and 'structural sin'. The need for structural social transformation is emphasised time and time again, as this is considered the only adequate strategy to overcome the epidemic. According to the theologians, one of the key social structures that is in urgent need of transformation is gender inequality or patriarchy. It is precisely on the issue of patriarchy that the theologians and the churches most fundamentally diverge in their approach to men and masculinities.

Transforming Masculinities within or beyond Patriarchy

As previously mentioned, Chitando criticises the Pentecostal engagement with masculinities in Zimbabwe as inadequate because it only focuses on individual behaviour. In his opinion, this does not take into account the powered structures of gender in which masculinities are embedded and that give rise to problematic male

---

[53] J. Hlatywayo, 'Dangerous Masculinities: An Analysis of the Misconception of "Real Manhood" and its Impact on Vulnerabilities to HIV among the Ndau of Chipinge in Zimbabwe', in E. Chitando and S. Chirongoma (eds), *Redemptive Masculinities: Men, HIV and Religion* (Geneva, 2012), 113–25; T.S. Maluleke, 'An African Theology Perspective on Patriarchy', in *The Evil of Patriarchy in Church, Society and Politics* (Cape Town, 2009), 31–6.

behaviour. Further exploring his critique, it appears that Chitando's real concern is that Pentecostal churches maintain and reinforce one of the main structures that in his opinion underlies the epidemic: patriarchy. Though the churches are praised for realising change in men's behaviour, their contribution to the transformation of masculinities towards gender justice, which Chitando considers necessary in view of HIV and AIDS, is considered negatively:

> While the Zimbabwean Pentecostal movement has sought to restructure masculinities and promote responsibility, there is need to adopt a more radical approach in the wake of the HIV epidemic. The Pentecostal approach is still rooted in the paradigm of the male as the leader. ... In essence, men are being asked to be more considerate towards women and children. Men are being asked to become benevolent dictators, and women to embrace the patriarchy of love. This does not promote gender justice in the HIV era.[54]

> Pentecostal teaching on men as breadwinners and heads of households can, inadvertently, sponsor gender-based violence. ... While Pentecostals encourage women to be economically empowered, they are not willing to challenge the myth of male headship. The HIV epidemic calls for courage in redefining gender roles.[55]

The criticism offered here can easily be applied to the two case studies presented in this book. As concluded above, NAOG as well as Regiment parish analyse and address men and masculinities first and foremost at the level of the individual. At this level they seek to change men, and they do so by promoting an alternative ideal of manhood. Central to their definitions of this ideal, indeed, are notions such as male headship and leadership. In other words, the churches engage in what Chitando calls 'the paradigm of the male as the leader' and they reinforce what he calls the 'myth of male headship'. According to Chitando, this does not promote gender justice but rather maintains patriarchy. Even though his evaluation is nuanced by discussions of a 'patriarchy of love', the critique is not softened.

With his rejection of concepts such as male headship and leadership in Christian discourses on masculinity, Chitando stands in the tradition of African women's theology. As early as 1979, Mercy Oduyoye presented the concept of headship as in crucial need of a feminist deconstruction.[56] Recently Sarojini Nadar, in her account of a South African men's movement (the Mighty Men's Conference),

---

[54] Chitando, *A New Man for a New Era?*, 122.

[55] Ibid., 124.

[56] M.A. Oduyoye, 'The Roots of African Christian Feminism', in J.S. Pobee and C.F. Hallencreutz (eds), *Variations in Christian Theology in Africa* (Nairobi, 1979), 42. According to Oduyoye, the concept of headship 'does not affect marital relations only; for the whole of human relations suffer because headship is still cast in the mould of ancient political systems with their despots and kings and queens'.

has engaged in such a deconstruction. She finds the discourse in this movement to be full of rhetoric of male headship and responsibility. As an African woman theologian she evaluates this from the viewpoint of her 'feminist hermeneutic of suspicion' in order to conclude:

> [A] theology of headship and submission is simply yet another way of promoting violence (in its varied forms) through the insidious myth that men as the stronger sex need to protect women, or to "defend the weak". This is what Mary Stewart van Leeuwen has called soft patriarchy[;] it seems innocent enough – i.e. "men taking responsibility" is hardly an unpalatable idea, but if "taking responsibility" means asserting dominating and coercive measures, including those in the religious domain, to maintain power, then our justice antennas have to be tuned in, so that we are not deceived by this palatable patriarchy, masquerading as "restoring masculinity".[57]

It is not clear to what extent the discourse in the Mighty Men's Conference corresponds to the discourse found in the case studies presented in this book. Yet it is clear that the case-study churches, just like the men's movement of Nadar and the Pentecostal movement in Zimbabwe that Chitando writes about, employ concepts such as male headship and responsibility and promote an ideology that can be labelled as 'soft patriarchy'. In other words, various Christian discourses that seek to change men and to transform masculinities do so within a context of patriarchy, upholding patriarchal concepts but redefining them in terms of responsibility, protection and love. Furthermore, it is clear that scholars such as Chitando and Nadar do not evaluate this strategy positively, because they envision a transformation of masculinity *beyond* patriarchy in order to bring about gender justice. This has to be understood from the fundamental critique of any patriarchal ideology by the theologians. One can think of the reference of Philomena Mwaura to patriarchy as a sin, Tinyiko Maluleke's statement on patriarchy as being evil, or Musa Dube's reference to patriarchy as 'violence normalized and inflicted daily on the souls of women and girls'.[58] These feminist political and theological views lead to the radical rejection of anything that smells of patriarchy. Most likely, this also implies a negative evaluation by the theologians of the types of masculinity promoted in Regiment parish and NAOG.

Regarding the divergences in the ways African theologians and the case-study churches analyse and reflect upon masculinities, this might be the most fundamental

---

[57] S. Nadar, 'Who's Afraid of the Mighty Men's Conference? Palatable Patriarchy and Violence against Wo/men in South Africa', in E. Chitando and S. Chirongoma (eds), *Redemptive Masculinities: Men, HIV and Religion* (Geneva, 2012), 361.

[58] Maluleke, *An African Theology Perspective on Patriarchy*, 1; M.W. Dube, *The HIV & AIDS Bible: Selected Essays* (Scranton, 2008), 140; P.N. Mwaura, 'Gender Mainstreaming in African Theology: An African Women's Perspective', *Voices from the Third World*, 24/1 (2001): 175.

one: the churches address men and seek to transform masculinities within an ideological frame that can be considered patriarchal, while the theologians aim at the 'liberation of men from patriarchy'[59] in order to achieve gender justice. According to the theologians, only a radical transformation is adequate enough to overcome the unequal structure of gender and power underlying the HIV epidemic. In their opinion, it is not just certain types of behaviour on the part of men that have to be changed, but the constructs of masculinity and the structures of gender that inform, facilitate and/or legitimate this behaviour. This radical and structural approach to the transformation of masculinities in the context of HIV is in line with the vision that African women theologians have presented earlier for the transformation of gender relations. As Nigerian theologian Rose Uchem states unequivocally:

> It must be clarified again that what has been said in this dissertation is not about individual women or men, but an analysis of a system of structural and cultural injustice against women, which also holds men in bondage. ... Sure, there are many nice men of goodwill who are truly good to women, but nice-ness is not enough. The subject at hand is a structural and systematic evil in a world, into which people are born, all set up for them. Therefore it needs more than personal and interpersonal nice-ness. Nice people need to have their social consciousness sharpened, learn how to recognize and question unjust social structures and how not to collude with unjust systems.[60]

It is clear that the churches in the case studies, like many other churches, do not engage in such a radical project as is articulated here. Therefore their efforts to transform masculinities will, in the end, be evaluated negatively by the theologians, even though it is recognised that these efforts may be preventive in the context of HIV. For the theologians, HIV (or any other concrete social problem) is not the primary concern that leads them into a quest for transformed masculinities. Their real concern is with what they call gender injustice or patriarchy. The HIV epidemic, in the words of Chitando, only 'provides an opportunity' to overcome the problem of patriarchy and to achieve gender justice.[61] Therefore for the gender-critical African theologians it is imperative that transformed versions of masculinity go beyond patriarchy. The churches, on the other hand, concerned with micro-ethics concerning men's behaviour rather than with structures of gender as such, do

---

[59] E. Chitando, *Troubled but not Destroyed* (Geneva, 2009), 92–3 and 96–7; Dube, *The HIV & AIDS Bible*, 139–40; M.A. Oduyoye, 'Acting to Construct Africa: The Agency by Women', in R. van Eijk and J. van Lin (eds), *Africans Reconstructing Africa* (Nijmegen, 1997), 38.

[60] R.N. Uchem, *Overcoming Women's Subordination: An Igbo African and Christian Perspective. Envisioning an Inclusive Theology with Reference to Women* (Enugu, 2001), 230.

[61] Chitando, *A New Man for a New Era?*, 122.

not see a problem in employing concepts such as male headship, leadership and responsibility as long as these are effective in bringing about a positive change among men and the transformation masculinities.

Understanding Gender from Creation versus Re-creation

The efforts of the churches to transform masculinities through some patriarchal notions, and the endeavour of the theologians to overcome patriarchy, are informed by their respective gender ideologies and the underlying theological foundations. In case of the churches, their gender ideology is strongly based on the theological doctrine of creation. More specifically, it is informed by a literal and normative reading of the Genesis creation stories. As mentioned above, this results in an ambiguous gender ideology that supports a notion of gender equality but simultaneously legitimates a hierarchical gender order. The churches not only teach that man and woman are created different (and therefore need to complement each other), but also that man was created first and therefore has a primary position in the order of the sexes. Following on from this, in both churches masculinity is defined by, or at least associated with, notions such as headship, leadership and a primary responsibility. These notions indicate a sense of male primacy, which is part and parcel of patriarchal gender ideology.

As already mentioned in Chapter 2, the African theologians under discussion also refer to the Genesis creation stories. Like the churches, they understand Genesis 1:27 as foundational for a theological account of gender equality. In their publications, time and time again it is stated that both women and men are created in the image of God. Different from the churches, the theologians do not limit their understanding of gender equality to a sense of equal human dignity that still allows a man to be the head in marriage. Rather they claim the full potential of the idea that men and women are created equally in the image of God.[62] Furthermore, the theologians differ from the churches in their biblical hermeneutics, as they present a fundamental critique of the creation story of Genesis 2 and its popular interpretation. Rather than taking this story as foundational to their theological understanding of gender, they criticise the story and/or its popular interpretations for being patriarchal and androcentric, and they call for a critical deconstruction and re-reading.[63] Most fundamentally, in contrast to the churches, the theologians do not understand gender from the theological doctrine of creation but from

---

[62] Cf. M.A. Oduyoye, *Introducing African Women's Theology* (Cleveland, 2001), 44–6.

[63] Most radically the text is denounced by Uchem, *Overcoming Women's Subordination*, 181. Some other scholars seem to be critical of the popular interpretations of the text rather than of the text itself (cf. A. Nasimiyu-Wasike, 'Genesis 1–2 and some Elements of Diversion from the Original Meaning of the Creation of Man and Woman', in M.N. Getui, K. Holter and V. Zinkuratire (eds), *Interpreting the Old Testament in Africa* (Nairobi, 2001), 177–8; T. Okure, 'Women in the Bible', in M.A. Oduyoye and V. Fabella

the idea of re-creation brought about by Jesus Christ, i.e. from Christology and eschatology. Indeed, in NAOG the perception of Jesus Christ as the second Adam also occurs, but this is understood in terms of a *restoration* of God's original intention: the image of 'biblical manhood' presented by Adam in Genesis 2 is thought to be restored and fully embodied in Jesus Christ. The theologians, however, understand the re-creation in Christ in terms of a *new creation*. See, for example, Isabel Phiri, who opposes a literalistic (mis)reading of the Genesis creation stories that subordinates women to men by pointing to 'the promise of Galatians 3:28'. This Bible verse states that in Christ there is neither male nor female. Phiri interprets it as a reference to 'the new life as God intended it to be, a life full of partnership between men and women'.[64] According to Phiri, through the re-creation in Christ a 'liberated community of men and women' will be established, and the church is to anticipate this future.[65] Likewise Rose Uchem envisions 'a new world order, modelled on Christ and not on androcentric ideologies justified with the Adamic myth'.[66] In this new order, she says, marriage is no longer defined by the headship model but by a partnership of equals and a shared leadership that does not serve the 'inherited privilege of one sex, the male sex'.[67] As appears from these quotations, the idea of a re-creation through Christ is employed by the theologians to overcome the patriarchal ideologies of gender informed by an account of creation. It provides them with a basis to call for a radical equality and justice in gender relations.

In gender theoretical terms, the difference between a perception of gender rooted in creation and one rooted in re-creation can be categorised with the concepts of essentialism and constructivism. The account of creation gives rise to an essentialist understanding of gender in the churches: as it is believed that God has created humankind differently as male and female and has attached distinct characteristics to both sexes, it is also assumed that there is something that can be qualified as a true essence of manhood and womanhood as part of the order of creation. The essentialist stance of the churches enables them to define a positive ideal of manhood (such as 'biblical manhood' in NAOG) promoted among men. In both case-study churches these ideals are based biblically on the creation story of Genesis 2. The theologians, on the other hand, consider gender as socially constructed rather than as designed by God. This enables them to deconstruct ideologies and structures of gender critically. Furthermore, due to their orientation towards re-creation, they do not consider gender constructions as fixed but rather as open for transformation. On the basis of the account of re-creation they articulate

---

(eds), *With Passion and Compassion: Third World Women Doing Theology* (Maryknoll, 1988), 48–52.

[64] I.A. Phiri, *Women, Presbyterianism and Patriarchy: Religious Experience of Chewa Women in Central Malawi* (Blantyre, 1997), 156.

[65] Ibid., 151–60.

[66] Uchem, *Overcoming Women's Subordination*, 189.

[67] Ibid., 228.

a broad vision for gender relations, captured in the concept of gender justice understood in terms of equality and partnership. However, they hardly define a specific positive ideal of masculinity. It may be easier to define masculinity on the basis of an essentialist understanding of gender as rooted in creation than on the basis of a critical perception of gender as in need of deconstruction and reconstruction.

Masculinity Politics and Biblical Hermeneutics

As appears from the above section, the case-study churches and the theologians deal with the Genesis creation stories in different ways. In the churches these stories are read literally and taken as normative for the understanding of gender and masculinity. The theologians on the other hand have a far more critical approach, not only to popular interpretations of Genesis 1–3 but also to the biblical text itself. As Phiri points out, 'African women theologians are re-reading the Genesis creation story in the light of source and redaction criticism. This has necessitated going beyond the texts as well as a literalistic reading of the passages.'[68] Presenting a similar critical approach, Uchem calls for revisiting the creation stories, in order to oppose readings that take the accounts as factual, literal and historical.[69] Explaining this, both Phiri and Uchem point to the way the stories have been foundational to the understanding of women as inferior beings, secondary to men.

The difference between the churches and the theologians in how they deal with the Genesis creation stories is illustrative of their diverging biblical hermeneutics.[70] From the case studies it is clear that the churches themselves differ in the way they use the Bible. In NAOG the Bible is often quoted in preaching as well as in conversations with church members, while in Regiment parish this happens only occasionally. Members of both churches indicate that the level of knowledge of the Bible is a major difference between Catholics and Pentecostals. However, the case-study churches correspond in their perception of the Bible as the holy and authoritative Word of God. This influences their hermeneutics, as it does not allow criticism of biblical texts. The theologians, on the other hand, have a somewhat different hermeneutical approach to the Bible. In the words of Oduyoye, they affirm 'the Bible as a source for God-word', which brings in a slight but significant nuance.[71] When the Bible is *a source for* the word of God, the task is to distinguish in the biblical text where God is speaking and where God is not speaking. As put by Oduyoye, the Bible needs to be read 'with a critical eye' in order to 'discover in it the Triune God as liberator of the oppressed, the rescuer of the marginalized and all who live daily in the throes of pain, uncertainty

---

[68] Phiri, *Women, Presbyterianism and Patriarchy*, 155.
[69] Uchem, *Overcoming Women's Subordination*, 179–80.
[70] In this context, I understand 'hermeneutics' basically as the principles and processes of understanding and interpreting the biblical text by readers and in relation to their context.
[71] Oduyoye, *Introducing African Women's Theology*, 48.

and deprivation'.[72] Though African women theologians have employed different hermeneutical concepts and approaches, their interpretation of the Bible is generally characterised by this quest for liberation and justice.[73] As outlined in Chapter 2, this hermeneutics results in a critical sensitivity to and deconstruction of patriarchal traditions in the biblical texts. The concrete implications of this are illustrated in the way the theologians deal with the Genesis account of creation, and in the way they look at the notion of male headship (and female submission) as mentioned in some of the Pauline epistles of the New Testament. Drawing from their critical biblical hermeneutics, the theologians clearly oppose and reject this notion. The churches, however, can hardly do so because they read the Bible as an authoritative text. Rather than rejecting it, they redefine the idea of male headship in order to dissociate it from its connotation of domination. As has been explored above, the theologians acknowledge this redefinition but evaluate it as not radical enough. Rather, they blame the churches, in the words of Sarojini Nadar, for their 'hermeneutical immobility' and state that 'more holistic, liberating ways of engaging with Scripture must be developed if the Church is to become a place of gender justice and equality'.[74] Clearly, biblical hermeneutics is a major area of divergence between the African theologians, who are concerned about gender issues, and the case-study churches (and, most likely, many other African churches).

It is clear that different hermeneutical approaches have direct implications for the way in which the Bible is used in the transformation of masculinities. When the Bible is read in a literal and normative way, it is easy, in the words of Banda, 'to discuss afresh from a biblical angle what fatherhood really means in our society' because 'the Bible gives such important guidelines'.[75] The theologians, having a far more critical approach focused on the deconstruction of patriarchal traditions, have more difficulty in deriving a positive ideal from the Bible. They make use of biblical texts to address critical issues among men – for example, the story of the rape of Tamar in order to address sexual violence – but these stories function as counter-examples rather than as constructive models.[76]

---

[72] Ibid., 50.

[73] Cf. M.W. Dube, 'Talitha Cum Hermeneutics of Liberation: Some African Women's Ways of Reading the Bible', in A.F. Botta and P.R. Andinach (eds), *The Bible and the Hermeneutics of Liberation* (Atlanta, 2009), 133–46; M.W. Dube, 'Circle Readings of the Bible/Scriptoratures', in J.A. Smit and P.P. Kumar (eds), *Study of Religion in Southern Africa: Essays in Honour of G.C. Oosthuizen* (Leiden, 2005), 77–96.

[74] S. Nadar, 'On Being Church: African Women's Voices and Visions', in I.A. Phiri and S. Nadar (eds), *On Being Church: African Women's Voices and Visions* (Geneva, 2005), 21–2.

[75] J. Banda, *Fatherhood in the 21st Century* – Part 1 (Lusaka, 2008).

[76] E.g., see G. West, 'The Contribution of Tamar's Story to the Construction of Alternative African Masculinities', in S.T. Kamionkowski and W. Kim (eds), *Bodies, Embodiment and Theology of the Hebrew Bible* (New York, 2010), 184–200. See also T.S.

Conclusion

It is often suggested that Pentecostal and Catholic types of Christianity are worlds apart. Indeed, the above discussion has shown that Catholicism and Pentecostalism in Africa have distinct characteristics, both sociologically and theologically. These differences impact on the ways in which men are addressed, how gender is thought about, and how masculinities are transformed. For example, in line with the general idea that Pentecostalism is more explicitly involved in 'modernity' and Catholicism with 'tradition', the case-study churches differ in the way they define their Christian type of masculinity in (dis)continuity with what they consider as traditional culture, and in a different orientation towards modern views and developments. Furthermore, as a church in the Pentecostal tradition of holiness, NAOG demands more commitment from its members to the church's moral standards; hence, it addresses male church members in a more explicit and radical discourse and promotes a stricter ideal of manhood compared with Regiment parish, which is in the Catholic tradition of an inclusive ecclesiology that does not strictly demarcate the boundaries between the church and 'the world'. In spite of these differences, the comparison has also revealed some striking convergences. Both churches address similar issues related to men's behaviour. They also promote a largely corresponding alternative ideal of masculinity. In both cases, the formulation of this ideal is inspired by the long tradition of thinking about gender in Christianity that takes as its anthropological starting point the theological account of creation. The view of the Bible as a book with divine authority leaves the churches with little space to read the creation stories or other biblical texts (on male headship, for example) more critically. As a consequence, the churches reflect the above-mentioned ambiguity about gender that is characteristic of much of Christianity. This ambiguity is reflected in the 'soft patriarchy' that characterises their ideals of masculinity and gender relations.

When comparing the churches and the theologians, the most important issue is the fundamental difference in the paradigms in which the churches on the one hand, and the theologians on the other, seek to transform masculinities. The churches are primarily concerned about the behaviour of men, which they seek to change by promoting alternative masculinities defined with certain patriarchal notions. The theologians are concerned about deeply rooted structures of gender inequality. They seek to 'liberate men from patriarchy' and to transform masculinities towards gender justice. Concretely, this fundamental divergence means that the theologians can only be suspicious and critical of the alternative, soft patriarchal types of masculinity that are promoted in the churches, built on notions such as male responsibility, headship and leadership. Even though they acknowledge that such ideals of masculinity can be helpful in combating HIV and gender-based violence, they still evaluate them negatively because in their opinion

---

Maluleke, 'Men and their Role in Community', in M.W. Dube (ed.), *Africa Praying. A Handbook on HIV/AIDS Sensitive Sermon Guidelines and Liturgy* (Geneva, 2003), 190–93.

a more radical transformation of masculinities is needed. The theologians aim at the deconstruction of patriarchy in order to achieve gender justice, which in their opinion is a theological imperative.

The conclusion that the churches and the theologians engage in different paradigms when it comes to their approach to men and masculinities may not be surprising. It is quite logical that the discursive practices in local church communities are different from the analyses and reflections of academic theologians. What is interesting, however, is that the latter, being aware of the different approach to masculinities by churches, evaluate this approach negatively. This may be a result of the so-called 'church-enabling task' that they have assigned themselves.[77] This task includes critically evaluating the praxis and preaching in churches as well as prophetically calling on churches when they – in the opinion of the theologians – do something wrong. I do not question this task, yet I want to raise some questions about the basis on which the theologians analyse transformations of masculinity in local churches and evaluate them as inadequate. The classic feminist concept of patriarchy, which appears to be the normative analytical frame in their work, may not be the most helpful concept to analyse and understand the ways in which local church communities effect change in men and contribute to a transformation of masculinities. This issue is explored in the following chapter, which also proposes an alternative approach.

---

[77] Cf. T.S. Maluleke, 'Half a Century of African Christian Theologies: Elements of the Emerging Agenda for the Twenty-first Century', in O.U. Kalu (ed.), *African Christianity: An African Story* (Pretoria, 2005), 474–5.

Chapter 6
Understanding Transformations of Masculinity: Patriarchy, Male Agency and Gender Justice

So far, in this book I have explored how African theologians envision a transformation of masculinities and how such a transformation takes place in local church communities. The differences between the theologians and the churches have been discussed at length in the previous chapter. In this concluding chapter I want to bring the discussion a step forward by raising some key conceptual and theoretical issues in the study of masculinities in African Christian and broader religious contexts. The central question here is how transformations of masculinity in religious contexts, such as in the case-study churches, can be understood by critical scholars of religion and gender, particularly of men, masculinities and religion. When I use an inclusive 'we' in this chapter, it relates to this body of scholarship.

Transforming Masculinities towards Gender Justice

The African theologians discussed in Chapter 2 present a vision to transform masculinities towards gender justice. Patriarchal masculinities, in their opinion, have to be deconstructed, and alternative ideals of 'redemptive' and 'liberating' masculinities have to be developed and promoted. With this proposal, these theologians make an important theological contribution to the debate on religion and masculinities in Africa. As Björn Krondorfer and Stephen Hunt recently pointed out, the study of men, masculinities and religion has not only an analytical or a deconstructionist but also a transformative agenda. They put it eloquently, saying:

> Following a transformative trajectory, the critical study of men and religion opens an academic venue that does not limit itself to describing *what is* but envisions *what may become*. Scholarly inquisitiveness can enrich and reconfigure the global canvas of religious and gendered becomingness.[1]

---

[1] B. Krondorfer and S. Hunt, 'Introduction: Religion and Masculinities – Continuities and Change', *Religion and Gender*, 2:2 (2012), 200–201.

It is against this background that I appreciate the theology of gender justice presented by African theologians. This theology opens up an alternative vision of gender relations, enabling us to think beyond the complexities and ambiguities that characterise the politics of religion and gender at grassroots level.

A crucial question, however, is how the vision of gender justice relates to the grassroots reality. In much of (pro)feminist scholarship in religion and theology the notion of gender justice tends to be understood in an a-historicised and a-contextualised way.[2] Its meaning is considered self-evident, as the term is often used without explanation or reflection. In fact, gender justice is often equated with a feminist notion of gender equality. An important lesson from intercultural theology is that theology is always a contextual practice and that there are no universal theological-ethical visions for our world. This implies that gender justice, as a theological-ethical concept, cannot have a universal meaning and cannot be equated, for example, with a single (modern Western) notion of gender equality.[3] From an intercultural theological perspective, the question as to what gender justice actually means remains an open one, to be raised and investigated constantly in view of concrete social, cultural and religious contexts and their specific issues and challenges. This question will be answered differently in the multiple contexts of contemporary African Christianity and world Christianity. Not only progressive academic theologians, such as the African theologians discussed in this book, develop contextual theologies of gender justice. The discourses in churches and faith communities, such as the case studies presented in this book, can also present us with local theologies of gender justice, though this concept may not be used explicitly and these theologies may not be articulated systematically. When gender becomes an explicit theme in religious discourse, out of a concern about current configurations of gender in society that are oppressive, and with the aim of transforming these configurations so that they become more life-giving and foster the human dignity of every person regardless of sex, then we can speak of a local theology of gender justice in practice.

For the African theologians, as discussed in Chapter 2, gender justice is a political project aiming for the liberation of women and the promotion of equality

---

[2] Cf. S. Coakley, 'Shaping the Field: A Transatlantic Experience', in D.F. Ford, B. Quash and J.M. Soskice (eds), *Fields of Faith: Theology and Religious Studies for the Twenty-first Century* (Cambridge, 2005), 50–51.

[3] For a discussion on (gender) justice from an intercultural theological perspective, see M.P. Aquino, 'Feminist Intercultural Theology: Towards a Shared Future of Justice', in M.P. Aquino and M.J. Rosado-Nunes (eds), *Feminist Intercultural Theology: Latina Explorations for a Just World* (Maryknoll, 2007), 9–28. Unfortunately, in this article Maria Pilar Aquino does not systematically reflect on the concept of gender justice itself. Though not including religious or theological perspectives, an insightful and critical discussion on the concept of gender justice from conceptual, contextual and strategic angles can be found in M. Mukhopadhyay and N. Singh (eds), *Gender Justice, Citizenship and Development* (Ottawa, 2007).

in gender relations. Their theology of gender justice is contextual in the sense that it is related to critical social realities in African contexts, such as the HIV epidemic. However, in a certain way it is also a-contextual, because gender justice often is understood in terms of a global feminist discourse about gender equality. Aside from the political project, for these theologians gender justice is also a key analytical and a normative evaluative concept. On the basis of their theological understanding of gender justice, the theologians strongly criticise churches for perpetuating patriarchy in their teaching, preaching and practices. The observation of anthropologist Saba Mahmood, that feminism is 'both an *analytical* and a *politically prescriptive* project', certainly also applies to the African theologians in their engagement with issues of gender and masculinities in the HIV context.[4] A direct consequence of this is that the theologians are hardly sensitive to the subtle changes in gender relations and gender identities taking place in local religious contexts, and to the specific discourses that enable and shape these changes. Following the above-mentioned intercultural theological approach to gender justice, for me the challenge is to identify (traces of) local theologies of gender justice in practice, for example in the case-study churches presented in Chapters 3 and 4. Clearly, these churches do not simply follow the African theologians in their deconstruction of patriarchy and in the promotion of gender equality. They continue to use language of male headship and male leadership – notions that the theologians consider obstacles to gender justice. Yet, a more flexible and contextual understanding of gender justice makes us sensitive to the complexity of religious gender discourse, such as that found in the case studies, and opens our eyes to the 'transformations of masculinity for the better' which they bring about at a grassroots level.

Framing Religious Discourse on Masculinity

If we are to analyse religious discourses on masculinity, searching for their transformative effects, what are the conceptual frames that can be used? Several theoretical concepts have been used to examine and evaluate religious gender discourse. In this section I will discuss three of them: patriarchy, soft patriarchy, and neo-traditionalism. Are these concepts helpful to understand the discourses found in the case-study churches, are they sensitive to the transformations taking place here?

Patriarchy

Patriarchy is the central concept used by the African theologians discussed in Chapter 2 as well as by scholars in the critical study of men, masculinities and

---

[4] S. Mahmood, *Politics of Piety: The Islamic Revival and the Feminist Subject* (Princeton, 2005), 10.

religion, and by (pro)feminist scholars in religion and theology. The concept of patriarchy is critically sensitive to the distribution of social and symbolic power in gender relations, to social structures of gender inequality, and to cultural and religious ideologies of male supremacy. Not surprisingly, in the study of religion the concept of patriarchy has been used to criticise religious institutions and religious beliefs for maintaining and reinforcing male dominance and the subordination of women. As mentioned in Chapter 1, patriarchal constructions of masculinities in the sphere of religion constitute a major theme in the critical study of men, masculinities and religion.[5] Religious discourses that use patriarchal language and themes to define masculinity or to appeal to men are criticised, for example by Joseph Gelfer in his study of mythopoetic, evangelical and Catholic men's movements in the United States.[6] According to Gelfer, the 'masculine spiritualities' promoted in these movements often have good underlying intentions, yet they reflect

> an all-too-familiar patriarchal spirituality. This patriarchal spirituality encourages a certain type of hegemonic masculinity that dominates women and subordinate [e.g. gay] masculinities; it does this chiefly by defining masculinity by archetypes, revising the definition of and depoliticising patriarchy.[7]

In a similar way, scholars in African theology criticise religious discourses on masculinity in contemporary African contexts. As mentioned in the previous chapter, Ezra Chitando acknowledges the good intentions of the Pentecostal movement in Zimbabwe in promoting new, more constructive forms of masculinity among men, but in the end his evaluation is still negative because Pentecostalism continues to promote patriarchal views such as male headship and leadership.[8] Clearly, similar criticism can be applied to the case studies presented in this book, if these are analysed within the framework of patriarchy. The detailed analysis in chapters 3 and 4 has revealed that both churches more or less explicitly support patriarchal forms of masculinity, defined in terms of headship, leadership and a primary responsibility of men. This is informed by their reading of patriarchal biblical texts about creation (Genesis 2) and marriage (Ephesians 5). An analysis in terms of patriarchy critically reveals the patriarchal discourse in which masculinity is often shaped in the churches. The conclusion of such an analysis could be that the case-study churches, in the words of Gelfer, may have good intentions but

---

[5] S.B. Boyd, 'Trajectories in Men's Studies in Religion: Theories, Methodologies, and Issues', *Journal of Men's Studies*, 7/2 (1999): 266; G.K. Baker-Fletcher, 'Critical Theory, Deconstruction and Liberation?', *Journal of Men's Studies*, 7/2 (1999): 277.

[6] For example, see J. Gelfer, *Numen, Old Men: Contemporary Masculine Spiritualities and the Problem of Patriarchy* (London, 2009).

[7] Ibid., 175.

[8] E. Chitando, 'A New Man for a New Era? Zimbabwean Pentecostalism, Masculinities and the HIV Epidemic', *Missionalia*, 35/3 (2007): 112–27.

that their trajectories and theologies to transform masculinities reflect the all-too-familiar story of patriarchy.

Though an analysis in terms of patriarchy is important because gender is always about power, the value of this analysis is limited. It confirms what the critical scholar already knows – that religion often perpetuates patriarchy – but it does give little new insight in the various and complex ways masculinities are shaped and possibly also reshaped in religious gender discourse. The concept of patriarchy focuses on a fixed structure of male dominance, but it ignores the variations, negotiations and subtle changes of patriarchal themes in specific discourses. In relation to the case studies, an analysis in terms of patriarchy makes us critically aware of patriarchal symbols such as male headship, but it assumes too easily that we already know the meaning of such a symbol: the idea is that male headship simply means male dominance, and the discourses that promote it are believed to reinforce religious forms of patriarchy. However, in the Northmead Assembly of God sermons, for example, Banda explicitly dissociates male headship from male dominance. He preaches:

> Male headship does not mean male domination. What we have seen most times is male domination. And it stinks in the nostrils of God. It is a distortion of God's order. Because male domination implies that the woman is less than the man, but that's not biblical.[9]

In this sermon, Banda tries to 'reconcile' and 'balance' his notion of male–female equality with 'the very difficult aspect of male headship'. The serious efforts to combine a notion of gender equality with the traditional theme of male headship already demonstrate the complexity of the religious gender discourse represented by Banda. Even with a feminist hermeneutics of suspicion, it is not satisfying to interpret such a discourse simply as a variation of the all-too-familiar story of patriarchy. Such an interpretation does not help us to understand the context-specific meaning of male headship in Banda's sermons, nor the political intentions with which it is employed, nor the transformations of masculinity it may bring about. In poststructuralist feminist theory and gender studies, the very concept of patriarchy has been critiqued for its monolithic portrayal and universalising account of gender relations and masculinities.[10] A more nuanced conceptual frame is needed to analyse religious discourse on masculinity.

---

[9] J. Banda, *Fatherhood in the 21st Century* – Part 6 (Lusaka, 2008), DVD.

[10] Cf. J. Butler, *Gender Trouble: Feminism and the Subversion of Identity*, 2nd edn (London, 2006), 48; S.M. Whitehead, *Men and Masculinities: Key Themes and New Directions* (Cambridge, 2002), 87–8.

Soft Patriarchy

The concept of soft patriarchy allows for some nuance in the conceptualisation of patriarchy in relation to men, masculinities and religion. Soft patriarchy has mainly been used to refer to men in evangelical Protestant circles in the United States.[11] The most elaborate account on soft patriarchy has been provided by sociologist Bradford Wilcox. He uses the concept to account for the subtle shifts in conservative Protestant gender discourses in America, such as the shift from a practical to a symbolic form of patriarchy, from 'male headship' to 'servant leadership', and to a greater emotional and practical involvement of men in the home.[12] Others have applied the label of soft patriarchy to the Promise Keepers, an evangelical men's movement that was enormously popular in the United States in the 1990s. In this movement, according to masculinity scholar Michael Kimmel, 'Masculine malaise, the search for meaning and community, is resolved by the assertion of a kinder, gentler patriarchal control.'[13] Where Wilcox uses 'soft patriarchy' in a sympathetic way to conceptualise subtle transformations of masculinity that are symbolically shaped in a patriarchal discourse,[14] other scholars use it as a more critical term to emphasise that, in spite of some discursive shifts, the 'new' forms of masculinity are still patriarchal. According to Kimmel, for example, the Promise Keepers represent 'the second coming of patriarchy'.[15] In this analysis, the promotion of soft patriarchy in evangelical American circles is a reactionary response to modern egalitarian impulses, an attempt to re-establish the patriarchal order in the home.

In Chapter 5, I have applied the term 'soft patriarchy' to the case-study churches and the ideals of masculinity they promote. I used the concept, like Wilcox, in a sympathetic way, to acknowledge that the churches, though they use traditional patriarchal language in relation to male headship and leadership, do not promote

---

[11] Mary Stewart van Leeuwen points to the emergence of forms of soft patriarchy in 'evangelical, Pentecostal, and fundamentalist Christian churches in many parts of the world', under the influence of trends in similar churches in Western nations, particularly the United States. Her comment that soft patriarchy has emerged 'despite (or perhaps in reaction to) three decades of feminist-led gains for women' shows that she mainly speaks of the United States, as not all other regions have a three-decade history of feminist movements. See M.S. van Leeuwen, 'Faith, Feminism, and the Family in an Age of Globalization', in M.L. Stackhouse with P.J. Paris (eds), *God and Globalization, Volume 1: Religion and the Powers of the Common Life* (New York, 2000), 213.

[12] W.B. Wilcox, *Soft Patriarchs, New Men: How Christianity Shapes Fathers and Husbands* (Chicago, 2004).

[13] M. Kimmel, *Misframing Men: The Politics of Contemporary Masculinities* (New Brunswick, 2010), 167.

[14] Joseph Gelfer (*Numen, Old Men*, 59) criticises Wilcox, saying that he 'promotes soft patriarchs'. This criticism is incorrect, however, as Wilcox uses soft patriarchy as an analytical term. It is not something he wants to promote, but what he observes.

[15] Kimmel, *Misframing Men*, 171.

a brutal form of male dominance but rather a form of male responsibility in the circles of marriage, the family and the community. There are many similarities between the discourse presented by Banda in Northmead Assembly of God and the discourse of 'soft patriarchy' found in American evangelical Protestant circles. Banda's 'balancing' of male–female equality and male headship can be considered an example of soft patriarchy, as can his redefinition of male headship from domination to responsibility and his emphasis on men serving their wives and families. In the other case study, in Regiment parish, there is not an explicit discourse that illustrates soft patriarchy. In a more implicit way, however, the ideals of masculinity in the parish can be considered soft patriarchal in the sense that people often hold patriarchal views that at least are tolerated by the church but which the church seeks to 'soften'. For example, the church leadership does not reject the idea of male headship, but emphasises that it should be practised in a responsible way with respect to the 'equal human dignity' of women. In a more symbolic way, the Catholic Church represents soft patriarchy in its institutional organisation: the 'fathers' who dominate the church hierarchy are *serving* the church, and they present a model for lay Catholic men who are *serving* the domestic church, that is, their family.

Although the concept of soft patriarchy can be applied to the case-study churches, this concept has its limitations for an analysis of the transformations of masculinity taking place here. In its sympathetic usage, the concept suggests that *in spite of* some patriarchal themes, religious discourse of soft patriarchy may yet allow for subtle changes in masculinities and gender relations. It does not lead to a greater understanding of how these changes are brought about precisely through the specific ways in which patriarchal themes are discursively employed. It its critical use, soft patriarchy has the same deficit as the concept of patriarchy outlined in the previous section. Of course, to say that the case-study churches promote soft patriarchal ideals of masculinity means that these ideals somehow still are patriarchal. But again, this only confirms what the critical scholar already expects, and it does not lead to a better understanding of the complex ways masculinities are (re)shaped through religious discourse.

Neo-traditionalism

In the study of religion and gender, the label of neo-traditionalism is often applied to evangelical Protestantism in the United States. In fact, the soft patriarchy promoted in evangelical circles exemplifies the neo-traditional character of evangelical Protestantism in North America. In a 1999 study among American evangelicals, the great majority were found to agree 'with a neotraditional rhetoric of gender and family responsibilities'.[16] According to the researchers, this rhetoric

---

[16] S.K. Gallagher and C. Smith, 'Symbolic Traditionalism and Pragmatic Egalitarianism: Contemporary Evangelicals, Families, and Gender', *Gender and Society*, 13/2 (1999): 217.

combines traditional and egalitarian themes and it emphasises men's headship – defined in terms of responsibility – 'as a core family value'.[17] They interpret the evangelical discourse as 'symbolic traditionalism' because male headship in reality is not so much about material provision and decision-making but about abstract qualities such as spiritual leadership and accountability.[18] Though the notion of headship entitles men to a greater power, at the same time male power is tempered and domesticated by the emphasis on men loving and respecting their wives and being involved in their families. A typical example of neo-traditional discourse in American evangelical Protestantism is represented by the Council on Biblical Manhood and Biblical Womanhood (CMBW). This organisation was established in 1987 out of a concern about the influence of feminism, not only in society at large but also in evangelical circles. In opposition to feminist egalitarianism, the founders articulated the complementary position, affirming that men and women are equal in the image of God but yet have different, complementary roles and functions:

> In the home, men lovingly are to lead their wives and family as women intelligently are to submit to the leadership of their husbands. In the church, while men and women share equally in the blessings of salvation, some governing and teaching roles are restricted to men.[19]

As feminist biblical scholar Susanne Scholz points out in her critical review of 'the Christian Right's discourse on gender and the Bible', the traditionalist position of the CMBW is a reactionary stance that exemplifies the struggle of conservative evangelicalism with modern life, which now focuses on modern gender practices.[20] Authors associated with the CMBW, such as John Piper, take the Bible as the authoritative source to understand 'biblical manhood' and 'biblical womanhood' as intended by God in the order of creation, and hence they criticise modern views of gender, including 'evangelical feminism'.

Like the CMBW, the Promise Keepers are often considered an example of neo-traditional Christian gender discourse. According to masculinity scholar Kenneth Clatterbaugh this is a conservative movement pushing towards traditional male roles:

> Grounding their view in biblical passages that suggest that women should follow men's lead in the family and in the church and that women should pledge

---

[17] Ibid.

[18] Ibid., 217–24.

[19] 'Home', website of The Council on Biblical Manhood and Biblical Womanhood, accessed 30 May 2012, http://www.cbmw.org.

[20] S. Scholz, 'The Christian Right's Discourse on Gender and the Bible', *Journal of Feminist Studies in Religion*, 21/1 (2005): 87.

subservience to their husbands, this movement sought to restore men to their rightful place in church, community and family.[21]

The label of neo-traditionalism is hardly applied to Catholic discourse on gender. Though the Catholic Church certainly does not simply follow modern liberal views of gender, it has more easily engaged with modern discourse. At first sight it seems that the Catholic Church, instead of providing a reactionary response to modernity à la conservative evangelicalism, has shaped its own version of modernity, for example in the call of the former Pope John Paul II for 'a new feminism'.[22] However, a closer look shows that Catholicism also presents a neo-traditional discourse, as it clearly opposes modern feminist views that, in the view of the church, do not recognise the fundamental difference between man and woman.[23] Like the evangelical discourse, Catholic thinking about gender is centred on the notion of complementarity of the sexes. This complementarity is often drawn in a subtly hierarchical way.[24] Yet, official Catholic documents do not use the typical neo-traditional evangelical language of a symbolic male headship. Rather, they emphasise the equal dignity of woman and man in creation, while calling for collaboration between both with respect for their difference.

With regard to the case studies presented in this book, at first sight the discourse in NAOG can be considered as neo-traditional. As mentioned in Chapter 4, Bishop Banda directly derives his definition of 'biblical manhood' from a typical American neo-traditionalist, John Piper. The meaning of male headship in the sermons *Fatherhood in the 21st Century* has many resemblances to evangelical Protestant discourse that defines headship in terms of servant leadership. Like the Promise Keepers, Banda employs biblical themes and texts in order to 'restore manhood' as it was intended by God in creation. In spite of the many similarities, however, it is difficult to apply the concept of neo-traditionalism to the case study of NAOG (or to Regiment parish). One reason is that using the concept in African contexts would be confusing, as in the study of religion in Africa the term neo-traditionalism is not used for Christianity – a 'modern' religion – but to new religious movements that (re)turn to indigenous religious beliefs and practices.[25] This already points to the second and more fundamental problem: Pentecostalism in Africa is involved in a completely different dynamic of 'tradition' and

---

[21] K. Clatterbaugh, 'Men's Rights', in M. Flood, J.K. Gardiner, B. Pease and K. Pringle (eds), *International Encyclopedia of Men and Masculinities* (New York, 2007), 433.

[22] John Paul II, *Evangelium Vitae* (Rome, 1995), no. 99.

[23] Cf. Congregation for the Doctrine of Faith, *Letter to the Bishops of the Catholic Church on the Collaboration of Men and Women in the Church and in the World* (Rome, 2004).

[24] A. Kalbian, *Sexing the Church: Gender, Power, and Ethics in Contemporary Catholicism* (Bloomington, 2005), 97–105.

[25] Cf. M. de Witte, 'Neo-traditional Religions', in E.K. Bongmba (ed.), *The Wiley-Blackwell Companion to African Religions* (Malden, 2012), 173–83.

'modernity' than is evangelical Protestantism in the United States. A discourse that can be neo-traditional in America or in Europe is not automatically neo-traditional in Zambia or elsewhere. The same type of discourse can even be modernising in an African context, as appears from the case study in NOAG. As explored in Chapter 5, Pentecostalism in Africa at least discursively breaks with the tradition of 'African culture' and presents Christianity as something new and different. The Catholic Church in Africa has a more positive view of 'African culture' and its compatibility with the Christian faith. However, the case study of Regiment parish shows that, also in a Catholic context, patterns of male dominance are often associated with African culture while Christianity is believed to promote a more equal relationship between man and woman. Thus, the term neo-traditionalism does not and actually cannot apply to the gender discourse found in the case-study churches, even when this discourse clearly resembles neo-traditional evangelical rhetoric. For example, when Banda in NAOG underlines 'the biblical principle' of male headship but explicitly dissociates it from the traditional connotation of domination, and rather 'balances' and 'reconciles' it with another 'biblical principle', the notion of male–female equality, this exemplifies the paradoxical yet modernising impulse of Pentecostal gender discourse in Africa.[26] Furthermore, when Banda uses the theme of headship to call on men to take responsibility for themselves, their wives and families and in society at large, this illustrates how rhetoric that at first sight seems conservative and traditional is used to bring about change in men and masculinities.

The various concepts discussed above are not helpful as a conceptual frame to analyse and understand the discourse on masculinity as found in the case-study churches. The concept of (soft) patriarchy is too limited to understand the complexities and ambiguities in religious gender discourse, and the concept of neo-traditionalism assumes a context of modern Western society and therefore cannot be unproblematically applied to Christian discourses in African contexts. Though the concepts of (soft) patriarchy and neo-traditionalism can be useful for a critical analysis of religious discourse on masculinity, they are not sensitive to the more or less subtle transformations of masculinity in specific discourses.

Religious Discourse and Male Agency

If we are to understand transformations of masculinity in African Christian contexts, we need an analytical frame that is more sensitive to the specific ways in which religion brings about change in men and masculinity. Religion is a major force in processes of personal and social transformation in African societies. As the Africanist scholars Stephen Ellis and Gerrie ter Haar point out, 'it is largely through religious ideas that Africans think about the world today, and ... religious

---

[26] Cf. J. Soothill, *Gender, Social Change and Spiritual Power: Charismatic Christianity in Ghana* (Leiden, 2007), 186–96.

ideas provide them with a means of becoming social and political actors'.[27] When this applies to personal and social transformation in general, it also applies to the issue of gender transformation, particularly the transformation of masculinities. As Lesotho theologian Paul Leshota writes, a transformation of the social systems of masculinity begins with men's personal *metanoia*, 'a change of the heart'.[28] The question, then, is how religious resources – separated by ter Haar into four categories: religious ideas, religious practices, religious organisation, and religious experiences[29] – bring about such a *metanoia*. How does religion provide men with the means to become social and political actors and, indeed, to take responsibility for their own lives and the lives of others? This question draws our attention to male agency and the way it is enabled and shaped by religious discourse.

Indeed, agency is a useful concept to analyse and understand transformations of masculinity in the sphere of religion, precisely because it enables us to go beyond a focus on a fixed structure of male domination. Even if religious discourse promotes (soft) patriarchal ideals of masculinity, we still have to examine what type of male agency is produced here (and how), because we cannot assume that we already know what power means.[30] The concept of patriarchy analyses gender in a binary scheme of male domination and female submission. In such a scheme, power is considered to be oppressive, hierarchically organised and unequally distributed. Subsequently, a notion such as male headship can only be understood as a symbol of gender hierarchy that enables men to exercise power over women. Male agency, in the conceptual frame of patriarchy, is inherently problematic because it is associated with this monolithic conceptualisation of power. Going beyond an analysis of male agency in terms of patriarchy therefore also requires a different understanding of power. A Foucauldian perspective allows for a more complex and nuanced understanding of power in gender relations. Here, power is not something with a singular intentionality, structure or location but, rather, is relational and circulatory, something that pervades life and produces new relations and subjectivities. This has two important implications for our discussion of gender and masculinities. First, the essentialist categories of women as 'the oppressed' and men as 'the oppressors' are decentred and, alternatively, attention is drawn to how people are agents in power relations.[31] Second, power in general, and men's

---

[27] S. Ellis and G. ter Haar, *Worlds of Power: Religious Thought and Political Practice in Africa* (London, 2004), 2.

[28] P. Leshota, 'The Spell of Discrete Islands of Consciousness: My Journey with Masculinities in the Context of HIV and AIDS', in E. Chitando and S. Chirongoma (eds), *Redemptive Masculinities: Men, HIV and Religion* (Geneva, 2012), 165.

[29] G. ter Haar, *How God Became African: African Spirituality and Western Secular Thought* (Philadelphia, 2009), 86.

[30] Cf. M. Mayblin, *Gender, Catholicism, and Morality in Brazil: Virtuous Husbands, Powerful Wives* (New York, 2010), 13.

[31] Cf. M. Kamitsuka, *Feminist Theology and the Challenge of Difference* (Oxford, 2007), 92–3.

power in particular is not only and not necessarily coercive but also productive. This insight makes it possible to reconsider an 'oppressive' notion such as male headship and to examine the type of power it produces in particular contexts and relations, and how it shapes men as agential subjects.

Informed by recent debates in gender studies, I understand agency as a critical-dynamic and contextual concept. Agency is *critical*, because I locate agency, in Judith Butler's terms, within the possibility of a variation on gender as a repetitive process.[32] In other words, I speak of male agency when men resist problematic norms of hegemonic masculinity and come to perform an alternative, more constructive type of masculinity. This variation is the beginning of transformation, and in a certain way the variation *is* the transformation taking place, because it makes men social and political actors. Agency is *dynamic* because the appearance of the variation on hegemonic norms of gender cannot be fixed. Neither can it be prescribed or postulated, particularly not by academic scholars from the West working in post-colonial contexts in our globalising world. African theologians may have a clear understanding of redemptive masculinities and may work to liberate men from patriarchy, but I prefer to examine how men in their specific social, cultural and religious contexts subtly transform the way they understand and embody their male identity. As I have argued elsewhere, in an African Pentecostal discourse the notion of male headship can enable agency among men, in the sense that it targets them for change rather than simply reinforcing the status quo of a patriarchal masculinity.[33] An example of this is the way in which Banda dissociates male headship from male domination, rejecting the latter while affirming the former, and how he then uses the notion of headship to call upon men to take up their 'God-given' responsibilities. This example shows that agency is always contextual, and the understanding of agency should therefore not be restricted by the normative assumptions and political ideals we have as critical scholars in the field of religion and gender. As Saba Mahmood points out,

> [I]f the ability to effect change in the world and in oneself is historically and culturally specific (both in terms of what constitutes "change" and the means by which it is effected), then the meaning and sense of agency cannot be fixed, but must emerge through an analysis of the particular concepts that enable modes of being, responsibility, and effectivity.[34]

---

[32] Butler, *Gender Trouble*, 198.

[33] See A.S, van Klinken, 'Male Headship as Male Agency: An Alternative Understanding of a "Patriarchal" African Pentecostal Discourse on Masculinity', *Religion and Gender*, 1/1 (2011): 104–24.

[34] S. Mahmood, *Politics of Piety: The Islamic Revival and the Feminist Subject* (Princeton, 2005), 14–15.

This applies as much to the men in the case studies presented in this book as to the women who participate in the Muslim piety movement in Egypt that is central in Mahmood's study, even though the ethnographic contexts are completely different.

In what follows I will analyse male agency as it is produced in and through religious discourse. My analysis will be informed by debates in the emerging field of the anthropology of Christianity, where the issue of (dis)continuity is a central theme. So far, these debates mainly focus on Pentecostal forms of Christianity in Africa and elsewhere. Much attention has been paid to the way Pentecostalism and its born-again discourse brings about 'a complete break with the past', which is often understood in terms of an engagement with modernity.[35] Joel Robbins rightly observes that the emphasis on discontinuity is characteristic of Protestant Christianity, particularly of evangelical and Pentecostal forms of Protestantism, while Catholicism has a greater emphasis on continuity.[36] This is relevant to my discussion here, because the theme of rupture is closely linked to a moral trajectory of 'change in one's self'.[37] Therefore in the following sections I will explore how Pentecostal and Catholic discourses (re)shape men as gendered, moral and social agents in (dis)continuity with the past, as a preliminary comparative exercise in the anthropology of Christianity. I will do so by focusing on the personal accounts of two men, one from each of the case-study churches.

Born-again Discourse and Pentecostal Masculinity[38]

The first portrait is of a man in his late 20s, let's call him Danny Mulenga, who is a member of Northmead Assembly of God and actively participates in the church's youth ministry. His story presents a typical example of born-again conversion as a break with the past.[39]

Mulenga originates from another part of the country and moved to Lusaka some years ago for professional purposes. His parents died during his childhood and youth years, after which he stayed with an older brother. However, his brother did not really look after him. Mulenga ended up having bad friends, stopped going

---

[35] B. Meyer, '"Make a Complete Break with the Past". Memory and Post-colonial Modernity in Ghanaian Pentecostalist Discourse', *Journal of Religion in Africa*, 28:3 (1998): 316–49. See also M. Engelke, 'Discontinuity and the Discourse of Conversion', *Journal of Religion in Africa*, 31/1–2 (2004): 82–109.

[36] J. Robbins, 'Continuity Thinking and the Problem of Christian Culture: Belief, Time, and the Anthropology of Christianity', *Current Anthropology*, 48/1 (2007): 16.

[37] Cf. F. Klaits, 'Introduction: Self, Other and God in African Christianities', *Journal of Religion in Africa*, 41:2 (2011), 143–53.

[38] This section is largely derived from my article 'Men in the Remaking: Conversion Narratives and Born-again Masculinity in Zambia', *Journal of Religion in Africa*, 42/3 (2012): 215–239.

[39] Interviews with Danny Mulenga were conducted in Lusaka on 6 and 13 November 2008.

to school, and one day found himself being arrested by the police. Looking back at this period, Mulenga said: 'All these things made me becoming self-reliant. I thought: I can live on my own. I don't have to depend on a person. I am a man.' Apparently, independence was a key notion of his male identity at that time. This changed when, after one incident in his life, he decided to give his life to Christ and became born again. Then he learned that in the period before his conversion, when he was playing around and doing all things he and his friends considered manly, he actually was not a real man:

> I wasn't yet a man. After receiving Christ and after reading the Word of God, now I think: Being a man is being responsible; it is about accepting responsibilities. Being responsible over yourself, over your surrounding and for other people's lives. For me, that is being a man now. ... I used to stay on my own, to do my own things. I used to drink, to smoke, to have girlfriends; I used to mess around. I couldn't call myself a man because I wasn't responsible over my life and the life of others, and the feelings of others. But when I changed I became responsible and started to say: When I do this, my family is not happy, when I smoke I may get sick; this is not good for me. That is when I became a man because I started doing what God has purposed me to do.

Clearly, this is a narrative of discontinuity. Mulenga narrates his break with the past, in particular the immediate past of a lifestyle which he now considers immoral and, interestingly, unmanly. Some scholars have suggested that for men, becoming born again is a threat to their male identity. Giving up drinking, womanising and other activities that – according to the popular norms of masculinity in their society – are considered 'manly', born-again men would run the risk of being looked at as 'sissies'.[40] However, in the case of Mulenga, his break with the past does not seem to have damaged his masculine self-image, which rather is reshaped and re-affirmed. Through 'receiving Christ' and 'reading the Word of God' he has gained a new understanding of manhood, and hence considers himself now a better man than before conversion and than his former friends still are. Even if others would not consider him a real man, he would not mind because he knows better. Mulenga's account shows that becoming born again is not a disembodied spiritual rebirth but involves and affects men as gendered and embodied beings. Mulenga put this eloquently, saying: 'You have to accept Christ, and that is when God is going to make a man out of you.' Clearly this applies to him personally. Being born again has not just made him a new individual, but a new man.

For Mulenga, the break with the past entails a break with the norms of masculinity popular among non-born-again young men. He phrases his new

---

[40] V. Brereton, *From Sin to Salvation: Stories of Women's Conversions, 1800 to the Present* (Bloomington, 1991), 98–101; H. Gooren, 'Conversion Narratives', in A.H. Anderson, M. Bergunder, A. Droogers and C. van der Laan (eds), *Studying Global Pentecostalism: Theories and Methods* (Berkeley, 2010), 103–5.

understanding of manhood as 'being responsible' and 'accepting responsibilities'. Apparently, in this narrative male agency is about responsibility. It can be questioned whether this really is a new concept. As anthropologist Paul Dover points out, in traditional settings in Zambia manliness is generally associated with notions such as responsibility and wisdom.[41] It could be argued, therefore, that the Pentecostal born-again discourse provides young men in modern urban settings, where traditional ways of learning masculinity have largely disappeared, with a new discursive *rite de passage* into mature manhood. For young men like Mulenga who have grown up without a father or other adult male figure, Pentecostalism not only provides them with a discourse but also with a social group in which they find role models, both of their own age and adults. Recall the youth pastor in NAOG who wants to be a father for youths living in a fatherless society, and recall Bishop Banda, who presents himself explicitly as an example of responsible manhood. Though the understanding of mature manhood in terms of taking responsibility may be more or less in line with traditional understandings in Zambia, Mulenga frames this understanding in a typical Christian way. Demonstrating that 'breaking with the past is not only the erasure of tradition but the inscription of another',[42] he refers to Genesis 2, particularly to the notion that Adam was instructed by God to watch over the earth and to name the animals. In his opinion this biblical passage underscores men's leadership in relation to women and demonstrates that 'a real man is supposed to be responsible'. This interpretation, which clearly echoes Banda's preaching on 'biblical manhood' (see Chapter 4), shows that in a Pentecostal discourse the rather patriarchal idea of a unique, primary position of men in the order of creation can be a religious resource that enables male agency in the form of responsibility.[43]

It is interesting to see what 'taking responsibility' concretely means for Mulenga. First, it means that he changed his lifestyle. Drinking, smoking and playing with girlfriends are the things he used to consider as manly. However, after conversion he learned that true manhood is reached through controlling personal conduct: 'That is when I became a man.' In contrast to his peers who cannot control themselves and just follow their desires, Mulenga as a born-again man believes that the ability to control the self is a way to prove male strength. Even before his born-again conversion he realised that, in the current era of AIDS, self-control is crucial: 'I used to be careless. I thought AIDS is just for those who are unfortunate. But when it was coming closer, to my family and to friends, I changed.' Now Pentecostalism seems to provide him with the means to discipline the bodily self. Interestingly, in the area of sexuality, bodily discipline for Mulenga

---

[41] Cf. P. Dover, 'Gender and Embodiment: Expectations of Manliness in a Zambian Village', in L. Ouzgane and R. Morrell (eds), *African Masculinities: Men in Africa from the Late Nineteenth Century to the Present* (New York, 2005), 173–88.

[42] M. Engelke, 'Past Pentecostalism: Notes on Rupture, Realignment, and Everyday Life in Pentecostal and African Independent Churches', *Africa*, 80/2 (2010): 179.

[43] Cf. Van Klinken, *Male Headship as Male Agency*.

is not only an issue of self-control but also one of respect for a woman: 'As a Christian, when I am in a relationship and I insist on sex, I am not respecting her body.' He knows through experience that some girls say: 'Christian boys are boring because they don't kiss us, they don't have sex with us, they don't take us out at night', but he says not to mind about that. Mulenga's new sense of responsibility has furthered his commitment to a new purpose in life: to bring together his fragmented family and to look after his cousins who are left orphaned because of AIDS. This shows that the theme of rupture does not necessarily entail a break with close relatives, as is sometimes suggested, but can result in a renewed concern about, and engagement with, the family.[44] Out of his sense of responsibility, Mulenga has also engaged in activities aimed at HIV prevention among the youth, after he witnessed several peers dying from AIDS. For him this is all part of doing what God has purposed him to do as a man, which illustrates his religious motivation. The references to AIDS in Mulenga's story show that his born-again conversion has to be understood against the background of the HIV epidemic. In his own words, 'AIDS has come very close' with friends and close relatives dying of the disease. His story illustrates the fact that men in present-day Zambia are living in the shadow of AIDS.[45] The epidemic has revealed the dangerous fragility of masculinity. Pentecostal Christianity, in particular its born-again discourse, provides Mulenga, and most likely other men, with a way to cope with this existential vulnerability.

Mulenga testifies to a radical change, not just in his way of living in general but in his life as a man and his perception of manhood. His account, like the stories of other men I interviewed in NOAG, shows how the programme of born-again conversion, which in the words of Ruth Marshall is a 'discursive regime',[46] creates not only a new type of *moral* subject but also a new *male gendered* subject. Through this regime, men can indeed make a break with the past, including its dangerous forms of masculinity. Empowered by God they become new male selves that no longer live lives that make them vulnerable to the dangers of HIV and AIDS. Recounting their breaks with the past and the changes in their lives, Mulenga and other men in NAOG did not so much speak about miraculous interventions of God in their lives.[47] Rather, their stories suggest that God is actively present, but in the background of their lives. God warns them, encourages them and gives them strength, but moral transformation first is the foremost task of the reborn self. However, because this process of transformation or sanctification is full of

---

[44] For a similar argument, see M. Lindhardt, '"If you are saved you cannot forget your parents": Agency, Power, and Social Repositioning in Tanzanian born-again Christianity', *Journal of Religion in Africa*, 40/3 (2010): 240–72.

[45] Cf. A. Simpson, *Boys to Men in the Shadow of AIDS: Masculinities and HIV Risk in Zambia* (New York, 2009).

[46] R. Marshall, *Political Spiritualities: The Pentecostal Revolution in Nigeria* (Chicago, 2009), 36.

[47] Ibid., 155.

challenges and temptations, men realise they cannot do it by themselves. 'Being a born-again man', as Mulenga puts it, 'is not something that you achieve on your own. It has to take God. ... I can't say: I am arrived. I have my mistakes. I am still a man in the making.' This confirms that *becoming* born-again may be an event of rupture, but *being* born-again 'is an ongoing existential project, not a state acquired once and for all, a project that is never fully achieved and always runs of the risk of being compromised'.[48] Born-again masculinity, it appears, is as unstable and fragile as all gender identities. However, it anchors itself in a strong belief in God's transformative power. Mulenga, as a singer in the church choir, experiences this power during church services and meetings, when he leads the congregation into ecstatic worship and voluble speaking in tongues. It is through these typical Pentecostal 'sensational forms' that he and other born-again men sense the presence of God that transforms their lives, including their male identities.[49]

Catholic Discourse and Saintly Masculinity

The second portrait is of a man in his 50s, whom I will call Marc Bwali, who is a parishioner of Regiment parish and is deeply involved in the St Joachim Catholic Men's Organization.[50] He told me that he had been a 'traditional Catholic' for a long time, attending Mass now and then but not really committed to the church and the faith. This changed when his son got sick and finally died. His wife sought solace in the faith and joined one of the lay movements in the parish. She encouraged her husband to do the same. After some time he decided to join the St Joachim group. He recalls how this decision had a great impact on his life:

> Before I joined St Joachim, I used not to go to SCC meetings and I used to drink a lot of beer. But immediately when I joined Joachim this began to change. The day I suited I felt so joyous that after that I became concerned with attending SCC meetings, going to church. Nowadays I come to Mass almost every day. And beer drinking changed as well. We also started eating together as a family, and we say prayers together as a family. So I became more of a family man, and that's the way it is supposed to be.

Clearly, a discontinuity is narrated here. This is a conversion story – not a conversion in terms of religious affiliation or belief (Bwali was a Catholic and continues to be a Catholic) but in terms of a new moral and spiritual lifestyle. In contrast to Mulenga in the previous section, Bwali does not frame his conversion in a typical born-again discourse of receiving or accepting Christ. His life changed

---

[48] Ibid., 131.

[49] B. Meyer, 'Aesthetics of Persuasion: Global Christianity and Pentecostalism's Sensational Forms', *The South Atlantic Quarterly*, 109/4 (2010): 741–64.

[50] The interview with Marc Bwali was conducted on 9 November 2008.

after he decided to join the St Joachim men's organisation, and in particular after he was suited. The suiting is the ceremony (preferably held on the 26th of July, the feast day of St Joachim) in which new members, after a probation and preparation period of six months, make their promises and are clothed for the first time in the organisation's uniform. For Bwali, the suiting was a day of joy that even further increased his motivation to live up to the promises he had made: to participate in church and SCC activities, to love and respect his wife, and to receive the sacraments of Reconciliation (confession) and Holy Communion regularly.[51]

The fact that Bwali mentions his suiting so explicitly in his conversion story highlights the central role of ritualism and symbolism in the production of subjectivity and agency in a Catholic context. As I have described in Chapter 3, the colours of the uniform are full of meaning, and the uniform as a whole symbolically expresses the new moral and spiritual orientation of the Joachim members. Bwali's account shows that wearing the heavenly blue uniform is not just an outward expression, but is a performative practice that reconstitutes the male self. That is also why, after suiting, the Joachim members receive a new name: from then on, they add 'Joa' before their first names, expressing their new identity. Thus, Bwali signed the consent form for the interview as 'Joa Marc Bwali'. Perhaps this name is typical of the Catholic position in the debate about Christianity and (dis) continuity. The Joachim members do not receive a completely new name, but an extra name that precedes their personal name, as if the moral trajectory initiated in the organisation does not aim at a radical break with the former self (as in Pentecostalism) but at a renewed sense and expression of the self.

Of course, the name 'Joa' refers to St Joachim, the patron saint of the organisation, who is promoted as the model of Catholic manhood. As outlined in Chapter 3, St Joachim is particularly modelled as a family man. Bwali's story exemplifies the 'hermeneutics of imitation' through which the values represented by the saint figure are interpreted by devotees and applied to their lives.[52] Retelling the story about St Joachim, Bwali emphasises that the saint was God-fearing and pious, a faithful husband and a caring father, prayerful both personally and with his family. These themes are echoed in the above quotation where Bwali describes the changes in his life: he now attends Mass, almost on a daily basis, and the SCC meetings; and he has become 'more of a family man', meaning concretely that now he shares meals with his family and leads his family in prayer. Being a family man also has a material dimension:

---

[51] Cf. *Constitution of St Joachim Catholic Men's Organization* (Lusaka, 2001), 9–10.

[52] For a general discussion about the hermeneutics of imitation in relation to saints, see J. Duyndam, 'Hermeneutics of Imitation: A Philosophical Approach to Sainthood and Exemplariness', in M. Poorthuis and J. Schwartz (eds), *Saints and Role Models in Judaism and Christianity* (Leiden, 2004), 7–24. For a more specific analysis of the hermeneutical process of imitation in the St Joachim men's organisation, see my article 'St. Joachim as a Model of Catholic Manhood in Times of AIDS: A Case Study of Masculinity in an African Christian Context', *CrossCurrents*, 61/4 (2011): 467–79.

> Since I joined St Joachim I have become a very responsible man: I support my family fully. My wife has now confidence in me that I bring all the money at home. Before I joined, I used to keep a part for drinking.

Interestingly, Bwali tells us that he has also acquired a new understanding of marriage, particularly the relationship between husband and wife. Here, he perceives a discontinuity between 'African culture' and Christianity:

> In the African context, some people think that the man must be always at the top; he is the head. Indeed he is the head according to the Bible, but the Bible also says that when you are married negotiation must be from both angles. But in the African context that aspect doesn't arrive. Unless you are a Christian and you pray. Because God will guide you. You will find that in certain families where there is no prayer, in such families you will find that a man is at his own and the wife and the children are on their own as well. But in our families we are together. We eat together. And in that way you bring your family together.

Bwali still upholds the 'traditional' notion of the man as head of the family, because in his opinion this is biblical. However, he combines this with a sense of mutuality and companionship that he also considers biblical but that is, of course, a rather modern concern. This egalitarian tendency subverts and subtly changes the practice of male headship, making it more symbolic. Agency, in Bwali's account, is shaped after St Joachim and means living up to the 'vocation' of being a family man. Joachim members invest their male identity in their marriage and family and in the church, which requires an emotional, spiritual and material commitment. This demonstrates the potential of saints to provide 'a space in which to think differently, to think [and to practise] against and outside socially normative patterns'.[53] Indeed, Joachim members state how they are different from other men in the community because they live up to an alternative and, in their opinion, higher ideal of manhood. Their motivation to do so is also related to the shadow of AIDS in their lives and the resulting sense of vulnerability. Like Mulenga, Bwali has lost several friends and relatives 'as a result of their lifestyle', which led him to a process of introspection.

Bwali's story shows that in the conversion process initiated by the imitation of St Joachim, the male self becomes a subject of moral transformation. This is not an easy process as it is full of challenges. Bwali says he still faces temptations, among others in the area of sexuality. However, when he feels tempted he prays the rosary or makes the sign of the cross. 'It has happened to me several times. I [made] the sign of the cross and said "Get off, Satan" and I found automatically my mind switching off to another thing.' Thus, the simple gesture of making the sign of the

---

[53] F. Meltzer and J. Elsner, 'Introduction', in F. Meltzer and J. Elsner (eds), *Saints: Faith Without Borders* (Chicago, 2011), ix.

cross is a spiritual means – in Foucauldian terms a 'technique of the self'[54] – to protect the body and the mind, which again underlines the importance of ritual practice as a means to discipline the self. In the context of the men's organisation, moral transformation is not only a personal but also a collective process. In their meetings, Joachim members sometimes share their weaknesses and the challenges they face, as a kind of confessional practice, and they encourage each other and pray together. The organisation offers men a social and spiritual space in which new and younger members are nurtured and supported by the senior Joachims. The importance of this group setting for men's moral transformation is underlined by Ellis and ter Haar when they write: 'The social element in transformation is at least as important as the personal one, since if others also perceive a transformation to have taken place, they may regard a transformed person as different from his or her previous self.'[55] This element of social recognition is also mentioned by Bwali, who proudly told me that othershave noticed changes in his life:

> Recently I have been elected as a vice chair in my section [SCC]. They trusted me, they said, because they have seen a change in my life. It gave me self-confidence and will make me still more committed to the church. Also my friends and colleagues noticed the change in my life, and some of them have started to attend the SCC, too.

Bwali's account shows that instead of a discursive regime, such as in Pentecostal forms of Christianity, Catholicism provides men with a social and spiritual space and a ritual practice to transform the male self. Clearly, this also produces male agency, in the sense that men become social and political actors representing a new form of masculinity that is modelled after a saint. The resulting 'saintly masculinity' deviates from popular notions of masculinity, but at the same time it gives the Joachim members the status of mature, responsible and wise men in the community.

Conclusion

The above analysis of the accounts of two Zambian Christian men in terms of agency reveals some of the significant transformations of masculinity taking place in and through religious discourse. Though none of them has been 'liberated from patriarchy', as the African theologians would like to see, they both testify to have become a 'new man'. Indeed, their understanding and practice of masculinity has changed, they have taken responsibility for their own lives and the lives of others, and they also express different and more positive attitudes towards women.

---

[54] M. Foucault, 'Technologies of the Self', in P. Rabinow (ed.), *Ethics: Subjectivity and Truth. Essential Works of Foucault, 1954–1984*, vol. 1 (London, 2000), 223–52.

[55] Ellis and ter Haar, *Worlds of Power*, 166–7.

Their stories exemplify the types of transformations in masculinity taking place at a grassroots level of African Christianities, in local church communities and Christian movements. The critical scholar of men, masculinities and religion can easily lose sight of these transformations when his or her analysis is primarily guided by the question of whether or not religious discourse echoes the old-and-too-familiar language of patriarchy. This question is certainly not irrelevant, but it cannot account for the complexities and ambiguities that characterise much of religious gender discourse and it is not sensitive to the more subtle changes that may take place. Religious discourse such as that found in the case studies presented in this book, even though it uses more or less patriarchal language – and sometimes precisely through its specific employment of some patriarchal themes – can bring about changes in men that are helpful in concrete social contexts, such as those of HIV and AIDS. In that sense, the case-study churches and the type of discourse they represent contribute to what the African theologians call 'redemptive masculinities', though these masculinities are not necessarily also 'liberative'. If we come to understand this, it also becomes possible to acknowledge that these discourses somehow are local theologies of gender justice in practice: they are concerned about current configurations of gender and aim to transform these for the better, using the theological resources available in their tradition.

My call for a more open and contextual understanding of gender justice is not intended as a relativist account in which every religious discourse can be considered as a local theology of gender justice in practice. I have emphasised that such a discourse has to bring about 'a transformation for the better' in gender relations and masculinities in order to be recognised as a local theology of gender justice. Of course, this immediately raises the question what can be considered as 'better'. My response would be that no general answer can be given to this question as the answer always depends on the challenges and issues in concrete social contexts. Moreover, although there is not one normative theological-ethical understanding of gender justice that can be universally applied but rather many local theologies of gender justice, all these theologies may claim to be normative and to have a general significance. This underlines the need for dialogue and critical discussion within contemporary world Christianity about the understanding of gender and the transformation of categories of femininity and masculinity so that they become more life-giving and foster the human dignity of every person regardless of sex. In fact, this book has organised just such a discussion by analysing and intersecting the discourses of progressive African theologians, a local Pentecostal church and a Catholic parish in Zambia.

This book has been written at the intersection of various perspectives and disciplines. It is located in the field of religious studies, which itself is an amalgam of different approaches. In this study I have combined theological, anthropological and gender-critical methods and concepts to analyse and reflect upon the question of the transformation of masculinities in contemporary African Christianity. At its best, the combination of these different perspectives has strengthened the argument and enriched the book, but I am aware of some of the tensions underlying this project. The questions of (1) the relation between redemptive and liberative masculinities and (2) the understanding and implications of gender justice remain critical and call for further study and discussion, within the fields of African theological studies, the critical study of men, masculinities and religion, and the study of gender in African and world Christianities. It was not my aim to provide the final answer, but rather to show the complexity of these questions and to suggest a way of how they can be engaged constructively. I hope this contributes to the quest for transformed masculinities in African Christian contexts and opens up new perspectives on how to think about the relation between religion and masculinities in the context of the HIV epidemic and beyond, inspired by a desire for gender justice in our globalising world.

Bibliography

Unpublished Material

Northmead Assembly of God Church Constitution – Excerpt of Key Articles (Lusaka, 2008).
Pre-marital Counselling Check List Form, Northmead Assembly of God.
Pre-marital Counselling General Guide, Marriage Ministry, Northmead Assembly of God.
Pre-marital Evaluation Questionnaire, Northmead Assembly of God.
Standard Liturgy for Wedding Service, Northmead Assembly of God.

Published Material

Addai-Mensah, P., *Mission, Communion and Relationship: A Roman Catholic Response to the Crisis of Male Youths in Africa* (New York: Peter Lang, 2009).
Ambasa-Shisanya, C., 'Widowhood and HIV Transmission in Siaya District, Kenya', in E. Chitando and N. Hadebe (eds), *Compassionate Circles: African Women Theologians Facing HIV* (Geneva: WCC Publications, 2009), 53–70.
Anane, M., 'The Soul is Willing: Religion, Men and HIV/AIDS in Ghana', in M. Foreman (ed.), *AIDS and Men: Taking Risks or Taking Responsibility?* (London: Zed Books, 1999), 79–94.
Antonio, E.P., 'Introduction: Inculturation and Postcolonial Discourse', in E.P. Antonio (ed.), *Inculturation and Postcolonial Discourse in African Theology* (New York: Peter Lang, 2006), 1–28.
Aquino, M.P., 'Feminist Intercultural Theology: Towards a Shared Future of Justice', in M.P. Aquino and M.J. Rosado-Nunes (eds), *Feminist Intercultural Theology: Latina Explorations for a Just World* (Maryknoll: Orbis Books, 2007), 9–28.
Arnfred, S., 'Re-thinking Sexualities in Africa: Introduction', in S. Arnfred (ed.), *Re-Thinking Sexualities in Africa* (Uppsala: Nordiska Afrika Institutet, 2004), 7–29.
Asamoah-Gyadu, J.K., 'Born of Water and the Spirit: Pentecostal/Charismatic Christianity in Africa', in O.U. Kalu (ed.), *African Christianity: An African Story* (Pretoria: Department of Church History, University of Pretoria, 2005), 388–409.
Asselin, J.P., 'Anne and Joachim, SS.', in B.L. Marthaler (ed.), *New Catholic Encyclopedia*, 2nd edn (Detroit: Gale, 2003), 468–70.

Ayanga, H., 'Religio-cultural Challenges in Women's Fight Against HIV/AIDS in Africa', in T.M. Hinga, A.N. Kubai, P. Mwaura and H. Ayanga (eds), *Women, Religion and HIV/AIDS in Africa: Responding to Ethical and Theological Challenges* (Pietermaritzburg: Cluster Publications, 2008), 34–48.

Baker-Fletcher, G.K., 'Critical Theory, Deconstruction and Liberation?', *Journal of Men's Studies*, 7/2 (1999), 275–80.

Banda, J.H.K., *Cultivating a Lifestyle of Truth – Part 3* (Lusaka: Northmead Assembly of God, 2005), DVD.

_____ *Cultivating a Lifestyle of Truth – Part 4* (Lusaka: Northmead Assembly of God, 2005), DVD.

_____ *Cultivating a Lifestyle of Truth – Part 5* (Lusaka: Northmead Assembly of God, 2005), DVD.

_____ *Cultivating a Lifestyle of Truth – Part 6* (Lusaka: Northmead Assembly of God, 2005), DVD.

_____ *Cultivating a Lifestyle of Truth – Part 7* (Lusaka, Northmead Assembly of God, 2005), DVD.

_____ *Cultivating a Lifestyle of Truth – Part 8* (Lusaka: Northmead Assembly of God, 2005), DVD.

_____ *Fatherhood in the 21st Century – Part 1* (Lusaka: Northmead Assembly of God, 2008), DVD.

_____ *Fatherhood in the 21st Century – Part 2* (Lusaka: Northmead Assembly of God, 2008), DVD.

_____ *Fatherhood in the 21st Century – Part 3* (Lusaka: Northmead Assembly of God, 2008), DVD.

_____ *Fatherhood in the 21st Century – Part 4* (Lusaka: Northmead Assembly of God, 2008), DVD.

_____ *Fatherhood in the 21st Century – Part 5* (Lusaka: Northmead Assembly of God, 2008), DVD.

_____ *Fatherhood in the 21st Century – Part 6* (Lusaka: Northmead Assembly of God, 2008), DVD.

_____ *HIV&AIDS and Stigma in the Church* (Lusaka: Northmead Assembly of God, 2008), DVD.

_____ 'Knowing God – Part 12', website of Northmead Assembly of God, publication date unknown; accessed 28 September 2009. http://www.northmeadassembly.org/index.php?option=com_content&view=article&id=269%3Atheme-knowing-god-part-12&catid=37%3Abible-study&showall=1.

_____ 'When the Grass Withers and the Flowers Fall', website of Northmead Assembly of God, publication date unknown; accessed 23 March 2009. http://www.northmeadassembly.org.zm/ddata/news/viewnews.cgi?category=3&id=1037458688.

_____ 'Between Two Worlds – Part II', website of Northmead Assembly of God, publication date unknown; accessed 24 March 2009. http://www.northmeadassembly.org.zm/ddata/news/viewnews.cgi?category=3&id=1041935291.

_____ *Making Relationships more Meaningful – Part 1* (Lusaka: Northmead Assembly of God, publication date unknown), DVD.

_____ *Making Relationships more Meaningful – Part 2* (Lusaka: Northmead Assembly of God, publication date unknown), DVD.

Bartkowski, J.P., *The Promise Keepers: Servants, Soldiers, and Godly Men* (New Brunswick: Rutgers University Press, 2004).

Baylies, C., 'Perspectives on Gender and AIDS in Africa', in C. Baylies and J. Bujra (eds), *AIDS, Sexuality and Gender in Africa: Collective Strategies and Struggles in Tanzania and Zambia* (London: Routledge, 2000), 1–24.

Beattie, T., 'Carnal Love and Spiritual Imagination: Can Luce Irigaray and John Paul II Come Together?', in J. Davies and G. Loughlin (eds), *Sex these Days: Essays on Theology, Sexuality and Society* (Sheffield: Sheffield Academic Press, 1997), 160–83.

Bediako, K., *Theology and Identity: The Impact of Culture upon Christian Thought in the Second Century and in Modern Africa* (Akropong-Akuapem: Regnum, 1992).

Boesten, J. and Poku, N.K., 'Gender, Inequalities and HIV/AIDS', in J. Boesten and N.K. Poku (eds), *Gender and HIV/AIDS: Critical Perspectives from the Developing World* (Farnham: Ashgate, 2009), 1–28.

Bond, G.C., 'Zambia: Peoples and Cultures', in J. Middleton (ed.), *Encyclopedia of Africa South of the Sahara – Part IV* (New York: Scribner's Sons, 1997), 414–17.

Boyd, S.B., 'Trajectories in Men's Studies in Religion: Theories, Methodologies, and Issues', *Journal of Men's Studies*, 7:2 (1999), 265–8.

Boyd, S.B., Longwood, W.M., and Muesse, M.W., 'Men, Masculinity and the Study of Religion', in S.B. Boyd, W.M. Longwood and M.W. Muesse (eds), *Redeeming Men: Religion and Masculinities* (Louisville: Westminster John Knox Press, 1996), xviii–xxii.

_____ 'Where Do We Go from Here? Some Concluding Remarks', in S.B. Boyd, W.M. Longwood and M.W. Muesse (eds), *Redeeming Men: Religion and Masculinities* (Louisville: Westminster John Knox Press, 1996), 285–93.

Brereton, V., *From Sin to Salvation: Stories of Women's Conversions, 1800 to the Present* (Bloomington: Indiana University Press, 1991).

Brusco, E.E., *The Reformation of Machismo: Evangelical Conversion and Gender in Colombia* (Austin: University of Texas Press, 1995).

Bujo, B., *African Theology in its Social Context* (Nairobi: Paulines Publications, 1992).

_____ *The Ethical Dimension of Community: The African Model and the Dialogue between North and South* (Nairobi: Paulines Publications, 1998).

Bujo, B. and Czerny, M. (eds), *AIDS in Africa: Theological Reflections* (Nairobi: Paulines Publications, 2007).

Bujra, J., 'Targeting Men for a Change: AIDS Discourse and Activism in Africa', in F. Cleaver (ed.), *Masculinities Matter! Men, Gender and Development* (London: Zed Books, 2002), 209–34.

Bujra, J. and Baylies, C., 'Responses to the AIDS Epidemic in Tanzania and Zambia', in C. Baylies and J. Bujra (eds), *AIDS, Sexuality and Gender in Africa: Collective Strategies and Struggles in Tanzania and Zambia* (London: Routledge, 2000), 25–58.

Butler, J., *Gender Trouble: Feminism and the Subversion of Identity*, 2nd edn (London: Routledge, 2006).

Cannell, F. 'The Anthropology of Christianity', in F. Cannell (ed.), *The Anthropology of Christianity* (Durham, NC: Duke University Press, 2006), 1–50.

Cartledge M.J. and D. Cheetham, 'Introduction', in M.J. Cartledge and D. Cheetham (eds), *Intercultural Theology: Approaches and Themes* (London: SCM Press, 2011), 1–10.

Catholic Bishops of Zambia, 'Called to be the Family of God: A Pastoral Letter from the Catholic Bishops of Zambia to Launch the Five Year African Synod Programme' (May 1996), in J. Komakoma (ed.), *The Social Teaching of the Catholic Bishops and Other Christian Leaders in Zambia: Major Pastoral Letters and Statements 1953–2001* (Ndola: Mission Press, 2003), 341–6.

———— 'Choose Life: The Sacred Value of Human Life and the Evil of Promoting Abortion: A Pastoral Letter from the Catholic Bishops' (30 November 1997), in J. Komakoma (ed.), *The Social Teaching of the Catholic Bishops and Other Christian Leaders in Zambia: Major Pastoral Letters and Statements 1953–2001* (Ndola: Mission Press, 2003), 370–89.

———— 'The Church as a Caring Family: A Pastoral Letter to all Catholics by the Bishops of Zambia on the 1997 Theme for the Synod Implementation' (21 March 1997), in J. Komakoma (ed.), *The Social Teaching of the Catholic Bishops and Other Christian Leaders in Zambia: Major Pastoral Letters and Statements 1953–2001* (Ndola: Mission Press, 2003), 353–67.

———— 'The Missionary Family: A Pastoral Letter to all Catholics from the Bishops of Zambia on the 1999 Theme for the Implementation of the African Synod' (25 March 1999), in J. Komakoma (ed.), *The Social Teaching of the Catholic Bishops and Other Christian Leaders in Zambia: Major Pastoral Letters and Statements 1953–2001* (Ndola: Mission Press, 2003), 400–409.

———— 'You Shall be My Witnesses: Pastoral Letter of the Catholic Bishops of Zambia to Mark 100 Years of Catholic Faith in Zambia' (9th July 1991), in J. Komakoma (ed.), *The Social Teaching of the Catholic Bishops and Other Christian Leaders in Zambia: Major Pastoral Letters and Statements 1953–2001* (Ndola: Mission Press, 2003), 237–58.

———— 'Have Life to the Full: A Pastoral Letter from the Catholic Bishops of Zambia on HIV/AIDS' (24 November 2002), in African Jesuit AIDS Network (ed.), *Catholic Bishops of Africa and Madagascar Speak Out on HIV & AIDS* (Nairobi: Paulines Publications, 2004), 91–4.

———— *A Call to Integrity: A Pastoral Letter from the Zambia Episcopal Conference on the Role of all Zambians to Work for the Common Good of our Nation* (Lusaka: Zambia Episcopal Conference, 2009), http://www.

catholiczambia.org.zm/index.php?option=com_docman&task=doc_down load&gid=15&Itemid=55 (accessed 10 June 2012).

_____ *That They May Have Abundant Life: A Pastoral Statement* (Lusaka: Zambia Episcopal Conference, 2012), http://www.catholiczambia.org.zm/index.php?option=com_docman&task=doc_download&gid=21&Itemid=55 (accessed 10 June 2012).

Cheyeka, A.M., 'Towards a History of the Charismatic Churches in Post-Colonial Zambia', in J.B. Gewald, M. Hinfelaar and G. Macola (eds), *One Zambia, Many Histories: Towards a History of Post-Colonial Zambi*a (Leiden: Brill, 2008), 144–63.

Chilufya, B.C., 'Christian Marriage: What is it?', *The Parish Newsletter*, 114 (19 November 2006), Regiment Parish, Lusaka.

Chirongoma, S., 'Women, Poverty, and HIV in Zimbabwe: An Exploration of Inequalities in Health Care', in I.A. Phiri and S. Nadar (eds), *African Women, Religion, and Health: Essays in Honor of Mercy Amba Ewudziwa Oduyoye* (Maryknoll: Orbis, 2006), 173–86.

Chitando, E., *Acting in Hope: African Churches and HIV/AIDS 2* (Geneva: WCC Publications, 2007).

_____ *Living with Hope: African Churches and HIV/AIDS 1* (Geneva: WCC Publications, 2007).

_____ 'A New Man for a New Era? Zimbabwean Pentecostalism, Masculinities and the HIV Epidemic', *Missionalia*, 35:3 (2007), 112–27.

_____ 'Religious Ethics, HIV and AIDS and Masculinities in Southern Africa', in R. Nicolson (ed.), *Persons in Community: African Ethics in a Global Culture* (Scottsville: University of KwaZulu-Natal Press, 2008), 45–63.

_____ *Troubled but not Destroyed* (Geneva: WCC Publications, 2009).

Chitando, E. and Chirongoma, S., 'Challenging Masculinities: Religious Studies, Men and HIV in Africa', *Journal of Constructive Theology*, 14:1 (2008), 55–69.

_____ 'Introduction', in E. Chitando and S. Chirongoma (eds), *Redemptive Masculinities: Men, HIV and Religion* (Geneva: WCC Publications 2012), 1–28.

Chitando, E. and Gunda, M.R., 'HIV and AIDS, Stigma and Liberation in the Old Testament', *Exchange: Journal of Missiological and Ecumenical Research*, 36:2 (2007), 184–97.

Clark, J.M., 'A Gay Man's Wish List for the Future of Men's Studies in Religion', *Journal of Men's Studies*, 7/2 (1999), 269–73.

Clatterbaugh, K., 'Men's Rights', in M. Flood, J.K. Gardiner, B. Pease and K. Pringle (eds), *International Encyclopedia of Men and Masculinities* (New York: Routledge, 2007), 430–33.

Colson, E., *Tonga Religious Life in the Twentieth Century* (Lusaka: Bookworld, 2006).

Congregation for the Doctrine of Faith, *Letter to the Bishops of the Catholic Church on the Collaboration of Men and Women in the Church and in the World* (Rome: The Vatican, 31 May 2004), http://www.vatican.va/roman_curia/

congregations/cfaith/documents/rc_con_cfaith_doc_20040731_collaboration_en.html (accessed 10 June 2012).
Constitution of St Joachim Catholic Men's Organization (Lusaka: Archdiocese of Lusaka, 2001).
Coakley, S., 'Shaping the Field: A Transatlantic Experience', in D.F. Ford, B. Quash and J.M. Soskice (eds), *Fields of Faith: Theology and Religious Studies for the Twenty-first Century* (Cambridge: Cambridge University Press, 2005), 39–55.
Coleman, S., 'Transgressing the Self: Making Charismatic Saints', in F. Meltzer and J. Elsner (eds), *Saints: Faith Without Borders* (Chicago: University of Chicago Press, 2011), 73–96.
Connell, R.W., *Masculinities*, 2nd edn (Berkeley: University of California Press, 2005).
Davison, J., *Gender, Lineage, and Ethnicity in Southern Africa* (Boulder: Westview Press, 1997).
De Witte, 'Neo-Traditional Religions', in E.K. Bongmba (ed.), *The Wiley-Blackwell Companion to African Religions* (Malden: Blackwell, 2012), 173–83.
Delooz, P., 'Towards a Sociological Study of Canonized Sainthood in the Catholic Church', in S. Wilson (ed.), *Saints and their Cults: Studies in Religious Sociology, Folklore and History* (Cambridge: Cambridge University Press, 1985), 189–216.
Deutch, J.G., Probst, P. and Schmidt, H. (eds), *African Modernities: Entangled Meanings in Current Debate* (Oxford: James Currey, 2002).
Dibeela, C., 'Men and the use of Power', in M.W. Dube (ed.), *Africa Praying: A Handbook on HIV/AIDS Sensitive Sermon Guidelines and Liturgy* (Geneva: WCC Publications, 2003), 193–5.
Dilger, H. and Offe, J., 'Making the Difference? Structure, Agency and Culture in Anthropological Research on Gender and Aids in Africa', *Curare*, 28:2–3 (2005), 266–80.
Ditchfield, 'Thinking with Saints: Sanctity and Society in the Early Modern World', in F. Meltzer and J. Elsner (eds), *Saints: Faith Without Border* (Chicago: University of Chicago Press, 2011), 157–89.
Dover, P., 'Gender and Embodiment: Expectations of Manliness in a Zambian Village', in L. Ouzgane and R. Morrell (eds), *African Masculinities: Men in Africa from the Late Nineteenth Century to the Present* (New York: Palgrave Macmillan, 2005), 173–88.
Dube, M.W., 'Grant Me Justice: Female and Male Equality in the New Testament', *Journal of Religion and Theology in Namibia*, 3 (2001), 82–115.
―――― 'Postcoloniality, Feminist Spaces, and Religion', in L.E. Donaldson and P.-L. Kwok (eds), *Postcolonialism, Feminism and Religious Discourse* (New York: Routledge, 2002), 100–120.
―――― 'Theological Challenges: Proclaiming the Fullness of Life in the HIV/AIDS & Global Economic Era', *International Review of Mission*, 91:363 (2002), 535–50.

_____ 'Culture, Gender and HIV/AIDS: Understanding and Acting on the Issues', in M.W. Dube (ed.), *HIV/AIDS and the Curriculum: Methods of Integrating HIV/AIDS in Theological Programmes* (Geneva: WCC Publications, 2003), 84–100.

_____ 'The Prophetic Method in the New Testament', in M.W. Dube (ed.), *HIV/AIDS and the Curriculum: Methods of Integrating HIV/AIDS in Theological Programmes* (Geneva: WCC Publications, 2003), 43–58.

_____ 'Service for/on Homosexuals', in M.W. Dube (ed.), *Africa Praying: A Handbook on HIV/AIDS Sensitive Sermon Guidelines and Liturgy* (Geneva: WCC Publications, 2003), 209–14.

_____ 'Grant Me Justice: Towards Gender-Sensitive Multi-Sectoral HIV/AIDS Readings of the Bible', in M.W. Dube and M.R.A. Kanyoro (eds), *Grant Me Justice! HIV/AIDS & Gender Readings of the Bible* (Pietermaritzburg: Cluster Publications, 2004), 3–26.

_____ 'Talitha Cum! Calling the Girl-Child and Women to Life in the HIV/AIDS & Globalization Era', in M. Degiglio-Bellemare and G.M. Garcia (eds), *Talitha Cum! The Grace of Solidarity in a Globalized World* (Geneva: WSCF Publications, 2004), 8–26.

_____ 'Circle Readings of the Bible/Scriptoratures', in J.A. Smit and P.P. Kumar (eds), *Study of Religion in Southern Africa: Essays in Honour of G.C. Oosthuizen* (Leiden: Brill, 2005), 77–96.

_____ 'Adinkra! Four Hearts Joined Together on Becoming Healer-Teachers of African Indigenous Religion/s in HIV & AIDS Prevention', in I.A. Phiri and S. Nadar (eds), *African Women, Religion, and Health: Essays in Honor of Mercy Amba Ewudziwa Oduyoye* (Maryknoll: Orbis, 2006), 131–56.

_____ 'Who Do You Say that I Am?', *Feminist Theology*, 15:3 (2007), 346–67.

_____ *The HIV & AIDS Bible: Selected Essays* (Scranton: University of Scranton Press, 2008).

_____ 'HIV and AIDS Research and Writing in the Circle of African Concerned African Women Theologians 2002–2006', in E. Chitando and N. Hadebe (eds), *Compassionate Circles: African Women Theologians Facing HIV* (Geneva: WCC Publications, 2009), 173–96.

_____ 'HIV+ Feminisms, Postcoloniality and the Global AIDS Crisis', in D.N. Hopkins and M. Lewis (eds), *Another World is Possible: Spiritualities and Religions of Global Darker People* (London: Equinox, 2009), 143–59.

_____ 'In the Circle of Life: African Women Theologians' Engagement with HIV and AIDS', in E. Chitando and N. Hadebe (eds), *Compassionate Circles: African Women Theologians Facing HIV* (Geneva: WCC Publications, 2009), 197–236.

_____ 'Talitha Cum Hermeneutics of Liberation: Some African Women's Ways of Reading the Bible', in A.F. Botta and P.R. Andinach (eds), *The Bible and the Hermeneutics of Liberation* (Atlanta: Society of Biblical Literature, 2009), 133–46.

Duyndam, J., 'Hermeneutics of Imitation: A Philosophical Approach to Sainthood and Exemplariness', in M. Poorthuis and J. Schwartz (eds), *Saints and Role Models in Judaism and Christianity* (Leiden: Brill, 2004), 7–24.

Ellis, S. and Ter Haar, G., *Worlds of Power: Religious Thought and Political Practice in Africa* (London: C. Hurst & Co, 2004).

Engelke, M., 'Discontinuity and the Discourse of Conversion', *Journal of Religion in Africa*, 31:1–2 (2004), 82–109.

_____ 'Past Pentecostalism: Notes on Rupture, Realignment, and Everyday Life in Pentecostal and African Independent Churches', *Africa*, 80:2 (2010), 177–99.

Epprecht, M., *Heterosexual Africa? The History of an Idea from the Age of Exploration to the Age of AIDS* (Athens: Ohio University Press, 2008).

Frederiks, M.T., 'Theologies of Anowa's Daughters: An African Women's Discourse', in F. Wijsen (ed.), *Global Christianity: Contested Claims* (Amsterdam: Rodopi, 2007), 177–97.

_____ 'HIV and Aids: Mapping Theological Responses in Africa', *Exchange: Journal of Missiological and Ecumenical Research*, 37:1 (2008), 4–23.

Foreman, M. (ed.), *AIDS and Men: Taking Risks or Taking Responsibility?* (London: Panos and Zed Books, 1999).

Foucault, M., 'Sexuality and Solitude', in P. Rabinow (ed.), *Ethics: Subjectivity and Truth. Essential Works of Foucault, 1954–1984*, vol. 1 (London: Penguin Books, 2000), 175–84.

_____ 'Technologies of the Self', in P. Rabinow (ed.), *Ethics: Subjectivity and Truth. Essential Works of Foucault, 1954–1984*, vol. 1 (London: Penguin Books, 2000), 223–52.

Gabaitse, R., 'Searching for Contextual Relevance: The Department of Theology and Religious Studies, University of Botswana's Response to HIV and AIDS', in E. Chitando (ed.), *Mainstreaming HIV and AIDS in Theological Education: Experiences and Explorations* (Geneva: WCC Publications, 2008), 33–48.

_____ 'Passion Killings in Botswana: Masculinity at Crossroads', in E. Chitando and S. Chirongoma (eds), *Redemptive Masculinities: Men, HIV and Religion* (Geneva: WCC Publications 2012), 305–21.

Gallagher, S.K. and Smith, C., 'Symbolic Traditionalism and Pragmatic Egalitarianism: Contemporary Evangelicals, Families, and Gender', in *Gender and Society*, 13:2 (1999), 211–33.

Garner, R.C., 'Safe Sects? Dynamic Religion and AIDS in South Africa', *The Journal of Modern African Studies*, 38:1 (2000), 41–69.

Gathogo, J.M., 'Chasing a Leopard Out of the Homestead: Mundurume's Task in the Era of HIV and AIDS', in E. Chitando and S. Chirongoma (eds), *Redemptive Masculinities: Men, HIV and Religion* (Geneva: WCC Publications 2012), 447–70.

Gelfer, J., 'Identifying the Catholic Men's Movement', *Journal of Men's Studies*, 16:1 (2008), 41–56.

_____ *Numen, Old Men: Contemporary Masculine Spiritualities and the Problem of Patriarchy* (London: Equinox, 2009).

_____ 'Evangelical and Catholic Masculinities in Two Fatherhood Ministries', *Feminist Theology*, 19:1 (2010), 36–53.

Gifford, P., 'Chiluba's Christian Nation: Christianity as a Factor in Zambian Politics 1991–1996', *Journal of Contemporary Religion*, 13:3 (1998), 363–81.

Gooren, H., 'Conversion Narratives', in A. Anderson, M. Bergunder, A. Droogers and C. van der Laan (eds), *Studying Global Pentecostalism: Theories and Methods* (Berkeley: University of California Press, 2010), 93–112.

Gunda, M.R., *The Bible and Homosexuality in Zimbabwe: A Socio-historical Analysis of the Political, Cultural and Christian Arguments in the Homosexual Public Debate with Special Reference to the use of the Bible* (Bamberg: University of Bamberg Press, 2010).

Gutmann, M.C., 'Trafficking in Men: The Anthropology of Masculinity', *Annual Review of Anthropology*, 26 (1997), 385–409.

Gutterman, D.S., 'Postmodernism and the Interrogation of Masculinity', in S. Whitehead and F.J. Barrett (eds), *The Masculinities Reader* (Cambridge: Polity Press, 2001), 56–71.

Haddad, B., 'Choosing to Remain Silent: Links between Gender Violence, HIV/AIDS and the South African Church', in I.A. Phiri, B. Haddad and M. Masenya (eds), *African Women, HIV/AIDS and Faith Communities* (Pietermaritzburg: Cluster Publications, 2003), 149–67.

_____ (eds), *Religion and HIV and AIDS: Charting the Terrain* (Scottsville: University of KwaZulu-Natal Press, 2011).

Hansen, K.T., *Keeping House in Lusaka* (New York: Columbia University Press, 1997).

Hinga, T.M., 'AIDS, Religion and Women in Africa: Theo-ethical Challenges and Imperatives', in T.M. Hinga, A.N. Kubai, P. Mwaura and H. Ayanga (eds), *Women, Religion and HIV/AIDS in Africa: Responding to Ethical and Theological Challenges* (Pietermaritzburg: Cluster Publications, 2008), 76–104.

Hirmer, O., *About the Killer Called AIDS* (Nairobi: Paulines Publications, 2001).

Hlatywayo, J., 'Dangerous Masculinities: An Analysis of the Misconception of "Real Manhood" and its Impact on Vulnerabilities to HIV among the Ndau of Chipinge in Zimbabwe', in E. Chitando and S. Chirongoma (eds), *Redemptive Masculinities: Men, HIV and Religion* (Geneva: WCC Publications 2012), 113–25.

Hock, K., 'Appropriated Vibrancy: 'Immediacy' as a Formative Element in African Theologies', in K. Koschorke (ed.), *African Identities and World Christianity in the Twentieth Century* (Wiesbaden: Harrassowitz Verlag, 2005), 113–26.

I Bought AIDS in a Bar, and Other True Stories (Nairobi: Paulines Publications, 2002).

Irvin, D.T., 'World Christianity: An Introduction', *The Journal of World Christianity*, 1:1 (2008), 1–26.

Isike, C. and Uzodike, U.O., 'Modernizing without Westernizing: Reinventing African Patriarchies to Combat the HIV and AIDS Epidemic in Africa', *Journal of Constructive Theology*, 14:1 (2008), 3–20.

Jenkins, P., *The New Faces of Christianity: Believing the Bible in the Global South* (Oxford: Oxford University Press, 2006).

―――― *The Next Christendom: The Coming of Global Christianity*, rev. edn (Oxford: Oxford University Press, 2007).

John Paul II. *Evangelium Vitae* (Rome: The Vatican, 25 March 1995), http://www.vatican.va/holy_father/john_paul_ii/encyclicals/documents/hf_jp-ii_enc_25031995_evangelium-vitae_en.html (accessed 10 June 2012).

―――― *Letter to Women* (Rome: The Vatican, 29 June 1995), http://www.vatican.va/holy_father/john_paul_ii/letters/documents/hf_jp-ii_let_29061995_women_en.html (accessed 10 June 2012).

―――― *Post-Synodal Apostolic Exhortation Ecclesia in Africa of the Holy Father John Paul II to the Bishops, Priests and Deacons, Men and Women Religious and all the Lay Faithful to the Church in Africa and its Evangelizing Mission Towards the Year 2000* (Yaoundé, 14 September 1995), http://www.vatican.va/holy_father/john_paul_ii/apost_exhortations/documents/hf_jp-ii_exh_14091995_ecclesia-in-africa_en.html (accessed 10 June 2012).

―――― *Man and Woman He Created them: A Theology of the Body* (Boston: Pauline Books & Media, 2006).

Kä Mana, 'Culture, Societé et Sciences Humaines Dans la Lutte Contre le VIH-SIDA en Afrique', in Kä Mana, J.-B. Kenmogne and H. Yinda (eds), *Religion, Culture et VIH-SIDA en Afrique: Un Hommage au Docteur Jaap Breetvelt* (Yaoundé: SHERPA, 2004), 66–83.

Kalipeni, E., Oppong, J. and Zerai, A., 'HIV/AIDS, Gender, Agency and Empowerment Issues in Africa', *Social Science and Medicine*, 64:5 (2007), 1015–18.

Kalu, O.U., *African Pentecostalism: An Introduction* (Oxford: Oxford University Press, 2008).

Kalbian, A.H., *Sexing the Church: Gender, Power, and Ethics in Contemporary Catholicism* (Bloomington: Indiana University Press, 2005).

Kalunga, S., 'Open Letter to My Future Wife', *Speak Out!* 26:3 (2009), 17.

Kamau, N., 'African Cultures and Gender in the Context of HIV and AIDS: Probing these Practices', in B. Haddad (ed.), *Religion and HIV and AIDS: Charting the Terrain* (Scottsville: University of KwaZulu-Natal Press, 2011), 257–72.

Kamitsuka, M., *Feminist Theology and the Challenge of Difference* (Oxford: Oxford University Press, 2007).

Kanyoro, M.R.A., *Introducing Feminist Cultural Hermeneutics: An African Perspective* (London: Sheffield Academic Press, 2002).

Kärkkäinen, V.M., *An Introduction to Ecclesiology: Ecumenical, Historical and Global Perspectives* (Downers Grove: InterVarsity Press 2002).

Klaits, F., 'Introduction: Self, Other and God in African Christianities', *Journal of Religion in Africa*, 41:2 (2011), 143–53.

King, U., 'Introduction: Gender and the Study of Religion', in U. King (ed.), *Religion and Gender* (Oxford: Blackwell Publishers, 1995), 1–38.

Kimmel, M., *Misframing Men: The Politics of Contemporary Masculinities* (New Brunswick: Rutgers University Press, 2010).

Kiura, J., *About Boys*, 4th reprint (Nairobi: Paulines Publications, 2007).

Kollman, P., 'Classifying African Christianities: Past, Present and Future: Part One', *Journal of Religion in Africa*, 40:1 (2010), 3–32.

Korte, A.-M., 'Paradise Lost, Growth Gained: Eve's Story Revisited. Genesis 2–4 in a Feminist Theological Perspective', in B. Becking and S. Hennecke (eds), *Out of Paradise: Eve and Adam and their Interpreters* (Sheffield: Sheffield Phoenix Press, 2010), 140–56.

Krondorfer, B., 'Who's Afraid of Gay Theology? Men's Studies, Gay Scholars, and Heterosexual Silence', *Theology and Sexuality*, 13:3 (2007), 257–74.

_____ 'Introduction', in B. Krondorfer (ed.), *Men and Masculinities in Christianity and Judaism: A Critical Reader* (London: SCM Press, 2009), xi–xxi.

_____ 'The Final Cause: The Cause of Causes – Editor's Introduction', in B. Krondorfer (ed.), *Men and Masculinities in Christianity and Judaism: A Critical Reader* (London: SCM Press, 2009), 3–4.

_____ *Male Confessions: Intimate Revelations and the Religious Imagination* (Stanford: Stanford University Press, 2010).

Krondorfer, B. and Culbertson, Ph., 'Men's Studies in Religion', in L. Jones (ed.), *Encyclopedia of Religion*, 2nd edn. Detroit and New York: Macmillan, 5861–5866.

Krondorfer, B. and Hunt, S., 'Introduction: Religion and Masculinities – Continuities and Change', *Religion and Gender*, 2/2 (2012), 194–206.

Küster, V., *Einführung in die Interkulturelle Theologie* (Göttingen: Vandenhoeck & Ruprecht, 2011).

Kwok, P.-L., *Postcolonial Imagination and Feminist Theology* (Louisville: Westminster John Knox Press, 2005).

Leshota, P., 'The Spell of Discrete Islands of Consciousness: My Journey with Masculinities in the Context of HIV and AIDS', in E. Chitando and S. Chirongoma (eds), *Redemptive Masculinities: Men, HIV and Religion* (Geneva: WCC Publications 2012), 149–70.

Let our Light Shine. Diamond Jubilee: Regiment Catholic Church 1939–1999 (Lusaka: Regiment parish, 1999).

Lindhardt, M., '"If you are saved you cannot forget your parents": Agency, Power, and Social Repositioning in Tanzanian born-again Christianity', *Journal of Religion in Africa*, 40:3 (2010), 240–72.

Lockhardt, W.H., '"We Are One Life", But Not of One Gender Ideology: Unity, Ambiguity, and the Promise Keepers', in R.H. Williams (ed.), *Promise Keepers and the New Masculinity: Private Lives and Public Morality* (Lanham: Lexington Books, 2001), 73–92.

Magesa, L., 'Christology, African Women and Ministry', *African Ecclesial Review*, 38:2 (1996), 66–88.

―――― *African Religion: The Moral Traditions of Abundant Life* (Maryknoll: Orbis, 1997).

―――― *Anatomy of Inculturation: Transforming the Church in Africa* (Maryknoll: Orbis, 2004).

―――― 'The Challenge of African Woman Defined Theology for the 21st Century', in N.W. Ndung'u and P.N. Mwaura (eds), *Challenges and Prospects of the Church in Africa: Theological Reflections of the 21st Century* (Nairobi: Paulines, 2005), 88–101.

Mahmood, S., *Politics of Piety: The Islamic Revival and the Feminist Subject* (Princeton: Princeton University Press, 2005).

Maimela, S., 'Seeking to be Christian in Patriarchal Society', *Journal of Black Theology in South Africa*, 9:2 (1995), 27–42.

Maluleke, T.S., 'The "Smoke Screens" Called Black and African Liberation Theologies – The Challenge of African Women Theology', *Journal of Constructive Theology*, 3:2 (1997), 39–63.

―――― 'African "Ruths", Ruthless Africas: Reflections of an African Mordechai', in M.W. Dube (ed.), *Other Ways of Reading. African Women and the Bible* (Atlanta: Society of Biblical Literature, 2001), 237–51.

―――― 'The Challenge of HIV/AIDS for Theological Education in Africa: Towards an HIV/AIDS Sensitive Curriculum', *Missionalia*, 29:2 (2001), 125–43.

―――― 'The Graveyardman, the "Escaped Convict" and the Girl-Child: A Mission of Awakening, an Awakening of Mission', *International Review of Mission*, 91:363 (2002), 550–57.

―――― 'Men and their Role in Community', in M.W. Dube (ed.), *Africa Praying: A Handbook on HIV/AIDS Sensitive Sermon Guidelines and Liturgy* (Geneva: WCC Publications, 2003), 190–93.

―――― 'Half a Century of African Christian Theologies: Elements of the Emerging Agenda for the Twenty-first Century', in O.U. Kalu (ed.), *African Christianity: An African Story* (Pretoria: Department of Church History, University of Pretoria, 2005), 469–93.

―――― 'An African Theology Perspective on Patriarchy', in *The Evil of Patriarchy in Church, Society and Politics* (Cape Town: Inclusive and Affirming Ministries, 2009), 31–6.

Maluleke, T.S. and Nadar, S., 'Breaking the Covenant of Violence against Women', *Journal of Theology for Southern Africa*, 114 (2002), 5–17.

Mane, P. and Aggleton, P., 'Gender and HIV/AIDS: What Do Men Have to Do with It?', *Current Sociology*, 49:6 (2001), 23–37.

Marshall, R., *Political Spiritualities: The Pentecostal Revolution in Nigeria* (Chicago: University of Chicago Press, 2009).

Martin, B., 'The Pentecostal Gender Paradox: A Cautionary Tale for the Sociology of Religion', in R.K. Fenn (ed.), *The Blackwell Companion to the Sociology of Religion* (Malden: Blackwell, 2001), 52–66.

Martin, D., *Pentecostalism: The World their Parish* (Malden: Blackwell Publishing, 2002).

───── *On Secularization: Towards a Revised General Theory* (Aldershot: Ashgate, 2005).

Martey, E., *African Theology: Inculturation and Liberation* (Maryknoll: Orbis, 1993).

Masenya, M., 'Trapped between Two "Canons": African–South African Christian Women in the HIV/AIDS Era', in I.A. Phiri, B. Haddad and M. Masenya (eds), *African Women, HIV/AIDS and Faith Communities* (Pietermaritzburg: Cluster Publications, 2003), 113–27.

Mate, R., 'Women as God's Laboratories: Pentecostal Discourses of Femininity in Zimbabwe', *Africa* 72:4 (2002), 549–68.

Maxwell, D., *African Gifts of the Spirit: Pentecostalism & the Rise of a Zimbabwean Transnational Religious Movement* (Oxford: James Currey/Harare: Weaver Press/Athens: Ohio University Press, 2006).

Mayblin, M., *Gender, Catholicism, and Morality in Brazil: Virtuous Husbands, Powerful Wives* (New York: Palgrave Macmillan, 2010).

Mbilinyi, M. and Kaihula, N., 'Sinners and Outsiders: The Drama of AIDS in Rungwe', in C. Baylies and J. Bujra (eds), *AIDS, Sexuality and Gender in Africa: Collective Strategies and Struggles in Tanzania and Zambia* (London: Routledge, 2000), 76–94.

Meltzer, F. and Elsner, J., 'Introduction', in F. Meltzer and J. Elsner (eds), *Saints: Faith Without Borders* (Chicago: University of Chicago Press, 2011), ix–xii.

Men and AIDS – A Gendered Approach (Geneva: UNAIDS, 2000).

Meyer, B., '"Make a Complete Break with the Past". Memory and Post-Colonial Modernity in Ghanaian Pentecostalist Discourse', *Journal of Religion in Africa*, 28:3 (1998), 316–49.

───── 'Christianity in Africa: From African Independent to Pentecostal-Charismatic Churches', *Annual Review of Anthropology*, 33 (2004), 447–74.

───── 'Aesthetics of Persuasion: Global Christianity and Pentecostalism's Sensational Forms', *The South Atlantic Quarterly*, 109/4 (2010), 741–64.

Miescher, S. and Lindsay, L.A., 'Introduction: Men and Masculinities in Modern Africa', in L.A. Lindsay and S. Miescher (eds), *Men and Masculinities in Modern Africa* (Portsmouth, NH: Heinemann, 2003), 1–29.

Morrell, R., 'The Times of Change: Men and Masculinity in South Africa', in R. Morrell (ed.), *Changing Men in Southern Africa* (Pietermaritzburg: University of Natal Press/London: Zed Books Ltd, 2001), 3–37.

Morrell, R. and Ouzgane, L., 'African Masculinities: An Introduction', in L. Ouzgane and R. Morrell (eds), *African Masculinities: Men in Africa from the Late Nineteenth Century to the Present* (New York: Palgrave Macmillan, 2005), 1–20.

Moyo, F.L., 'The AIDS Crisis: A Challenge to the Integrity of the Church in Malawi', in K.R. Ross (ed.), *Faith at the Frontiers of Knowledge* (Blantyre: CLAIM, 1998), 94–110.

——— 'Religion, Spirituality and being a Woman in Africa: Gender Construction within the African Religio-cultural Experiences', *Agenda*, 61 (2004), 72–8.

——— '"When the Telling itself is a Taboo": The Phoebe Practice', in I.A. Phiri and S. Nadar (eds), *On Being Church: African Women's Voices and Visions* (Geneva: WCC Publications, 2005), 184–202.

——— 'Sex, Gender, Power and HIV/AIDS in Malawi: Threats and Challenges to Women being Church', in I.A. Phiri and S. Nadar (eds), *On Being Church: African Women's Voices and Visions* (Geneva: WCC Publications, 2005), 127–45.

——— 'Navigating Experiences of Healing: A Narrative Theology of Eschatological Hope as Healing', in I.A. Phiri and S. Nadar (eds), *African Women, Religion and Health: Essays in Honor of Mercy Amba Ewudziwa Oduyoye* (Maryknoll: Orbis, 2006), 243–57.

——— 'A Quest for Women's Sexual Empowerment through Education in an HIV and AIDS Context. The Case of Kukonzekera Chinkhoswe Chachikhristu (KCC) among aMang'Anja and aYao Christians of t/a Mwambo in Rural Zomba, Malawi.' PhD thesis, University of KwaZulu-Natal, 2009.

——— 'The Making of Vulnerable, Gyrating and Dangerous Menstruating Women through *Chinamwali* Socialization', in E. Chitando and N. Hadebe (eds), *Compassionate Circles: African Women Theologians Facing HIV* (Geneva: WCC Publications, 2009), 35–52.

Mpundu, T.G., 'Men, Take Up the Challenge!', *The Parish Newsletter*, 254 (19 July 2009), Regiment Parish, Lusaka.

Mugala-Ng'Ambi, M., 'An Open Letter to My Future Husband', *Speak Out!* 26:2 (2009), 8.

Mukhopadhyay and N. Singh (eds), *Gender Justice, Citizenship and Development* (Ottawa: International Development Research Centre, 2007).

Musonda, D., 'General Introduction: Moral and Pastoral Issues', in J. Komakoma (ed.), *The Social Teaching of the Catholic Bishops and Other Christian Leaders in Zambia: Major Pastoral Letters and Statements 1953–2001* (Ndola: Mission Press, 2003), 14–21.

Mutambara, M., 'African Women Theologies Critique Inculturation', in E.P. Antonio (ed.), *Inculturation and Postcolonial Discourse in African Theology* (New York: Peter Lang, 2006), 173–91.

Mwaura, P.N., 'Gender Mainstreaming in African Theology: An African Women's Perspective', *Voices from the Third World*, 24:1 (2001), 165–79.

——— 'Stigmatization and Discrimination of HIV/AIDS Women in Kenya: A Violation of Human Rights and its Theological Implications', *Exchange: Journal of Missiological and Ecumenical Research*, 37:1 (2008), 35–51.

Nadar, S., 'On Being Church: African Women's Voices and Visions', in I.A. Phiri and S. Nadar (eds), *On Being Church: African Women's Voices and Visions* (Geneva: World Council of Churches, 2005), 16–28.

_____ 'Palatable Patriarchy and Violence against Wo/men in South Africa – Angus Buchan's Mighty Men's Conference as a Case Study on Masculinism', *Scriptura*, 102:3 (2009), 551–61.

_____ 'Towards a Feminist Missiological Agenda: A Case Study on the Jacob Zuma Rape Trial', *Missionalia*, 37:1 (2009), 85–102.

_____ 'Who's Afraid of the Mighty Men's Conference? Palatable Patriarchy and Violence against Wo/men in South Africa', in E. Chitando and S. Chirongoma (eds), *Redemptive Masculinities: Men, HIV and Religion* (Geneva: WCC Publications 2012), 355–72.

Nasimiyu-Wasike, A., 'Genesis 1–2 and some Elements of Diversion from the Original Meaning of the Creation of Man and Woman', in M.N. Getui, K. Holter and V. Zinkuratire (eds), *Interpreting the Old Testament in Africa* (Nairobi: Acton Publishers, 2001), 175–80.

_____ 'Imagining Jesus Christ in the African Context at the Dawn of a New Millennium', in N.W. Ndung'u and P.N. Mwaura (eds), *Challenges and Prospects of the Church in Africa: Theological Reflections of the 21st Century* (Nairobi: Paulines Publications, 2005), 102–18.

National HIV and AIDS Strategic Framework 2006–2010 (Lusaka: National HIV/AIDS/STI/TB Council, 2006).

Newton, J.L., *From Panthers to Promise Keepers: Rethinking the Men's Movement* (Oxford: Rowman and Littlefield, 2005).

Nganda, C.N., *Boys Growing Up*, 5th reprint (Nairobi: Paulines Publications, 2007).

Njoroge, N.J., *Kiama Kia Ngo: An African Christian Feminist Ethic of Resistance and Transformation* (Accra: Legon Theological Studies, 2000).

_____ 'AIDS: The Disease that Speaks Multiple Languages and Thrives on Other Pandemics', *Journal of Constructive Theology*, 10:2 (2004), 3–20.

_____ 'Beyond Suffering and Lament: Theology of Hope and Life', in D.C. Marks (ed.), *Shaping a Global Theological Mind* (Aldershot: Ashgate, 2008), 113–20.

_____ *Gender Justice, Ministry and Healing: A Christian Response to the HIV Pandemic* (London: Progressio, 2009).

Ochieng, M., *About True Love Waits*, 4th reprint (Nairobi: Paulines Publications, 2006).

Oduyoye, M.A., 'The Roots of African Christian Feminism', in J.S. Pobee and C.F. Hallencreutz (eds), *Variations in Christian Theology in Africa* (Nairobi: Uzima Press, 1979), 32–44.

_____ *Hearing and Knowing: Theological Reflections on Christianity in Africa* (Maryknoll: Orbis, 1986).

_____ 'The Circle', in M.A. Oduyoye and M.R.A. Kanyoro (eds), *Talitha, Qumi! Proceedings of the Convocation of African Women Theologians* (Ibadan: Daystar Press, 1990), 1–26.

_____ 'The Search for a Two-winged Theology: Women's Participation in the Development of Theology in Africa. The Inaugural Address', in M.A. Oduyoye and M.R.A. Kanyoro (eds), *Talitha, Qumi! Proceedings of the Convocation of African Women Theologians* (Ibadan: Daystar Press, 1990), 27–48.

_____ *Daughters of Anowa: African Women and Patriarchy* (Maryknoll: Orbis, 1995).

_____ 'Acting to Construct Africa: The Agency by Women', in R. van Eijk and J. van Lin (eds), *Africans Reconstructing Africa* (Nijmegen: Theologische Faculteit KU-Nijmegen, 1997), 27–44.

_____ *Introducing African Women's Theology* (Cleveland: The Pilgrim Press, 2001).

_____ 'Gender and Theology in Africa Today', *Journal of Constructive Theology*, 8:2 (2002), 35–46.

Oduyoye, M.A. and Amoah, E., 'The Christ for African Women', in M.A. Oduyoye and V. Fabella (eds), *With Passion and Compassion: Third World Women Doing Theology* (Maryknoll: Orbis, 1988), 35–46.

Okure, T., 'Women in the Bible', in M.A. Oduyoye and V. Fabella (eds), *With Passion and Compassion. Third World Women Doing Theology* (Maryknoll: Orbis, 1988), 47–59.

Oloo, N.O., *About Drinking*, rev. edn (Nairobi: Paulines Publications, 2007).

Orobator, A.E., *The Church as Family: African Ecclesiology in its Social Context* (Nairobi: Paulines Publications, 2000).

_____ *From Crisis to Kairos: The Mission of the Church in the Time of HIV/AIDS, Refugees, and Poverty* (Nairobi: Paulines Publications, 2005).

Owino, K., '"Maleness" and its Possible Influence on Abuse and Domestic Violence in South Africa: A Critique of Some Expressions of Evangelical Theology', *Journal of Constructive Theology*, 16:2 (2010), 146–68.

Paolini, A.J., *Navigating Modernity: Postcolonialism, Identity, and International Relations* (London: Lynne Rienner Publishers, 1999).

Pemberton, C., *Circle Thinking: African Women Theologians in Dialogue with the West* (Leiden: Brill, 2003).

Peterson, A.L., Vasquez, M.A. and Williams, P.J., 'The Global and the Local', in A.L. Peterson, M.A. Vasquez and P.J. Williams (eds), *Christianity, Social Change, and Globalization in the Americas* (Piscataway: Rutgers University Press, 2001), 210–28.

Phiri, I.A., *Women, Presbyterianism and Patriarchy: Religious Experience of Chewa Women in Central Malawi* (Blantyre: CLAIM, 1997).

_____ 'Life in Fullness: Gender Justice. A Perspective from Africa', *Journal of Constructive Theology*, 8:2 (2002), 69–81.

_____ 'Why does God Allow our Husbands to Hurt Us? Overcoming Violence against Women', *Journal of Theology for Southern Africa*, 114 (2002), 19–30.

_____ 'African Women of Faith Speak Out in an HIV/AIDS Era', in I.A. Phiri, B. Haddad and M. Masenya (eds), *African Women, HIV/AIDS and Faith Communities* (Pietermaritzburg: Cluster Publications, 2003), 3–22.

_____ 'HIV/AIDS: An African Theological Response in Mission', *The Ecumenical Review*, 56:4 (2004), 422–31.

_____ 'A Theological Analysis of the Voices of Teenage Girls on Men's Role in the Fight against HIV/AIDS in KwaZulu-Natal, South Africa', *Journal of Theology for Southern Africa*, 120 (2004), 34–45.

_____ 'Major Challenges for African Women Theologians in Theological Education (1989–2008)', *International Review of Mission*, 98:1 (2009), 105–19.

Phiri, I.A. and Nadar, S. (eds), *On being Church: African Women's Voices and Visions* (Geneva: WCC Publications, 2005).

_____ 'Introduction: "Treading Softly but Firmly"', in I.A. Phiri and S. Nadar (eds), *African Women, Religion and Health: Essays in Honor of Mercy Amba Ewudziwa Oduyoye* (Maryknoll: Orbis, 2006), 1–16.

Piper, J., 'A Vision of Biblical Complementarity: Manhood and Womanhood Defined According to the Bible', in J. Piper and W. Grudem (eds), *Recovering Biblical Manhood and Womanhood: A Response to Evangelical Feminism* (Wheaton: Crossway Books, 1991), 31–59.

Rasing, T., *The Bush Burnt, the Stones Remain: Female Initiation Rites in Urban Zambia* (Münster: Lit Verlag, 2002).

Reeser, T.W., *Masculinities in Theory: An Introduction* (Malden: Blackwell, 2010).

Report on the Global AIDS Epidemic 2010 (Geneva: UNAIDS, 2010).

Robbins, J., 'Continuity Thinking and the Problem of Christian Culture: Belief, Time, and the Anthropology of Christianity', *Current Anthropology*, 48:1 (2007), 5–38.

_____ 'Anthropology of Religion', in A. Anderson, M. Bergunder, A. Droogers and C. van der Laan (eds), *Studying Global Pentecostalism: Theories and Methods* (Berkeley: University of California Press, 2010), 156–78.

Ruether, R.R., *Sexism and God-talk: Towards a Feminist Theology* (Boston: Beacon Press, 1983).

_____ 'Patriarchy', in L.M. Russell and J.S. Clarkson (eds), *Feminist Dictionary of Feminist Theologies* (Louisville: Westminster John Knox Press, 1996), 205–7.

Sadgrove, J., '"Keeping Up Appearances": Sex and Religion Amongst University Students in Uganda', *Journal of Religion in Africa*, 37:1 (2007), 116–44.

Schmid, B., 'AIDS Discourses in the Church: What We Say and What We Do', *Journal of Theology for Southern Africa*, 125 (2006), 91–103.

Scholz, 'The Christian Right's Discourse on Gender and the Bible', *Journal of Feminist Studies in Religion*, 21:1 (2005), 83–104.

Schreiter, R.J., *Constructing Local Theologies* (Maryknoll: Orbis, 1985).

Shefer, T., Ratele, K., Strebel, A. and Shabalala, N., 'Masculinities in South Africa: A Critical Review of Contemporary Literature on Men's Sexuality', in

D. Gibson and A. Hardon (eds), *Rethinking Masculinities, Violence and AIDS* (Amsterdam: Het Spinhuis, 2005), 73–86.

Shisanya, C.R.A., 'The Impact of HIV/AIDS on Women in Kenya', in M.N. Getui and M.M. Theuri (eds), *Quests for Abundant Life in Africa* (Nairobi: Acton, 2002), 45–64.

―――――― 'Today's Lepers: Experiences of Women Living with HIV/AIDS in Kenya', in T.M. Hinga, A.N. Kubai, P. Mwaura and H. Ayanga (eds), *Women, Religion and HIV/AIDS in Africa: Responding to Ethical and Theological Challenges* (Pietermaritzburg: Cluster Publications, 2008), 144–66.

Simpson, A., *Boys to Men in the Shadow of AIDS: Masculinities and HIV Risk in Zambia* (New York: Palgrave Macmillan, 2009).

Soothill, J.E., *Gender, Social Change and Spiritual Power: Charismatic Christianity in Ghana* (Leiden: Brill, 2007).

Ter Haar, G., *How God Became African: African Spirituality and Western Secular Thought* (Philadelphia: University of Pennsylvania Press, 2009).

Teteki Abbey, R., 'Rediscovering Ataa Naa Nyonmo – the Father Mother God', in N.J. Njoroge and M.W. Dube (eds), *Talitha Cum! Theologies of African Women* (Pietermaritzburg: Cluster Publications, 2001), 140–57.

The Girl Child, Women, Religion and HIV/AIDS in Africa: Gender Perspectives. Report of the 4th Pan African Conference of the Circle of Concerned African Women Theologians. Yaoundé, Cameroun, September 2–8, 2007 (Circle of Concerned African Women Theologians, 2008).

The Pontifical Council for the Family, *The Truth and Meaning of Human Sexuality: Guidelines for Education within the Family* (Rome: The Vatican, 8 December 1995), http://www.vatican.va/roman_curia/pontifical_councils/family/documents/rc_pc_family_doc_08121995_human-sexuality_en.html (accessed 10 June 2012).

Togarasei, L., 'Paul and Masculinity: Implications for HIV and AIDS Responses among African Christians', in E. Chitando and S. Chirongoma (eds), *Redemptive Masculinities: Men, HIV and Religion* (Geneva: WCC Publications 2012), 229–45.

Trinitapoli, J. and Regnerus, M.D., 'Religion and HIV Risk Behaviors among Married Men: Initial Results from a Study in Rural Sub-Saharan Africa', *Journal for the Scientific Study of Religion*, 45:4 (2006), 505–28.

Uchem, R.N., *Overcoming Women's Subordination: An Igbo African and Christian Perspective. Envisioning an Inclusive Theology with Reference to Women* (Enugu: Snaap Press, 2001).

Van Dijk, R., 'Time and Transcultural Technologies of the Self in the Ghanaian Pentecostal Diaspora', in A. Corten and R. Marshall-Fratani (eds), *Between Babel and Pentecost: Transnational Pentecostalism in Africa and Latin America* (Bloomington: Indiana University Press, 2001), 216–34.

―――――― 'Modernity's Limits: Pentecostalism and the Moral Rejection of Alcohol in Malawi', in D.F. Bryceson (ed.), *Alcohol in Africa: Mixing Business, Pleasure, and Politics* (Portsmouth: Heinemann, 2002), 249–64.

Van Klinken, A.S., 'St. Joachim as a Model of Catholic Manhood in Times of AIDS: A Case Study on Masculinity in an African Christian Context', *CrossCurrents*, 61:4 (2011), 467–79.

———— 'Male Headship as Male Agency: An Alternative Understanding of a "Patriarchal" African Pentecostal Discourse on Masculinity', *Religion and Gender*, 1:1 (2011), 104–24.

———— 'The Homosexual as the Antithesis of "Biblical Manhood"? Heteronormativity and Masculinity Politics in Zambian Pentecostal Sermons', *Journal of Gender and Religion in Africa*, 17:2 (2011), 129–42.

———— 'The Ongoing Challenge of HIV and AIDS to African Theology: A Review Article', *Exchange: Journal of Missiological and Ecumenical Research*, 39:1 (2011), 89–107.

———— 'Transforming Masculinities towards Gender Justice in an Era of HIV and AIDS: Plotting the Pathways', in B. Haddad (ed.), *Religion and HIV and AIDS: Charting the Terrain* (Scottsville: University of KwaZulu-Natal Press, 2011), 275–96

———— 'Men in the Remaking: Conversion Narratives and Born-again Masculinity in Zambia', *Journal of Religion in Africa* 42:3 (2012), 215–39.

Van Klinken, A.S. and Gunda, M.R., 'Taking Up the Cudgels against Gay Rights? Trends and Trajectories in African Christian Theologies on Homosexuality', *Journal of Homosexuality*, 59:1 (2012), 114–38.

Van Leeuwen, M.S., 'Faith, Feminism, and the Family in an Age of Globalization', in M.L. Stackhouse with P.J. Paris (eds), *God and Globalization, Volume 1: Religion and the Powers of the Common Life* (New York: T&T Clark, 2000), 184–230.

Walligo, J.M., *Struggle for Equality: Women and Empowerment in Uganda* (Eldoret: AMECEA Gaba Publications, 2002).

Walls, A.F., *The Cross-cultural Process in Christian History: Studies in the Transmission and Appropriation of Faith* (Maryknoll: Orbis, 2002).

Ward, K., 'Same-sex Relations in Africa and the Debate on Homosexuality in East African Anglicism', *Anglican Theological Review*, 84/1 (2002), 81–111.

West, G., 'The Contribution of Tamar's Story to the Construction of Alternative African Masculinities', in S.T. Kamionkowski and W. Kim (eds), *Bodies, Embodiment and Theology of the Hebrew Bible* (New York: T&T Clark, 2010), 184–200.

West, G. and Zengele, B., 'Reading Job 'Positively' in the Context of HIV/AIDS in South Africa', *Concilium*, 4 (2004), 112–24.

West, G. and Zondi-Mabizela, P., 'The Bible Story that Became a Campaign: The Tamar Campaign in South Africa (and Beyond)', *Ministerial Formation*, 103 (2004), 5–13.

Whaling, F., 'Theological Approaches', in P. Connolly (ed.), *Approaches to the Study of Religion* (London: Cassell, 1999).

Whitehead, S.M., *Men and Masculinities: Key Themes and New Directions* (Cambridge: Polity Press, 2002).

Whitehead, S. and Barrett, F.J., 'The Sociology of Masculinity', in S. Whitehead and F.J. Barrett (eds), *The Masculinities Reader* (Cambridge: Polity Press, 2001), 1–26.

Wilcox, W.B., *Soft Patriarchs, New Men: How Christianity Shapes Fathers and Husbands* (Chicago: University of Chicago Press, 2004).

———— 'Religion and the Domestication of Men', *Contexts*, 5:4 (2006), 40–44.

What Does the Church Social Teaching Say about Gender Equality? (Lusaka: Jesuit Centre for Theological Reflection, 2008).

Zambia – Country Situation (Geneva: UNAIDS, 2008).

Websites

Council on Biblical Manhood and Womanhood, 'About us', website of The Council on Biblical Manhood and Womanhood, publication date unknown; accessed 7 May 2012. http://www.cbmw.org/About-Us.

———— 'Home', website of The Council on Biblical Manhood and Biblical Womanhood, publication date unknown; accessed 30 May 2012. http://www.cbmw.org.

'Council Members', website of The Council on Biblical Manhood and Womanhood, publication date unknown; accessed 7 May 2012. http://www.cbmw.org/Council-Members.

Northmead Assembly of God, 'Biographical Profile of Bishop Joshua H.K. Banda', website of Northmead Assembly of God, publication date unknown; accessed 6 January 2009. http://northmeadassembly.org/index.php?option=com_content&task=view&id=13&Itemid=27.

———— 'Choosing Hope', website of Northmead Assembly of God, publication date unknown; accessed 23 February 2012. http://www.northmeadassembly.org/index.php?option=com_content&view=article&id=263:about-choosing-hope&catid=57:choosing-hope&Itemid=53.

———— 'Church Ministries', website of Northmead Assembly of God, publication date unknown; accessed 18 March 2009. http://www.northmeadassembly.org.zm/ministry.html.

———— 'The Liberating Truth', website of Northmead Assembly of God, publication date unknown; accessed 23 February 2012. http://www.northmeadassembly.org/index.php?option=com_content&view=article&id=246:the-liberating-truth&catid=51:liberating-truth&Itemid=43.

———— 'Missions', website of Northmead Assembly of God, publication date unknown; accessed 23 February 2012. http://www.northmeadassembly.org/index.php?option=com_content&view=article&id=240&Itemid=29.

Worldwide Marriage Encounter, 'Sacramental Marriage', website of Worldwide Marriage Encounter, publication date unknown; accessed 27 December 2011. http://www.wwme.org/sacramental-marriage.html.

Index

Addai-Mensah, Peter, 156, 159, 162
African Christianity (study of), 9–12, 16–18, 199–200
African theology/theologians, 11–12, 25–9
  critical task of, 11–12, 178
  and HIV and AIDS, 37–47
  on masculinities, 9, 47–57, 166–76, 179–81, 182
  study of gender in, 25–37, 88n122, 179–81
African traditional religion/s, 6, 7, 20, 31, 34, 38
African women's theology, 25–7, 29, 39–47, 170; *see also* Circle of Concerned African Women Theologians
agency
  of men, 5, 6, 135, 141, 188–91, 193, 196, 197, 198
  of women, 3, 99
alcohol, 71–2, 84, 102, 106, 112–14, 137, 140, 149, 151, 156
anthropology
  of Christianity, 12–13, 17–18, 135, 161, 163, 191
  theological, 34, 47, 86–90, 130–34, 153–5
Assemblies of God, 11, 103, 104, 160n29

Baker-Fletcher, Garth Kasimu, 15, 58
Banda, bishop Joshua H.K., 103–47, 151, 153, 159, 163–5, 176, 183, 185, 187–8, 190, 193
Bible, 175–177; *see also* hermeneutics (biblical)
  as a resource to transform masculinities, 51, 53, 54, 55, 56, 103, 144
biblical manhood, 106, 110, 112, 117–30, 131, 133, 140, 142, 145–6, 157, 161, 165, 174; *see also* Council on Biblical Manhood and Biblical Womanhood
born again, 134–6
  and a change in lifestyle, 106, 112, 116, 120, 129–30, 138, 140–42, 156, 158, 159, 161, 191–5
Brusco, Elizabeth, 152
Bujo, Bénézet, 91, 94
Butler, Judith, 154, 190

Catholic bishops of Zambia, 62, 64, 67–8, 69, 74, 86–7, 90, 151
Catholicism, 92, 96–7, 157, 187, 191, 198
  in relation to tradition vs. modernity in Africa, 159–62, 164, 188
Chitando, Ezra, 37, 42, 47, 48–57, 158, 166, 167, 168, 169–70, 182
Christology, *see* Jesus Christ
Circle of Concerned African Women Theologians, 26, 47; *see also* African women's theology
circumcision, male (metaphor), 1–2, 130
Coleman, Simon, 144n192, 165
colonialism, 16–17, 20, 31
complementarity of the sexes, 82, 88n122, 89, 112, 124, 128, 131–2, 153–5, 186–7
condoms, 4, 7, 19, 49, 68, 83, 150
continuity (and discontinuity), 157, 162, 177, 191, 192, 195–7
conversion, 55, 111, 117, 135, 191–7
Council on Biblical Manhood and Biblical Womanhood, 118, 146, 186
creation, 77, 86–90, 112, 115, 118–19, 130–32, 153–5, 173–5, 187
  in the image of God, 34, 39, 47, 74, 86–8, 115, 123, 132, 154, 173, 186
  order of, 34, 112, 122, 124, 131–2, 153, 155, 163, 173–4, 186, 193

culture(s), African, 159–60, 161–2, 164, 188
   African (women) theologians on, 27, 31, 43–6, 49, 51
   men and masculinity in, 49, 69, 78, 80, 110, 116, 123, 125, 152–3, 197

decision-making (in marital/sexual relationships), 3, 41, 44–5, 49, 67, 73, 81, 115, 128, 146, 186
domination of men over women, 6, 44, 54, 73–4, 115–16, 123, 145, 152, 162, 183, 189
Dube, Musa W., 29–30, 34, 38–9, 40, 41, 43, 46, 52, 53, 55, 171

ecclesiology, 37, 155–7, 158, 177
   of the church as family of God, 62, 75, 90–92
eschatology, 35–6, 109, 101, 138
   and divine judgement, 101, 137–8, 145
Evangelicalism, 126n111, 133, 145–6, 152, 153n7, 161, 184–8, 191
Evangelical Fellowship of Zambia, 20, 104

family
   church as family of God, see Ecclesiology
   churches' concern with, 64–5, 72, 105, 113, 156, 159–60
   extended, 77–8, 108, 121, 146, 160–61
   men's role in the, 71–4, 77–80, 85, 90–3, 113–14, 117, 120–28, 186, 194, 195–7
   nuclear, 121, 146, 159–60
fatherhood, 74, 79–80, 116, 128, 144, 185, 193, 196
feminism/feminist theory, 16, 181, 183
   in African theology, 26n3, 33, 47, 57–9, 88n122, 170–71, 181
   churches on, 88, 92, 124, 154, 163, 187
   evangelical, 146, 186
   and the study of men, masculinities and religion, 13–16, 58
Foucault, Michel, 21n67, 83, 85, 129, 135, 198

Gelfer, Joseph, 58, 91, 92, 101–2, 153n7, 182, 184n14
gender
   essentialist perception of, 16, 48, 71, 89, 110, 150, 153–4, 174–5, 189
   and HIV and AIDS, 2–3, 39–43
   as a social construct, 4–5, 14, 29–30, 46, 51, 154, 174
gender equality
   African theologians on, 32, 34, 47, 173–4, 180–81
   churches on, 86–8, 90, 123–4, 132, 153, 154, 162–3, 173, 183, 185–8
gender justice, 32–7, 40, 46–7, 56–7, 74, 170–72, 179–81, 199
globalisation, 11, 146, 161n33, 163
God, 33–4, 36, 38–9, 80, 105, 136–8, 142, 145, 194–5
   as Creator, see Creation

Haddad, Beverley, 56, 166
headship (male)
   African theologians on, 32, 44, 59, 170–71, 174, 176
   as understood in/by churches, 73, 80–82, 90–92, 115, 121–4, 132, 146–7, 152–3, 163, 183–90
hegemonic masculinity, 4, 6–8, 48–50, 57, 120, 146, 155, 166–7, 190
hermeneutics
   African women theologians', 27, 30, 34, 171, 175–6
   biblical, 34, 81, 173, 175–6
   gender-critical/feminist, 30, 58, 171, 183
heterosexuality, 3, 15–16, 41–2, 131, 154–55
HIV and AIDS
   African theologians on, 37–47
   and gender, 2–3, 39–43
   and masculinities, 3–8, 48–50, 59, 168–9
   as a motivation for men to change, 100–101, 144–5
   response of churches to, 38–9, 62, 68–9, 83, 105, 109, 138, 150–51

holiness (ideal of), 93–4, 136–7, 156, 165, 177
Holy Spirit, 97, 113, 135–7
homosexuality, 16, 42–3, 111–12, 131, 138, 155

imitation, 93–4, 196, 144n192, 197
inculturation, 27, 162, 164

Jesus Christ, 34–5, 135, 174
   as a model of manhood, 54–5, 81, 92, 95, 119–20, 123, 125, 127, 133
   as the second Adam, 127, 132–4, 145, 174
Joachim, St
   Catholic men's organisation, 61–2, 64–6, 74, 79, 84–5, 98, 101–2, 152, 195–8
   as a model of manhood, 61, 65–6, 78, 85–7, 93–4, 157, 165, 144
John Paul II, 87–9, 95n153, 187
Joseph, St, 87, 92, 94–5, 144, 157
Justice, 36, 39–40, 43, 63, 74, 169, 176; *see also* gender justice

Kanyoro, Musimbi, 27, 30, 31, 34
Krondorfer, Björn, 14–15, 85n107, 179

leadership (male)
   African theologians on, 32, 50, 54, 170
   churches on, 85, 92, 117, 120–21, 126–28, 132–3, 153, 170
   religious, 164–5
liberation theology, 27, 33, 38–9, 43, 52, 169

machismo, 48–9, 152, 167
Magesa, Laurenti, 28, 32–3, 36, 88n122, 155n12
Mahmood, Saba, 59n186, 181, 190–91
Maluleke, Tinyiko S., 11, 28–9, 31, 37, 38, 43, 45, 50, 54
marriage, 6, 10
   African theologians on, 32, 44–5, 173–4
   churches on, 64–5, 69, 72–3, 79–82, 86, 89, 94, 108, 112, 115–16, 121–4, 131, 152–5

Marriage Encounter, 64, 79, 81–2, 86, 90, 162
Marshall, Ruth, 135, 194
Martin, Bernice, 146–7, 151
Martin, David, 124, 157, 159
masculinity/ies
   Catholic ideal of, 76–86, 97, 101–2, 152, 157–9, 197
   and HIV and AIDS, 3–8, 48–50, 59, 168–9
   liberating, 48, 52, 179, 190, 199
   messianic, 119–20, 127
   Pentecostal ideal of, 117–30, 157–8, 161, 177; *see also* biblical manhood
   redemptive, 53–4, 179, 190, 199
   as social constructs, 4–5, 14, 51, 89, 174–5 Maxwell, David, 129n123, 160n29
Meyer, Birgit, 161
model of manhood
   Adam as, 6, 103, 112, 118–19, 122, 126–8, 130–33, 134n147, 174, 193
   fathers as, 72, 144, 161, 193; *see also* fatherhood
   Jesus as, see Jesus Christ
   religious leaders as, 143, 164–5, 185
   saints as, 92–6, 157, 165; *see also* Joachim, St; Joseph, St
modernity, 13, 159–64, 187–8, 191
Moyo, Fulata L., 35, 37–8, 41, 44–7, 49, 51, 166
Mwaura, Philomena N., 28, 32, 33, 171

Nadar, Sarojini, 27, 43, 45, 50, 170–71, 176
Njoroge, Nyambura, 32, 40, 43, 45–6

Oduyoye, Mercy Amba, 25–6, 30, 31, 34, 35, 36–7, 170, 175

patriarchy, 6–7, 14–16, 102, 146–7, 169–73, 181–3
   African theologians on, 25, 28–32, 34–6, 44–6, 49–50, 52, 54–5, 57–8, 170–72
   soft, 153, 171, 184–5
peer pressure, 49, 64, 71, 82–3, 84

Pentecostalism, 104, 145–7, 156, 157–8, 167–8, 169–71, 191–5
  in relation to tradition vs. modernity in Africa, 161, 163, 188
Performativity, 94, 102, 196
Phiri, Isabel A., 26, 29, 31, 33, 35–6, 39, 42, 47–8, 59, 174, 175
Piper, John, 118, 131, 146, 161, 186–7
Postcoloniality, 16–17, 190
power
  constructive use of, 54–5, 92, 153, 186
  gender and, 3, 15–16, 29–31, 41–2, 49, 91, 115–16, 169, 172, 182, 189–90
  poststructuralist understanding of, 189–90
  transformative power of God/Jesus Christ, 133–4, 135, 142, 195
Promise Keepers, 146–7, 184, 186–7
provider (men as), 73, 77, 80, 113, 116, 121, 124–6, 163–4

regime, discursive/epistemic, 135, 154–5, 194, 198
responsibility
  as a notion of masculinity, 55, 59, 76–8, 118–21, 132–3, 137, 142, 151–3, 193–4
  men's lack of, 72–4, 116–17
Robbins, Joel, 191
Roman Catholic Church, *see* Catholicism

saints, 92–5, 144n192, 165, 197; *see also* Joachim, St; Joseph, St
self-control, 53, 82–4, 100n174, 101, 110, 129–30, 137, 140, 143, 193–4
sexuality, 3–4, 7, 35n60, 37–8, 41–7, 49, 68–71, 78, 83–4, 109–11, 129–30, 137, 150–51; *see also* homosexuality
Simpson, Anthony, 4, 6, 7, 8

Soothill, Jane, 17–18, 124n100, 126n111, 145, 156, 161, 163n40
stigmatisation
  of people living with HIV, 2, 38, 40, 50, 53, 105
subjectivity, 17–18, 85n107, 136, 189–90, 194, 196–7

technology/ies of the self, 83, 129, 143, 198
theology, 12; *see also* African theology
  contextual, 12, 37, 58, 180–81
  feminist, 14, 26n3, 57–9, 154, 180
  intercultural, 12–13, 180–81

violence against women, 41–2, 43–5, 48, 49–50, 74, 114–5, 166, 171

Walls, Andrew, 10
West, Gerald, 38, 53, 56
Wilcox, W. Bradford, 152, 184
women; *see also* domination of men over women; African women's theology
  (dis)empowerment of, 30, 44, 45, 46–7, 68
  and HIV and AIDS, 2–3, 39–41, 43–5
  on men/masculinities, 22, 71, 73, 79, 80, 81, 98, 115, 116, 121, 122, 139, 143
  Zambian Catholic bishops on, 67–8, 74, 82, 86–7, 90
world Christianity (study of), 10, 12, 17, 161n33, 180, 199–200

Zambia, 18–21, 65, 79, 80, 81, 106, 111, 113, 128, 132, 149, 151–3, 163, 164n40, 193–4
Zambian Episcopal Conference, 20, 62; *see also* Catholic Bishops of Zambia

For Product Safety Concerns and Information please contact our EU
representative GPSR@taylorandfrancis.com
Taylor & Francis Verlag GmbH, Kaufingerstraße 24, 80331 München, Germany

www.ingramcontent.com/pod-product-compliance
Lightning Source LLC
Chambersburg PA
CBHW071353290426

44108CB00014B/1528